COVID-19 Pandemic, Mental Health and Neuroscience - New Scenarios for Understanding and Treatment

Edited by Sara Palermo and Berend Olivier

Published in London, United Kingdom

COVID-19 Pandemic, Mental Health and Neuroscience - New Scenarios for Understanding and Treatment
http://dx.doi.org/10.5772/intechopen.100841
Edited by Sara Palermo and Berend Olivier

Contributors
Amr Ahmed, Amr Ghit, Mahmoud Elkazzaz, Asmaa Houjak, Shoji Nakamura, Jawza F. Alsabhan, Tahani K. Alshammari, Swapan Kumar Chatterjee, Snigdha Saha, Shahin Muhammed T. K., Ole Boe, Samir Rawat, Priya Joshi, Abhijit P. Deshpande, Andrzej Piotrowski, Derebe Madoro, Nixon M. Abraham, Meenakshi Pardasani, Diana Araja, Angelika Krumina, Uldis Berkis, Modra Murovska, Zaiga Nora-Krukle, Margot Gage Witvliet, Kanwar Hamza Shuja, Arfa Mubeen, Sania Mazher, Shazia Tariq, Fernanda Dreux M. Fernandes, Maria Vitoria do Amaral, Cibelle La Higuera Amato, Harpreet Kaur, Asmita Kaundal, John Teibo, Abolaji Olagunju, Titilade Teibo, Olabode Omotoso, Festus Atiba, Ahmad Babalghith, Gaber Batiha, Serefnur Ozturk, Fettah Eren, Chika Eze, Nneka Okafor, Emelda I. Emmanuel, Chinecherem Iloka, Dragana Komnenov, Yusuuf Tunde Gbonjubola, Adesola Oyinkansola Abiodun, Mary Olamide Akinwola, Shinichiro Maeshima, Koki - Kawamura, Aiko Osawa, Hidenori Arai, Robabe Khalili, Leila Karimi, Sara Palermo, Alessandro Giannandrea, Luisa Sist, Monica Martoni, Lara Colombo, Annalisa Grandi, Margherita Zito, Vicenzo Russo, Berend Olivier, Megan E. Breuer, Christiaan H. Vinkers, Jocelien D.A. Olivier

First published in London, United Kingdom, 2023 by IntechOpen
IntechOpen is the global imprint of INTECHOPEN LIMITED, registered in England and Wales, registration number: 11086078, 5 Princes Gate Court, London, SW7 2QJ, United Kingdom

British Library Cataloguing-in-Publication Data
A catalogue record for this book is available from the British Library

Additional hard and PDF copies can be obtained from orders@intechopen.com

COVID-19 Pandemic, Mental Health and Neuroscience - New Scenarios for Understanding and Treatment
Edited by Sara Palermo and Berend Olivier
p. cm.
Print ISBN 978-1-80355-090-9
Online ISBN 978-1-80355-091-6
eBook (PDF) ISBN 978-1-80355-092-3

For EU product safety concerns:
IN TECH d.o.o., Prolaz Marije Krucifikse Kozulić 3, 51000 Rijeka, Croatia,
info@intechopen.com or visit our website at intechopen.com.

Meet the editors

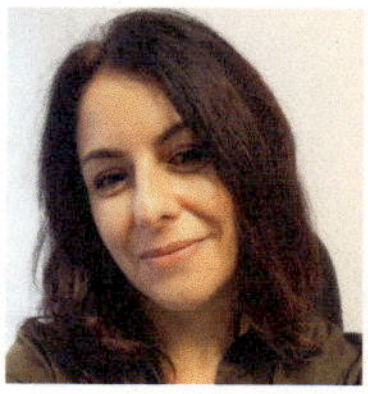

Sara Palermo has an MSc in Clinical Psychology and a Ph.D. in Experimental Neuroscience. She is an assistant professor in the Department of Psychology, University of Turin, Italy; the assistant specialty chief editor of *Frontiers in Psychology – Neuropsychology*; and the scientific director of the Istituto Nazionale di Filantropia – Filantropolis, Italy. She is also a scientific consultant at the Neuroradiologic Unit – Diagnostic and Technology Department, IRCCS Istituto Neurologico Carlo Besta, Italy. She is a member of the American Psychological Association, Italian Society of Neuropsychology, Italian Association of Psychogeriatrics, Italian Society of Neurology for Dementia, and International Society for Interdisciplinary Placebo Studies.

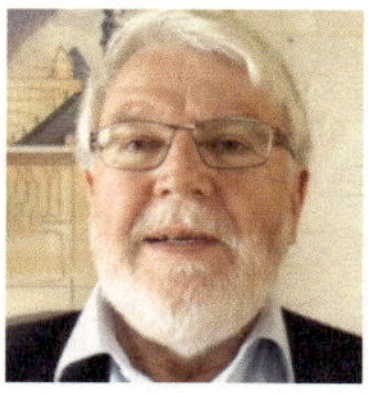

Berend Olivier obtained a Ph.D. in Neurobiology from Groningen University, the Netherlands. He worked at Solvay Pharmaceuticals for 22 years leading the research and development of new antidepressants, antipsychotics, anxiolytics, and serenics. He was heavily involved in the research and development of fluvoxamine, a marketed antidepressant, anxiolytic, and anti-OCD medication. From 1999 to 2001, he worked in New York to start a biotech company called PsychoGenics Inc., which develops psychiatric and neurological (genetic) models to screen, find, and develop new central nervous system drugs. From 1992 to 2014, he was a Professor of CNS Pharmacology at Utrecht University, the Netherlands, performing research on animal models, brain mechanisms, and pharmacology of psychiatric disorders. Since 2014, he has been developing animal models of male sexual disorders in the hope of finding new medicines for premature and delayed ejaculation.

Contents

Preface

The pandemic has created a global mental health crisis, fueling short- and long-term stress and undermining the mental health of millions. Estimates calculate an increase in both anxiety and depressive disorders of more than 25% during the first year of the pandemic. Although data are mixed, younger age, female gender, and pre-existing health conditions have often been reported risk factors. At the same time, mental health services have been severely disrupted and the treatment gap for mental health conditions has widened. The European Organization for Economic Co-operation and Development (OECD) report "Health at a Glance: Europe 2022" confirmed that as the pandemic evolved, people's mental health fluctuated with the intensity of the wave of infection and with the severity of the confinement measures. Mental healthcare services have been disrupted at all levels, with hospitalizations declining and many in-person consultations canceled or postponed, particularly during the early stages of the virus's circulation. According to the OECD, unmet needs for mental health care increased both during and after the pandemic with 23% of adults reporting unmet mental health needs in spring 2022, up from 20% in the spring of 2021.

Furthermore, COVID-19 is associated with manifold diseases of the peripheral and central nervous systems that may be affected during and after the disease. Brain imaging should be considered in the diagnostic workup of those COVID-19 patients who present with neurological symptoms. Indeed, typical and atypical neuroimaging features have been observed, which in turn were associated with motor, cognitive, and behavioral phenotypic manifestations. Hence the definition "NeuroCovid," which alludes to the acute and chronic disorders that can arise in people who have developed the disease, such as dizziness, headache, loss of smell and taste, confusion, reduced concentration cognitive fog, states of anxiety and depression, hallucinations, psychiatric symptoms, and memory loss. In addition, peripheral nervous system involvement with polyneuropathies has been observed. Numerous studies have documented these neurological and neuropsychic complications, and the effects of COVID-19 on the nervous system are becoming better defined.

Equally relevant are the consequences resulting from the extraordinary nature of the present times. It is likely that a variety of habits, rhythms, and arrangements will have to be altered/modified in order to cope with the COVID-19 pandemic and contain the infection (lockdowns and "physical distancing"). The pandemic has caused a series of other cascading effects that will probably be much more difficult to mitigate and that exposes us to complex consequences. The past years have brought many challenges, particularly for healthcare professionals, students, family members of COVID-19 patients, people with mental disorders, the frail, the elderly, and more generally those in disadvantaged socioeconomic conditions and workers whose livelihoods have been threatened. Indeed, the substantial financial impact of the pandemic may hamper progress towards economic growth as well as progress towards social inclusion and mental well-being.

With the aim of understanding and understanding the profound nature of the long-term problems for mental health derived from the pandemic, there are numerous studies underway all over the world that combine the work of multidisciplinary research groups.

This volume explores the complex relationship between COVID-19, mental health, acquired data, and possible interventions with a multidisciplinary approach encompassing physiological and cognitive mechanisms, medical treatment, psychosocial interventions, and self-management. The reader is taken through an excursus that moves from the virus-brain interactions to associated clinical conditions to possible treatments. Ample space is also given to social and geopolitical issues according to a biopsychosocial approach to physical and mental health.

The volume consists of twenty-one chapters divided into four thematic sections: "Coronavirus, Biochemical Signals and the Nervous System"; Mid- and Long-Term Sequelae of COVID-19: Clinical Conditions and Proposed Approaches"; Uncovering Pandora's Box: Challenges for Health Systems and Society"; and "Daily Life, Work and Well-Being: Impact, Resilience and Adaptation."

Sara Palermo
Department of Psychology,
University of Turin,
Turin, Italy

Neuroradiology Unit,
Diagnostic and Technology Department,
Fondazione Istituto di Ricovero e Cura a Carattere Scientifico (IRCCS)
Istituto Neurologico Carlo Besta,
Milan, Italy

Berend Olivier
Department of Psychopharmacology,
Utrecht Institute for Pharmaceutical Sciences (UIPS),
Utrecht University,
Utrecht, The Netherlands

Department of Psychiatry,
Yale University School of Medicine,
New Haven, USA

Section 1

Coronavirus, Biochemical Signals and the Nervous System

Chapter 1

Neurotropic SARS-CoV-2: Causalities and Realities

Meenakshi Pardasani and Nixon M. Abraham

Abstract

Evidences for the dysfunctions of central nervous system (CNS) caused by SARS-CoV-2 infection have accumulated since the beginning of pandemic. The clinical and experimental evidences on viral entry routes to CNS lead to several open questions. While the neurological impairments caused by the virus stay as a reality under Long COVID, dissecting the causality underlying these problems continues to be an intensely studied topic. Extensive reports of olfactory dysfunctions including anosmia, hyposmia, and parosmia due to infections during 2020–2021, led to the hypothesis of virus' CNS invasion through the olfactory nerve. Some of the investigations using animal models of cellular factors mediating the viral entry also suggest potential neurotropism. Conversely, recent studies proved the absence of viral particles in olfactory sensory neurons and olfactory bulb, hence leading to the deliberation on viral entry route. Here, we summarize the findings on the debated neurotropic characteristics of the virus, including clinical observations and the results from animal models. Further, we emphasize on the need of tracking olfactory and cognitive fitness in the post-COVID-19 era.

Keywords: SARS-CoV-2, olfactory fitness, neurotropism, cognitive impairments, neuro-COVID

1. Introduction

The Coronavirus disease 2019 (COVID-19) pandemic poses an unparalleled challenge to the public health in dealing with long-term adverse effects of the infection. Several neurological complications have been reported to be associated with COVID-19. At the beginning of pandemic, in one of the early correspondences on autopsy studies published in the New England Journal of Medicine reported the presence of SARS-CoV-2 in multiple organs including the brain [1]. Recently published brain imaging data from subjects who were scanned before and after infection show structural abnormalities in the central nervous system (CNS). Significant changes were found in the brain areas that are functionally connected to the primary olfactory cortex, orbitofrontal cortex, and olfactory tubercle. This suggests possible long-term cognitive impairments due to COVID-19 infection in the central nervous system (CNS) that may happen through olfactory mucosa [2]. These findings support early reports on the presence of SARS-CoV-2 RNA and protein in the nasopharynx [3]. However, the postmortem studies of olfactory and respiratory mucosa confirmed sustentacular and ciliated cells as the targets for SARS-CoV-2 infection. There were no evidences found in this study for the presence of viral particles in the olfactory sensory neurons (OSNs) or olfactory bulb (OB), questioning the neurotropism shown by the virus [4]. These contrasting results prompt us to carry out a narrative literature review on the reported causalities and realities on the neurotropic characteristics of SARS-CoV-2.

One of the virus entry routes, i.e., binding of viral spike (S) protein to the human angiotensin-converting enzyme 2 (hACE2) receptor and the S protein priming by host cell transmembrane protease, serine 2 (TMPRSS2) was uncovered at the beginning of pandemic [5]. These cellular factors are present in the non-neuronal cells of human olfactory epithelium, cortical neurons, Purkinje neurons, cerebellar and cortical astrocytes, etc. [6, 7]. Another receptor type that can mediate the infection, Neuropilin-1 (NRP1), is abundantly found in the neurons, olfactory epithelial cells, and endothelial cells [8, 9]. Other potential route can be through the ACE2 receptors present on the endothelial cells, thereby using the vascular system to attack the blood-brain barrier and to get access to the CNS [10]. Thus, despite the entry route to CNS being a debated topic, these evidences can be used to explain the pathophysiology of neurological impairments and long-term cognitive dysfunctions caused by COVID-19 infection. In this chapter, we are summarizing the evidences for the debated topic of SARS-CoV-2 neurotropism, the importance of quantifying olfactory and cognitive fitness in the context of Neuro-COVID and the studies in model systems that suggest neurotropism. To this end, we have carried out the literature review using a combination of keywords such as "SARS CoV2 entry routes to brain" and "Olfactory and cognitive impairments due to COVID-19" and "animal models of CoV-2." We have mostly used Google Scholar and PubMed to search for the articles. As we are aiming to provide a narrative overview on the debated topic of Neurotropic SARS-CoV-2, we are summarizing only the selected and relevant findings on this topic.

2. Entry routes of SARS-CoV-2

To investigate the pathophysiology associated with SARS-CoV-2 infection, one of the critical steps is to mechanistically discern the routes of its entry into the host. Unprecedented research is underway, since the beginning of the COVID-19-induced pandemic to tease out the different entry points of the novel SARS-CoV-2 in the human body. It has been confirmed that CoV-2 virus presents the spike glycoprotein to the cell membrane for binding to the human angiotensin-converting enzyme 2 (hACE2) receptor [11, 12]. It is famously referred to as the SARS-CoV functional receptor [13]. One of the imperative functions of hACE2 protein is maintaining the neural homeostasis by regulating the renin-angiotensin signaling (RAS) system [14]. A seamless entry into the cell is warranted by the cleavage of S2' site of the virus by the TMPRSS2 after engaging with hACE2 at the membrane [5, 15, 16]. In the endosomal compartments of the cell, the cleavage is mediated by Cathepsin L protease, which initiates formation of the fusion pores [17, 18]. Inside Golgi apparatus, Furin protease cleaves the virus into S1 and S2 compartments [19]. After successful entry and proteolytic cleavage, viral machinery is assembled and activated to spread the infection [16].

Importantly, the agents that allow SARS-CoV-2 entry, specifically, human-ACE2 (hACE2) are present across different bodily tissues including the brain [14]. Such a widespread expression in the body would allow for conjecturing several routes by which virus can enter and invade. Indeed, the repertoire of symptoms associated with

COVID-19 is a testimony to the tropism of virus in different cell types and tissues. Studies involving bulk and single-cell RNA sequencing revealed ACE2-TMPRSS2 expression in the different cell-types such as the sustentacular (SUS) cells, respiratory ciliated and secretory cells as well as the horizontal basal cells of the respiratory and olfactory epithelium (RE and OE) of human nasal mucosa [20, 21]. Other peripheral routes include that of the eye and oral tissues [22, 23]. Virus specimen was found to be present in the conjunctivital and tear swab of patients [24, 25]. Indeed, the viral entry machinery components, ACE2 and TMPRSS2, are present in conjunctivital epithelium and the epithelial and endothelial parts of the cornea [26]. Oral cavity also allows viral entry due to the enrichment of the entry proteins in the epithelial cells of the salivary glands and mucosae found in the single-cell RNA sequencing data of human samples [27]. Entry via oral route suggests correlation of salivary viral titer with the taste loss observed in COVID-19 patients [27, 28].

CoV-2 virus can potentially breach the blood-brain barrier (BBB) as a result of the barrier instability caused due to the increased number of inflammatory cytokines upon infection [10, 29]. Viral invasion of the brain areas by gaining entry from the circumventricular organs (CVOs) and brainstem structures could also serve as plausible routes in the patients who suffer from massive cytokine storm or those having compromised health prior to the infection [30]. One of the cytokines, tumor necrosis factor-α (TNF-α) can enter the BBB or in CVOs (structures lining the ventricles with accessible vasculature), which can activate downstream microglia and astrocytes [31]. The activated cells, in turn, can cause damage to the neurons via excitotoxicity and thereby impair the signaling processes of the brain [30]. Fecal-oral routes are yet another proposed route of viral dissemination in the body [32]. It is, however, not confirmed that this transmission route is responsible for gastrointestinal symptoms associated with COVID-19. It has been hypothesized that movement via vagal and spinal axonal fibers can allow viral invasion of the GI tract. Occurrence of syncope in patients with normal electrocardiogram assessment hints toward changes in the neural control of blood pressure changes [33, 34]. In one study, patients with syncope indeed had a significantly lower increase in the compensatory heart rate compared with those non-syncope ones, which suggested plausible impairment in the baro-reflexive control. Such an acute hypocapnic hypoxemia could have occurred due to CoV-2-mediated ACE2 internalization in specific midbrain and medullary nuclei, which can lead to impairments in baroreflex and chemoreceptor responses [33]. Malfunctioning of brain-lung axis can be indicated as severe lung and chest CT abnormalities and defects observed in neuroimaging analysis. The sensory neurons lining the airways can sense the virus induced inflammatory responses in the lungs and provide feedback to the brain [35, 36]. The carotid body sinus nerves innervating this organ can profoundly play a role in the retrograde transport of the virus to the brain. Carotid body invasion by virus due to local expression of ACE2 can cause impaired peripheral arterial chemoreception leading to hypoxic and hypercapnic conditions with changes in pH [37]. Separately, the mucosal immune system, which comprises the lymphoid tissues of the gut and the lungs, provides the clue for dissociating the components of gut-lung axis in mediating dysfunctions associated with the COVID-19 infection. Translocation of the active immune cells from gut to lungs can exacerbate inflammation, even causing lung injuries and respiratory distress. Within the gut, CoV-2 can downregulate ACE2 expression causing microbial dysbiosis and further affecting lungs via the gut-lung axis. Finally, neural control of the cardiovascular processes under COVID-19 infectious condition is yet another axis via which the virus can act and affect these organ systems [38]. Cardiac arrhythmias in COVID-19

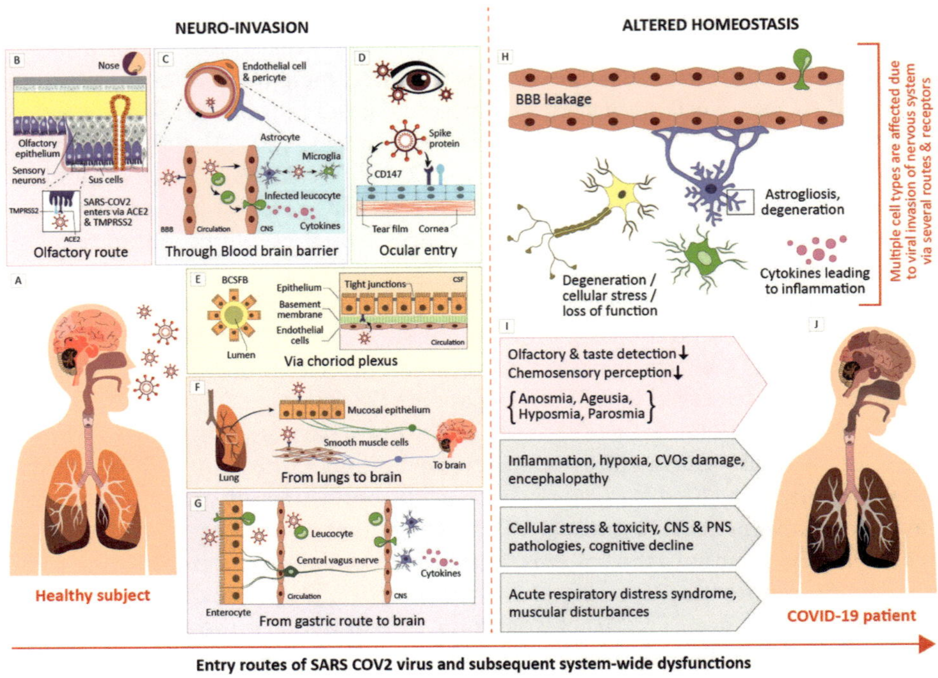

Figure 1.
Neuroinvasion by SARS-CoV-2 and subsequent dysfunctions. (A) Infection of a healthy subject by SARS-CoV-2 leads the entry of virus into different organ systems. (B–G) Routes and cell-types through which the virus can enter and invade the nervous system, i.e., via, olfactory route, via blood-brain barrier, eye, choroid plexus, blood-cerebrospinal fluid (CSF) barrier, via lungs to the brain and through the gastric enterocytes to the central nervous system [7, 40–42]. (H) Altered homeostasis can occur as a result of neuroinvasion by CoV-2 virus leading to detrimental effects at multiple cell types of the nervous system, i.e., neuron (yellow), astrocyte (blue) and microglia (green) [43]. (I) System-wide dysfunctions ranging from cellular to olfactory to CNS and PNS pathologies have been reported in COVID-19 patients. (J) An infected COVID-19 patient with different bodily systems affected due to the viral tropism.

patients are mostly occurring due to direct myocardial damage by CoV-2 infection or via the systemic inflammatory responses [39]. Arrythmias can also indirectly be caused by dysfunctional neural control of the heart rate. There are feedback mechanisms to the brain for maintenance of the cardiac rhythm and for dampening the production of cytokines and other inflammatory mediators in case of infection [38]. It could be that the severe CoV-2 infection can alter the neural feedback mechanisms of cardiovascular control. Apart from the olfactory route, these three axes i.e., the lung-brain, gut-lung, and heart-brain may also serve as the routes of transmission and invasion by the virus leading to multiple organs dysfunctions and manifestation of a variety of symptoms and conditions (**Figure 1**).

3. SARS-CoV-2: neurotropic or not?

The CNS is an immune privileged system of the body, owing to the highly protective brain-cerebrospinal fluid barrier, blood-brain barrier as well as surveillance by innate immune sentinels [44, 45]. Viral adaptations can allow multiple entry routes, either via the peripheral nerves or through the hematogenous routes. This can lead to neural and endothelial destruction causing CNS dysfunctions [46]. A variety of neuropathological viruses are the respiratory viruses belonging to the categories of the influenza virus (IV), the coronaviruses (CoV), human metapneumovirus (hMPV), and human respiratory syncytial virus (hRSV) [47–49]. They are known to enter the CNS through various routes and mechanisms and invade the system leading to long-term neurological sequalae in the patients [49]. Such viral infections, under severe conditions, usually lead to neurological impairments such as encephalitis, seizures, epilepsy, and other encephalopathies [50–52]. In subsequent section of the chapter, we review the neuroinvasive nature of CoVs and how studying them over the years has helped us understand the SARS CoV-2-mediated complications better. We will also highlight the ongoing debate about the neurotropic nature of the SARS-CoV-2 in the upcoming subsections.

3.1 Neuro-invasive capabilities of coronaviruses

The three kinds of epidemic-causing CoVs, the SARS CoV-1, Middle East Respiratory Syndrome (MERS) CoV, and the currently prevailing SARS CoV-2, have all been demonstrated to exhibit neurological invasive capabilities [53, 54]. Viral encephalitis, i.e., lesions in the brain parenchyma including neuronal damage caused due to virus, has been confirmed in COVID-19 patients [55]. Genomic sequencing of viral particles in the CSF of the patient verified the case of encephalitis [56]. In fact, encephalitis, polyneuropathy, and aortic ischemic stroke were also commonly observed in severe cases of SARS-CoV epidemic that occurred in 2003 [53]. SARS CoV-2 shares 79.5% genetic similarity with SARS-CoV virus, and hence, finding out the mechanisms of neurological impairments by CoV-2 might be more tractable [57]. Acute viral infection causing hypoxia, systemic toxemia, and other metabolic disorders can result in toxic encephalopathy. It is mainly characterized by cerebral edema and symptoms include headache, delirium, dysphoria, and in extreme cases, lead to loss of consciousness, coma, and paralysis [58]. COVID-19 patients often suffer from hypoxia, viremia, and even headache and disturbed consciousness, which can potentially lead to acute toxic encephalopathy. In extreme cases of COVID-19, enhanced cytokine storm, increased levels of D-dimer, and reduced platelet count can even allow viral-induced cerebrovascular events to occur [59]. Multiple reports of confirmed viral infection in the brain have been narrated since the beginning of the pandemic outbreak. MRI scan of a young COVID-19 female patient with mild symptoms and normal chest CT showed significant cortical hyperintensity in the right gyrus rectus and subtle hyperintensity in the OBs suggestive of viral invasion in these brain regions [60]. In autopsies assessment of brains of six patients who suffered from COVID-19, brainstem neural damage, meningitis, and pan-encephalitis were reported [61, 62]. HCoV-OC43, HCoV-229E, and SARS-CoV-1 are the human-infecting CoVs, which are capable of infecting the neurons directly, apart from causing CNS damage due to immunological and inflammatory responses [63, 64]. HCoV-OC43 has been associated with multiple sclerosis (MS) with its RNA detected in the CSF of 12 of 22 patients suffering with MS [65]. MERS-CoV, although, enters via a dipeptidyl peptidase receptor and has affected only ~2500 individuals since 2012, it also has been shown to generate neurological impairments such as seizures, headaches, and perceiving confusion [66]. Cases of Guillain-Barrè syndrome (GBS), axonal neuropathy, and Bickerstaff brainstem encephalitis have been reported under MERS-CoV infection [67]. This virus, however, was never detected in the human CSF. In case of COVID-19 as well, electromyography and other assessments had confirmed occurrence of GBS and axonal neuropathy in infected patients as well [68–70].

3.2 Pathogenic studies and mechanisms in favor of neurotropic nature of the SARS CoV-2

Reports associated with neurological impairments induced by CoV-2 in acute as well as post-acute infection stages have been accumulated since early 2020 [71, 72]. Whether these effects are occurring as a result of the neuroinvasive nature of the virus or due to the overt immune responses is not yet fully understood. A recent study in medRxiv reveals that in comparison to increased inflammatory and cytokine storm markers found in the serum of COVID-19 patients, their levels are rather low in the CSF. This was corroborated by comparing and contrasting the insignificant neuroinflammatory changes in these patients' CSF compared with CSF of patients with autoimmune pathologies that displayed very high neuroinflammation. On the contrary, a significant increase in CSF Neurofilament-L (NF-L) in critical cases suggests neuroaxonal injury and strengthens the neurotropic nature of the virus [73]. The olfactory transmucosal pathway has been an established port of entry for CoV-2 virus, but we only have a limited knowledge about the virus-host interactions [3]. The human sequencing data point toward the role of supporting cells of OE in the viral entry. This is because of the expression of ACE2 and TMPRSS2 proteins in these cells that serve as the entry factors [5]. The immunohistochemical analysis of the SARS-CoV-2 S protein, however, revealed a characteristic granular, perinuclear expression pattern in olfactory mucosal cell types, which were of neuronal origin (revealed by expression of Tuj1, Neurofilament 200, and Olfactory Marker Protein) obtained from the autopsy samples of the COVID-19-infected patients [3]. Additionally, presence of CoV-2 particles was confirmed in the CNS regions including the OB [74]. This questions the current understanding of non-neuronal vs. neuronal viral infection occurring in COVID-19. Generally, neurotropic viruses access the peripheral regions to gain entry into the CNS [75]. Whether the CoV-2 is causing neuronal pathogenesis directly or indirectly is not fully understood. We also do not have a complete understanding of the virus' pathway to the OB and other CNS regions. In an attempt to investigate the pathogenic mechanisms of the virus, an in vitro study of generating human sensory neurons from the human embryonic stem cell lines was carried out. These peripheral sensory neurons were shown to express ACE2 and were indeed receptive to the virus, which is in contrast with the reported non-neuronal expression of ACE2. One hour after the incubation with the virus, intracellular expression of nsp-14, S protein, RdRp, and nucleocapsid phosphoprotein viral genes was substantially upregulated in the infected neurons [76]. The molecular pathologies relating to chemosensory perception were specifically affected in the infected peripheral neurons. The human induced pluripotent stem cells (hIPSCs)-derived midbrain dopaminergic neurons were shown to be selectively permissible to the CoV-2 infection. Further, inflammatory and cellular senescence responses were observed in these neurons both in vitro and upon transplantation in vivo as well [77]. In another attempt to investigate if human neurons are a direct target of this virus, three-dimensional human brain organoids system was utilized. Preferred tropism to mature neurons of the cortical plate in relatively older brain organoids (day 60) was found out. The virus has relatively lesser influence on the actively proliferating neural precursor cells of the ventricular zone of young (day 15) organoids. Moreover, CoV-2-infected neurons displayed mislocalized Tau protein in their soma, which can potentially cause cellular stress reactivity and toxicity [78].

3.3 Evidences of SARS CoV-2 tropism beyond neurons: the other side of the coin

Conflicting results paired with the promiscuous entry routes of the virus stirs the ongoing debate on the neuronal vs. non-neuronal routes of invasion and tropism of SARS-CoV-2 virus. Those who are opposing the axonal hopping of the virus primarily point to the technical limitations of the studies *per se*. Meinhardt and colleagues critically evaluated the imaging data of virus nucleoproteins found at the OE, between the olfactory nerve layer and OB [3]. The axons of OSNs reaching to OB are highly entwined with the ACE2-expressing supporting cells processes, and they reasoned that the immunolabeled imaging may not convincingly reveal whether the virus is present in OSNs or in the wrappings of the sustentacular cells. Nevertheless, ultrastructural assessment using electron microscopy (EM) has also been done both in autoptic human samples and the animal models. Virus-like particles were detected in the cortex of K18-hACE2 mice, and pyknotic cells and abnormal mitochondrial ultra-structures in infected hamsters were observed using Transmission EM (TEM) [79]. A virus cytoplasmic inclusion body was also identified in the OB of an autotoptic patient sample observed using TEM [74]. However, TEM investigations are also subject to aberrant observations as virion-like vesicular bodies can act as decoys for pathologists and that direct neuronal infections cannot be confirmed by using this technique [80]. Post CoV-2 inoculation in rhesus monkey, one group carried out the transcriptomic profiling of the infected cells. Downregulation of genes involved in mitochondrial dysfunctions (ND3, ATP6, and COX3) was observed in the mature neurons, hippocampal microglia, endothelial vascular cells, and oligodendrocytes [81]. This is suggestive of dysfunctions happening in various cell types of the brain, which are collectively leading to CNS abnormalities. Hijacking the lipoprotein metabolism of susceptible cells of the brain barriers (BBB and BSCFB) suggests hematogenous route of entry [82]. Firstly, transcellular route, i.e., entering via ACE2 receptors of the choroid plexus epithelial cells, pericytes, astrocytes lining the endothelial cells followed by weakening of the tight junctions between the vascular endothelial cells of the BBB (called the paracellular modes) and finally utilizing the lipid vesicles and exosomes as the “Trojan horses” to breach the barrier while escaping the host’s immune oversight constitutes the non-neuronal mode of entry of the virus [82].

4. Neuro-COVID: neurological consequences of COVID-19 disease

Reports of neurological complications during COVID-19 infection and their persistence after the recovery have accumulated since the early outbreak. These impairments are broadly categorized as Neuro-COVID. Early investigation in China estimated that 36% of the COVID-positive patients had neurological disturbances [83]. Case test studies from France, performed in March–April 2020, also highlighted the occurrence of encephalopathy, state of confusion, and agitation as well as corticospinal tract symptoms in COVID-19 patients admitted to the hospital due to Acute Respiratory Distress Syndrome (ARDS) [84]. Since then, numerous reports and case studies from across different countries have confirmed the prevalence of mild-to-severe neurological and neuropsychiatric in the CoV-2-infected individuals. The neurological impact correlated with the severity of the infection and distributed across the categories of CNS pathologies, peripheral nervous system (PNS) diseases, and/or skeletal muscular disturbances. A cohort-based longitudinal study by the UK Biobank involving multimodal brain imaging before and after the CoV-2 infections showed emergence of virus-related abnormalities in specific brain regions and cognitive decline upon infection [2]. Using diffusion imaging-based changes as a readout for brain tissue damage upon infection, they observed detrimental effects in regions including the olfactory-limbic areas, the anterior olfactory nucleus, olfactory tubercle, and the anterior piriform cortex. Profound decrease in the gray matter thickness and contrast was also observed in parahippocampal gyrus and lateral orbitofrontal cortex of the patients. Brain abnormalities were more pronounced in hospitalized patients; however, cognitive decline associated with damage to crus II lobule of the cerebellum was found in majority of the individuals who turned positive for the CoV-2 in this longitudinal study [2]. As virus takes the olfactory route, chemosensory impairments are often seen in a large number of infective cases. These impairments, primarily, anosmia and ageusia, have not only served as the robust predictors of the CoV-2 infection, but also affected quality of life of the patients, recovered individuals, and healthcare workers [85, 86]. We will focus on different aspects that influence the severity and durability of the Neuro-COVID symptoms in the following subsections.

4.1 Effect of age and comorbidities on the neurological sequalae

The neurological symptoms tend to vary between older (>60 years of age) and younger (<18 years of age) cohorts. While delirium, myalgia, and fatigue were predominant in older cohorts, the younger cohorts primarily reported smell and taste issues, frequent headaches, and infrequently, seizures [66]. This also hinted toward the possibility of comorbidities playing a role in increasing the severity of the effect of the viral infection and tropism. Patients with preexisting neurological conditions had a higher occurrence of hospitalization, in-hospital mortality, enhanced delirium states, and more overall complications upon suffering from COVID-19 [87, 88]. In fact, social isolation and loneliness associated with the pandemic-induced quarantine added to the mental toll of elderly patients [89]. Symptoms worsened with quarantine in 67.5% patients suffering from Parkinson's disease in a Spanish cohort study [90]. Acute encephalopathy due to infection was more commonly observed in older patients with comorbidities and associated with greater critical care and 30-day mortality chances [87, 91]. Across different levels of the neurological impairments upon CoV-2 infection, age has been shown to be positively correlated with the disease severity [92]. Comorbid conditions including de-myelinating disease, acute encephalopathy, and cerebrovascular disease (CVD) were all positively correlated with the severity of the COVID-19 disease [93]. Patients suffering from Alzheimer's, Parkinson's, and other neurodegenerative disorders are at higher risk from infection and can suffer from greater respiratory, olfactory, and cognitive impairments than others [89, 94]. Elderly individuals also suffer from compromised immunity and increased signs of inflammation (increased cytokines, hormonal changes, decrease in growth factors production) leading to physical and mental frailty [92]. Such multiple dysregulations can lead to age-dependent morbid effects of CoV-2 infection.

4.2 Chemosensory and cognitive impairments: neuro-COVID to Long COVID

Among many neurological impairments, olfactory functioning changes in COVID-19 has highest odds ratio in non-hospitalized cases [86, 95]. These have also become common in healthcare workers. In a study comprising 700 workers, by utilizing a chemosensory perception test, over 80% displayed olfactory and gustatory impairments and ~48% had lowered trigeminal sensitivity. The reduced sensitivity remained in over 40% of the individuals with olfactory and gustatory impairments and ~23% in those with trigeminal issues [85]. "COVID & Cognition" cross-sectional study continually aims to understand the cognitive deficits in Long COVID [96]. Long COVID comprises long-lasting symptoms and difficulties arising due to COVID-19. Post-acute COVID persists between 3 and 12 weeks while chronic COVID is when the symptoms persist beyond 12 weeks [72]. Cognitive deficits are expected based on the loss of gray matter in specific regions prevalent in COVID-19. A small cohort study of hospitalized patients displayed gray volume reductions in the hippocampus, right amygdala, and left cingulate cortex. Cognitive deficits are thereby likely to occur, and the extent of it depends on the location and mechanism of the neural damage [97]. A multi-domain impact of the infection on human cognition was also observed in a large population, questionnaire-based study using British Intelligence tests. The cognitive deficits in reasoning, problem-solving, spatial planning, and target detection tasks were substantial and persisted post-infection suggesting that cognitive deficits are indeed prevalent in Long COVID [98]. Cognitive blunting, from mild-to-severe, also referred to as "brain fog" has also been observed in Long COVID. Fluorodeoxyglucose-PET study from two COVID-19 patients with confirmed brain fog and cognitive deficits confirmed abnormal hypometabolic regions in anterior cingulate cortex. Hypometabolisms are also observed in other neurological disorders and psychiatric diseases [99]. The prevalence of chemosensory deficits suggests that they can act as predictors of the COVID-19 infection, which has been elaborated upon, in the next section. The advancements in precisely determining neurocognitive deficits along with sensory impairments non-invasively are also explained.

5. Using "olfaction" to detect COVID-19 and the subsequent sensory-cognitive deficits

Having been one of the first symptoms to be affected in COVID-19, our sense of smell became an important and a robust tool to be utilized for detecting if an individual is infected [100]. This became much more beneficial in detecting "asymptomatic" or "paucisymptomatic" patients, i.e., those who did not develop other visible symptoms of the disease [101–103]. Since 2020, many empirical tests that could previously assess olfactory detection and sensitivity and acted as biomarker indicators of neurodegenerative disorders, have been also utilized as early screening tools for COVID-19. Brief Smell Identification test (BSIT), a revised version of University of Pennsylvania Smell Identification test (UPSIT), was among the first self-administered tests, which was utilized during first wave of COVID-19 [104, 105]. Briefly, it consisted of 12 scented strips (encapsulated odors), which are to be scratched by a pencil to release the odor. It is a forced-choice test, and the subject needed to choose one of the four choices which smelled like the tested odor. A high score indicated normal olfactory performance. Using this test, olfactory dysfunction was observed in 40% of the patients. Indeed, in those patients with just olfactory-related problems, other symptoms flared up ~2 days later [105]. Another study used the Persian version of the full 40-odor UPSIT and found out that 98% of the 60 patients had olfactory dysfunctions. In total, 58% of these were either anosmic or severly microsmic [106]. Hummel's quick olfactory sniffing Sticks (q-Sticks) test was also administered in COVID-19 patients, which consisted of asymptomatic individuals as well [107]. This test consisted of recognition of groups of three odors emanating from refill sticks. Although only 14% of the total patients reported smell loss before the test administration, q-Sticks test revealed that 81% of total patients suffered from anosmia or hyposmia [108]. Since the outbreak, such objective tests that can quantitatively measure olfactory detection, such as Quick-Smell Identification test (Q-SIT), SAFER scent cards, *SCENTinel* 1.0 among others have gained traction [109–111]. However, these traditional tests offer simplistic handle on determining odor detection abilities.

Based on the neurotropic potential of CoV-2, olfactory dysfunctions cannot just be restricted to sensory detection and threshold capacities. Rather, COVID-19 can cause both sensory and cognitive deficits, and efforts are being made to diagnose those too. To this end, highly automated tests with precise stimulus delivery are important.

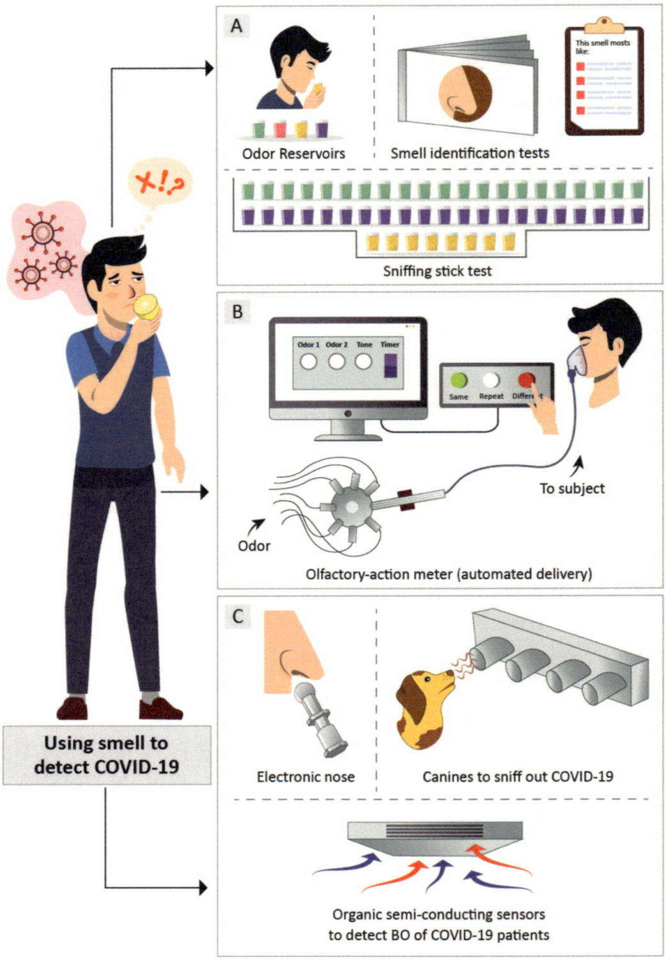

Figure 2.
"Olfaction" as a tool to detect COVID-19. (A) Objective tools such as University of Pennsylvania Smell Identification test (UPSIT), Sniffing stick tests among others have been utilized to evaluate the olfactory detection and discrimination capabilities. These tests consist of delivery of odors to the subject via reservoirs/pen refills/ microencapsulations [104, 106, 115]. (B) An automated odor delivery system, Olfactory-action meter (OAM) has been utilized to precisely calculate odor detection at the threshold levels and olfactory matching skills, i.e., both sensory and cognitive capabilities of symptomatic, asymptomatic, and healthy individuals [101, 112]. (C) Sense of smell, i.e., electronic noses, trained canines, and organic semiconducting sensors are also deployed to using the body odor (BO) of individuals to detect COVID-19 [116–119].

Olfactory-action meter (OAM), an automated machine with custom-written software that can generate odor pulses of varying complexities, has been utilized to assess olfactory detection abilities at differing concentration ranges as well as olfactory matching skills in asymptomatic carriers, symptomatic patients, and those who have recovered from the disease [101, 112, 113]. Compared with normal healthy subjects, up to 81% of the asymptomatic carriers failed at detecting odors at low concentrations (9% (v/v)). In total, 65% of these carriers depicted significantly lower detection at three low-concentration ranges (9–23.1%). Upon administering an olfactory matching task of determining whether the two odors delivered at a set inter-stimulus interval of 5 s are "same" or "different," they found out olfactory working memory deficits in the patients [101]. Not only that, upon carrying out this test with individuals who had recovered from COVID-19 (4–18 months after infection), persistent sensory-cognitive deficits were found out when this paradigm was employed over 5 days [112]. These studies point to the persistence of sensory-cognitive impairments in long-haulers (those suffering from Long-COVID) and also calls for further interrogation of CNS functioning. This also exhibits the importance of monitoring neurocognitive skills during post-infection periods in a pandemic-struck world. These results display the necessity of developing accurate noninvasive methods, which can precisely quantify cognitive deficits in Long COVID [112, 114].

Usage of electronic noses (eNoses) also became popular in detecting COVID-19-infected individuals. eNoses are machines that can mimic animal olfaction and can thus be applied as specific smell detectors of target volatile organic compounds. Usage of an eNose at a drive-through testing station that can detect COVID-19 in real time using body odor that has a nasal passage carried out in an attempt to use them as fast, reliable detectors of this disease [118]. Organic semiconducting sensors could also capture the scent of the asymptomatic carriers of the diseases, suggesting that they can also be deployed at large scale [119]. Finally, dogs can supposedly be our best friends, even during a pandemic. Multiple studies have reported using canines to detect the body odors of the infected patients. Axillary sweat samples of patients may well be successfully discriminated from the normal subjects at a success rate of 76–100% for trained dogs [117]. All these studies thus indicate that sense of smell can be utilized at different levels and scales for diagnosing COVID-19 and furthering the research on cognitive blunting due to this disease (**Figure 2**).

6. Using animal models for mechanistic understanding of entry, invasion, and destruction of nervous system

For a closer interrogation of the role of OE infection by CoV-2, gene expression patterns were studied in the mouse whole olfactory mucosa (WOM) and purified olfactory sensory neurons (OSNs). Single-cell sequencing of mouse WOM uncovered the expression of ACE2 and TMPRSS2 in the dorsally located SUS cells, basal globose cells as well as in a small fraction of the stem cells. Mouse OSNs, however, did not show the expression of the CoV-2 entry genes [6]. Within the OB as well, sequencing did not reveal any neuronal expression of these genes while the immunostaining displayed their expression in the pericytes of OB blood vessels. Postmortem magnetic resonance imaging (MRI) and histopathological examination confirmed microvascular injuries in the OB and brain stem of COVID-19-infected patients [120]. Such studies confirmed the olfactory trans-mucosal pathway of entry of CoV-2 virus into the body [3].

Using the hamster infection model of CoV-2 invasion, nucleoprotein expression was found out in Tuj1-positive infected OSNs and OMP staining also confirmed infection in mature OSNs [121]. Along with local inflammation of OE, SARS-CoV-2 infected the Tuj-1 positive immature OSNs, which appeared to be phagocytosed by the Iba1 and CoV-2-positive immune cells. In fact, global chromatin rearrangements occurred at day 3 post infection, which persisted even after the virus was cleared (10 days post infection) [122]. Whether the interferon response in the OSNs can bring about such chromatin changes in CoV-2 scenario remains an open question. It is also yet to be deciphered if other actively dividing cells are also prone to such disruptions and if not, then what makes certain cell types more unique and susceptible to viral-induced genomic modifications [123].

Nasal irrigation of virus in Golden Syrian Hamsters once again revealed the neuronal invasion. The OMP positive neuronal cilia were vanished in the virus-induced damaged epithelium of the animals. Both neuronal and non-neuronal cells were found out to be positive for cleaved caspase-3 after 4 days of infection, which was suggestive of cell death. Additionally, CoV-2 nucleoprotein was found at the junction of olfactory nerve and the OB and also in previously uncharacterized cells of the glomerular layer of the OB, suggestive of, invasion of the bulb by the virus [124]. Finally, to grasp the molecular underpinnings of the olfactory impairment upon viral infection, transcriptional changes in OE cells of the infected hamsters were studied. A significant reduction in the OR genes, i.e., the genes responsible for olfaction, was observed. At genomic level, they found out a drastic change in the long-range interactions of the OR genes with enhancer/activators 1 day post infection in a non-cell-autonomous fashion.

7. Conclusions

In this chapter, we have discussed the neurotropic nature of the SARS-CoV-2 virus. Using human and animal model studies, research groups across the globe have found out that neuroinvasion can occur by multiple routes, leading to dysfunctions of multiple cell types in the nervous system. The impairments that arise due to infection, which are collectively referred to as the Neuro-COVID, have also been summarized. Some of these symptoms persist in recovered individuals pointing to long-lasting consequences of the infection, which encompass the term Long COVID. We conclude that the virus can play havoc at multiple scales of the nervous system functioning, and the severity depends upon several factors such as the route and extent of infection, variant of the virus, and comorbidities in the patients. Finally, the under-appreciated sense of smell has indeed come into limelight, and the need for quantifying the olfactory and cognitive fitness has become vital during the pandemic. We, hereby, conclude that olfaction can be efficiently used in detecting the infection as well as providing a tool for investigating the cognitive capacities of human beings.

Acknowledgements

We thank Laboratory of Neural Circuits and Behaviour (LNCB) members for fruitful discussions and comments on the Manuscript.

This work was supported by the DST-Cognitive Science Research Initiative, (DST/CSRI/2017/271 to N.A.), DBT/Wellcome Trust India Alliance intermediate grant (IA/I/14/1/501306 to N.A.), and IISER-Pune Fellowship (M.P.).

Conflict of interest

The authors declare that they have no known competing financial interests or personal relationships that could have appeared to influence the work reported in this manuscript.

Notes/thanks/other declarations

We thank Rutuja Chalke for helping with the illustrations.

Author details

Meenakshi Pardasani* and Nixon M. Abraham*
Laboratory of Neural Circuits and Behaviour (LNCB), Department of Biology, Indian Institute of Science Education and Research (IISER), Pune, Maharashtra, India

*Address all correspondence to: nabraham@iiserpune.ac.in
and meenakshi.pardasani@gmail.com

References

[1] Puelles VG, Lütgehetmann M, Lindenmeyer MT, Sperhake JP, Wong MN, Allweiss L, et al. Multiorgan and renal tropism of SARS-CoV-2. New England Journal of Medicine. 2020;**383**:590-592

[2] Douaud G, Lee S, Alfaro-Almagro F, Arthofer C, Wang C, McCarthy P, et al. SARS-CoV-2 is associated with changes in brain structure in UK biobank. Nature. 2022;**604**:697-707

[3] Meinhardt J, Radke J, Dittmayer C, Franz J, Thomas C, Mothes R, et al. Olfactory transmucosal SARS-CoV-2 invasion as a port of central nervous system entry in individuals with COVID-19. Nature Neuroscience. 2021;**24**:168-175

[4] Khan M, Yoo S-J, Clijsters M, Backaert W, Vanstapel A, Speleman K, et al. Visualizing in deceased COVID-19 patients how SARS-CoV-2 attacks the respiratory and olfactory mucosae but spares the olfactory bulb. Cell. 2021;**184**:5932-5949

[5] Hoffmann M, Kleine-Weber H, Schroeder S, Krüger N, Herrler T, Erichsen S, et al. SARS-CoV-2 cell entry depends on ACE2 and TMPRSS2 and is blocked by a clinically proven protease inhibitor. Cell. 2020;**181**:271-280

[6] Brann DH, Tsukahara T, Weinreb C, Lipovsek M, den Berge K, Gong B, et al. Non-neuronal expression of SARS-CoV-2 entry genes in the olfactory system suggests mechanisms underlying COVID-19-associated anosmia. Science Advances. 2020;**6**:eabc5801

[7] Fodoulian L, Tuberosa J, Rossier D, Boillat M, Kan C, Pauli V, et al. SARS-CoV-2 receptors and entry genes are expressed in the human olfactory neuroepithelium and brain. iScience. 2020;**23**:101839

[8] Cantuti-Castelvetri L, Ojha R, Pedro LD, Djannatian M, Franz J, Kuivanen S, et al. Neuropilin-1 facilitates SARS-CoV-2 cell entry and infectivity. Science. 1979;**2020**(370):856-860

[9] Kyrou I, Randeva HS, Spandidos DA, Karteris E. Not only ACE2—The quest for additional host cell mediators of SARS-CoV-2 infection: Neuropilin-1 (NRP1) as a novel SARS-CoV-2 host cell entry mediator implicated in COVID-19. Signal Transduction and Targeted Therapy. 2021;**6**:1-3

[10] Huang X, Hussain B, Chang J. Peripheral inflammation and blood–brain barrier disruption: Effects and mechanisms. CNS Neuroscience & Therapeutics. 2021;**27**:36-47

[11] Heald-Sargent T, Gallagher T. Ready, set, fuse! The coronavirus spike protein and acquisition of fusion competence. Viruses. 2012;**4**:557-580

[12] Whittaker GR, Daniel S, Millet JK. Coronavirus entry: How we arrived at SARS-CoV-2. Current Opinion in Virology. 2021;**47**:113-120

[13] Li W, Moore MJ, Vasilieva N, Sui J, Wong SK, Berne MA, et al. Angiotensin-converting enzyme 2 is a functional receptor for the SARS coronavirus. Nature. 2003;**426**:450-454

[14] Gheblawi M, Wang K, Viveiros A, Nguyen Q, Zhong J-C, Turner AJ, et al. Angiotensin-converting enzyme 2: SARS-CoV-2 receptor and regulator of the renin-angiotensin system: Celebrating the 20th anniversary of the

discovery of ACE2. Circulation Research. 2020;**126**:1456-1474

[15] Glowacka I, Bertram S, Müller MA, Allen P, Soilleux E, Pfefferle S, et al. Evidence that TMPRSS2 activates the severe acute respiratory syndrome coronavirus spike protein for membrane fusion and reduces viral control by the humoral immune response. Journal of Virology. 2011;**85**:4122-4134

[16] Jackson CB, Farzan M, Chen B, Choe H. Mechanisms of SARS-CoV-2 entry into cells. Nature Reviews. Molecular Cell Biology. 2022;**23**:3-20

[17] Huang I-C, Bosch BJ, Li F, Li W, Lee KH, Ghiran S, et al. SARS coronavirus, but not human coronavirus NL63, utilizes cathepsin L to infect ACE2-expressing cells. Journal of Biological Chemistry. 2006;**281**:3198-3203

[18] Bayati A, Kumar R, Francis V, McPherson PS. SARS-CoV-2 infects cells after viral entry via clathrin-mediated endocytosis. Journal of Biological Chemistry. 2021;**296**:100306

[19] Whittaker GR. SARS-CoV-2 spike and its adaptable furin cleavage site. Lancet Microbe. 2021;**2**:e488-e489

[20] Sungnak W, Huang N, Bécavin C, Berg M, Queen R, Litvinukova M, et al. SARS-CoV-2 entry factors are highly expressed in nasal epithelial cells together with innate immune genes. Nature Medicine. 2020;**26**:681-687

[21] Klingenstein M, Klingenstein S, Neckel PH, Mack AF, Wagner AP, Kleger A, et al. Evidence of SARS-CoV2 entry protein ACE2 in the human nose and olfactory bulb. Cells, Tissues, Organs. 2020;**209**:155-164

[22] Collin J, Queen R, Zerti D, Dorgau B, Georgiou M, Djidrovski I, et al. Co-expression of SARS-CoV-2 entry genes in the superficial adult human conjunctival, limbal and corneal epithelium suggests an additional route of entry via the ocular surface. The Ocular Surface. 2021;**19**:190-200

[23] Sakaguchi W, Kubota N, Shimizu T, Saruta J, Fuchida S, Kawata A, et al. Existence of SARS-CoV-2 entry molecules in the oral cavity. International Journal of Molecular Sciences. 2020;**21**:6000

[24] Kaya H, Çalışkan A, Okul M, Sarı T, Akbudak İH. Detection of SARS-CoV-2 in the tears and conjunctival secretions of Coronavirus disease 2019 patients. The Journal of Infection in Developing Countries. 2020;(14):977-981

[25] Casagrande M, Fitzek A, Spitzer MS, Püschel K, Glatzel M, Krasemann S, et al. Presence of SARS-CoV-2 RNA in the cornea of viremic patients with COVID-19. JAMA Ophthalmology. 2021;**139**:383-388

[26] Zhou L, Xu Z, Castiglione GM, Soiberman US, Eberhart CG, Duh EJ. ACE2 and TMPRSS2 are expressed on the human ocular surface, suggesting susceptibility to SARS-CoV-2 infection. The Ocular Surface. 2020;**18**:537-544

[27] Huang N, Pérez P, Kato T, Mikami Y, Okuda K, Gilmore RC, et al. SARS-CoV-2 infection of the oral cavity and saliva. Nature Medicine. 2021;**27**:892-903

[28] Brandini DA, Takamiya AS, Thakkar P, Schaller S, Rahat R, Naqvi AR. Covid-19 and oral diseases: Crosstalk, synergy or association? Reviews in Medical Virology. 2021;**31**:e2226

[29] Al-Dalahmah O, Thakur KT, Nordvig AS, Prust ML, Roth W, Lignelli A, et al. Neuronophagia and microglial nodules in a SARS-CoV-2 patient with cerebellar hemorrhage. Acta Neuropathologica Communications. 2020;**8**:1-7

[30] Boldrini M, Canoll PD, Klein RS. How COVID-19 affects the brain. JAMA Psychiatry. 2021;**78**:682-683

[31] Liddelow SA, Guttenplan KA, Clarke LE, Bennett FC, Bohlen CJ, Schirmer L, et al. Neurotoxic reactive astrocytes are induced by activated microglia. Nature. 2017;**541**:481-487

[32] Guo M, Tao W, Flavell RA, Zhu S. Potential intestinal infection and faecal–oral transmission of SARS-CoV-2. Nature Reviews. Gastroenterology & Hepatology. 2021;**18**:269-283

[33] Canetta C, Accordino S, Buscarini E, Benelli G, la Piana G, Scartabellati A, et al. Syncope at SARS-CoV-2 onset. Autonomic Neuroscience. 2020;**229**:102734

[34] Baker J, Incognito A, v, Wilson RJA, Raj SR. Syncope and silent hypoxemia in COVID-19: Implications for the autonomic field. Autonomic Neuroscience. 2021;**235**:102842

[35] Mahammedi A, Ramos A, Bargalló N, Gaskill M, Kapur S, Saba L, et al. Brain and lung imaging correlation in patients with COVID-19: Could the severity of lung disease reflect the prevalence of acute abnormalities on neuroimaging? A global multicenter observational study. American Journal of Neuroradiology. 2021;**42**:1008-1016

[36] Zhou D, Wang Q, Liu H. Coronavirus disease 2019 and the gut–lung axis. International Journal of Infectious Diseases. 2021;113:300-307

[37] Porzionato A, Emmi A, Stocco E, Barbon S, Boscolo-Berto R, Macchi V, et al. The potential role of the carotid body in COVID-19. American Journal of Physiology-Lung Cellular and Molecular Physiology. 2020;**319**:L620-L626

[38] Lionetti V, Bollini S, Coppini R, Gerbino A, Ghigo A, Iaccarino G, et al. Understanding the heart-brain axis response in COVID-19 patients: A suggestive perspective for therapeutic development. Pharmacological Research. 2021;**168**:105581

[39] Nishiga M, Wang DW, Han Y, Lewis DB, Wu JC. COVID-19 and cardiovascular disease: From basic mechanisms to clinical perspectives. Nature Reviews. Cardiology. 2020;**17**:543-558

[40] Bauer L, Laksono BM, de Vrij FMS, Kushner SA, Harschnitz O, van Riel D. The neuroinvasiveness, neurotropism, and neurovirulence of SARS-CoV-2. Trends in Neurosciences. May 2022;**45**(5):358-368

[41] Jakhmola S, Indari O, Chatterjee S, Jha HC. SARS-CoV-2, an underestimated pathogen of the nervous system. SN Comprehensive Clinical Medicine. 2020;**2**:2137-2146

[42] Armstrong L, Collin J, Mostafa I, Queen R, Figueiredo FC, Lako M. In the eye of the storm: SARS-CoV-2 infection and replication at the ocular surface? Stem Cells Translational Medicine. 2021;**10**:976-986

[43] Tremblay M-E, Madore C, Bordeleau M, Tian L, Verkhratsky A. Neuropathobiology of COVID-19: The role for glia. Frontiers in Cellular Neuroscience. 2020;**14**:592214

[44] Barker CF, Billingham RE. Immunologically privileged sites. Advances in Immunology. 1978;**25**:1-54

[45] Han HS, Suk K. The function and integrity of the neurovascular unit rests upon the integration of the vascular and inflammatory cell systems. Current Neurovascular Research. 2005;**2**:409-423

[46] Ludlow M, Kortekaas J, Herden C, Hoffmann B, Tappe D, Trebst C, et al. Neurotropic virus infections as the cause of immediate and delayed neuropathology. Acta Neuropathologica. 2016;**131**:159-184

[47] Kapila CC, Kaul S, Kapur SC, Kalayanam TS, Banerjee D. Neurological and hepatic disorders associated with influenza. British Medical Journal. 1958;**2**:1311

[48] Nichols WG, Peck Campbell AJ, Boeckh M. Respiratory viruses other than influenza virus: Impact and therapeutic advances. Clinical Microbiology Reviews. 2008;**21**:274-290

[49] Bohmwald K, Gálvez NMS, Ríos M, Kalergis AM. Neurologic alterations due to respiratory virus infections. Frontiers in Cellular Neuroscience. 2018;**12**:386

[50] Wallace SJ, Zealley H. Neurological, electroencephalographic, and virological findings in febrile children. Archives of Disease in Childhood. 1970;**45**:611-623

[51] Ann Yeh E, Collins A, Cohen ME, Duffner PK, Faden H. Detection of coronavirus in the central nervous system of a child with acute disseminated encephalomyelitis. Pediatrics. 2004;**113**:e73-e76

[52] Webster DL, Gardner AH, Dye TJ, Chima RS. Status epilepticus: A possible association with human metapneumovirus infection. Pediatrics. 2014;**133**:e747-e750

[53] Desforges M, le Coupanec A, Dubeau P, Bourgouin A, Lajoie L, Dubé M, et al. Human coronaviruses and other respiratory viruses: Underestimated opportunistic pathogens of the central nervous system? Viruses. 2019;**12**:14

[54] Jha NK, Ojha S, Jha SK, Dureja H, Singh SK, Shukla SD, et al. Evidence of coronavirus (CoV) pathogenesis and emerging pathogen SARS-CoV-2 in the nervous system: A review on neurological impairments and manifestations. Journal of Molecular Neuroscience. 2021;**71**:2192-2209

[55] Ye M, Ren Y, Lv T. Encephalitis as a clinical manifestation of COVID-19. Brain, Behavior, and Immunity. 2020;**88**:945

[56] Zhou Z, Kang H, Li S, Zhao X. Understanding the neurotropic characteristics of SARS-CoV-2: From neurological manifestations of COVID-19 to potential neurotropic mechanisms. Journal of Neurology. 2020;**267**:2179-2184

[57] di Mauro G, Scavone C, Rafaniello C, Rossi F, Capuano A. SARS-Cov-2 infection: Response of human immune system and possible implications for the rapid test and treatment. International Immunopharmacology. 2020;**84**:106519

[58] Wu Y, Xu X, Chen Z, Duan J, Hashimoto K, Yang L, et al. Nervous system involvement after infection with COVID-19 and other coronaviruses. Brain, Behavior, and Immunity. 2020;**87**:18-22

[59] Fan H, Tang X, Song Y, Liu P, Chen Y. Influence of COVID-19 on cerebrovascular disease and its possible mechanism. Neuropsychiatric Disease and Treatment. 2020;**16**:1359

[60] Politi LS, Salsano E, Grimaldi M. Magnetic resonance imaging alteration of the brain in a patient with coronavirus disease 2019 (COVID-19) and anosmia. JAMA Neurology. 2020;**77**:1028-1029

[61] von Weyhern CH, Kaufmann I, Neff F, Kremer M. Early evidence of pronounced brain involvement in fatal

COVID-19 outcomes. The Lancet. 2020;**395**:e109

[62] Mehta S, Bhandari S, Mehta S. Brain autopsies in fatal COVID-19 and postulated pathophysiology: More puzzling than a Rubik's cube. Journal of Clinical Pathology. 2021;**74**:612-613

[63] Veleri S. Neurotropism of SARS-CoV-2 and neurological diseases of the central nervous system in COVID-19 patients. Experimental Brain Research. 2022;**240**:9-25

[64] Bergmann CC, Lane TE, Stohlman SA. Coronavirus infection of the central nervous system: host–virus stand-off. Nature Reviews. Microbiology. 2006;**4**:121-132

[65] Murray RS, Brown B, Brain D, Cabirac GF. Detection of coronavirus RNA and antigen in multiple sclerosis brain. Annals of Neurology: Official Journal of the American Neurological Association and the Child Neurology Society. 1992;**31**:525-533

[66] Sharifian-DorcheM,HuotP,OsherovM, Wen D, Saveriano A, Giacomini PS, et al. Neurological complications of coronavirus infection; A comparative review and lessons learned during the COVID-19 pandemic. Journal of the Neurological Sciences. 2020;**417**:117085

[67] Kim J-E, Heo J-H, Kim H, Song S, Park S-S, Park T-H, et al. Neurological complications during treatment of Middle East respiratory syndrome. Journal of Clinical Neurology. 2017;**13**:227-233

[68] Reichard RR, Kashani KB, Boire NA, Constantopoulos E, Guo Y, Lucchinetti CF. Neuropathology of COVID-19: A spectrum of vascular and acute disseminated encephalomyelitis (ADEM)-like pathology. Acta Neuropathologica. 2020;**140**:1-6

[69] Ameres M, Brandstetter S, Toncheva AA, Kabesch M, Leppert D, Kuhle J, et al. Association of neuronal injury blood marker neurofilament light chain with mild-to-moderate COVID-19. Journal of Neurology. 2020;**267**:3476-3478

[70] el Otmani H, el Moutawakil B, Rafai M-A, el Benna N, el Kettani C, Soussi M, et al. Covid-19 and Guillain-Barré syndrome: More than a coincidence! Revue Neurologique (Paris). 2020;**176**:518

[71] Xiong W, Kwan P, Zhou D, del Felice A, Duncan JS, Sander JW. Acute and late neurological complications of COVID19: The quest for evidence. Brain. 2020;**143**:e99-e99

[72] Nalbandian A, Sehgal K, Gupta A, Madhavan MV, McGroder C, Stevens JS, et al. Post-acute COVID-19 syndrome. Nature Medicine. 2021;**27**:601-615

[73] Garcia, Maria A, et al. Cerebrospinal fluid in COVID-19 neurological complications: Neuroaxonal damage, anti-SARS-Cov2 antibodies but no evidence of cytokine storm. Journal of the Neurological Sciences. 2021;**427**:117517

[74] Morbini P, Benazzo M, Verga L, Pagella FGM, Mojoli F, Bruno R, et al. Ultrastructural evidence of direct viral damage to the olfactory complex in patients testing positive for SARS-CoV-2. JAMA Otolaryngology—Head & Neck Surgery. 2020;**146**:972-973

[75] Koyuncu O, Hogue I, Enquist L. Virus infections in the nervous system. Cell Host & Microbe. 2013;**13**:379-393

[76] Lyoo K-S, Kim HM, Lee B, Che YH, Kim S-J, Song D, et al. Direct neuronal

infection of SARS-CoV-2 reveals cellular and molecular pathology of chemosensory impairment of COVID-19 patients. Emerging Microbes & Infections. 2022;**11**:406-411

[77] Han Y, Yang L, Kim TW, Nair MS, Harschnitz O, Wang P, et al. SARS-CoV-2 infection causes dopaminergic neuron senescence. Research Square. 2021. DOI: 10.21203/rs.3.rs-513461/v1

[78] Ramani A, Müller L, Ostermann PN, Gabriel E, Abida-Islam P, Müller-Schiffmann A, et al. SARS-CoV-2 targets neurons of 3D human brain organoids. The EMBO Journal. 2020;**39**:e106230

[79] Zhang L, Zhou L, Bao L, Liu J, Zhu H, Lv Q, et al. SARS-CoV-2 crosses the blood–brain barrier accompanied with basement membrane disruption without tight junctions alteration. Signal Transduction and Targeted Therapy. 2021;**6**:1-12

[80] Hopfer H, Herzig MC, Gosert R, Menter T, Hench J, Tzankov A, et al. Hunting coronavirus by transmission electron microscopy—A guide to SARS-CoV-2-associated ultrastructural pathology in COVID-19 tissues. Histopathology. 2021;**78**:358-370

[81] Jiao L, Yang Y, Yu W, Zhao Y, Long H, Gao J, et al. The olfactory route is a potential way for SARS-CoV-2 to invade the central nervous system of rhesus monkeys. Signal Transduction and Targeted Therapy. 2021;**6**:1-11

[82] Lam SM, Huang X, Shui G. Neurological aspects of SARS-CoV-2 infection—Lipoproteins and exosomes as Trojan horses. Trends in Endocrinology & Metabolism. Aug 2022;**33**(8):554-568

[83] Mao L, Jin H, Wang M, Hu Y, Chen S, He Q, et al. Neurologic manifestations of hospitalized patients with coronavirus disease 2019 in Wuhan, China. JAMA Neurology. 2020;**77**:683-690

[84] Helms J, Kremer S, Merdji H, Clere-Jehl R, Schenck M, Kummerlen C, et al. Neurologic features in severe SARS-CoV-2 infection. New England Journal of Medicine. 2020;**382**:2268-2270

[85] Bussière N, Mei J, Lévesque-Boissonneault C, Blais M, Carazo S, Gros-Louis F, et al. Chemosensory dysfunctions induced by COVID-19 can persist up to 7 months: A study of over 700 healthcare workers. Chemical Senses. 1 Jan 2021;**46**:bjab038. DOI: 10.1093/chemse/bjab038

[86] Gerkin RC, Ohla K, Veldhuizen MG, Joseph PV, Kelly CE, Bakke AJ, et al. Recent smell loss is the best predictor of COVID-19 among individuals with recent respiratory symptoms. Chemical Senses. 1 Jan 2021;**46**:bjaa081. DOI: 10.1093/chemse/bjaa081.

[87] Chou SH-Y, Beghi E, Helbok R, Moro E, Sampson J, Altamirano V, et al. Global incidence of neurological manifestations among patients hospitalized with COVID-19—A report for the GCS-NeuroCOVID consortium and the ENERGY consortium. JAMA Network Open. 2021;**4**:e2112131-e2112131

[88] Jindal HA, Sahoo SS, Jamir L, Kedar A, Sharma S, Bhatt B. Higher coronavirus disease-19 mortality linked to comorbidities: A comparison between low-middle income and high-income countries. Journal of Education Health Promotion. 2021;**10**:377

[89] Palermo S. "Neurocovid": An analysis of the impact of Covid-19 on the older adults. Evolving psychological and neuropsychological understanding. In: Fighting the COVID-19 Pandemic. IntechOpen; 2021. p. 215

[90] Santos-García D, Oreiro M, Pérez P, Fanjul G, Paz González JM, Feal Painceiras MJ, et al. Impact of coronavirus disease 2019 pandemic on Parkinson's disease: A cross-sectional survey of 568 Spanish patients. Movement Disorders. 2020;**35**:1712-1716

[91] Shah VA, Nalleballe K, Zaghlouleh ME, Onteddu S. Acute encephalopathy is associated with worse outcomes in COVID-19 patients. Brain, Behavior, & Immunity—Health. 2020;**8**:100136

[92] Palermo S. Covid-19 pandemic: Maximizing future vaccination treatments considering aging and frailty. Frontiers of Medicine (Lausanne). 2020;**7**:558835

[93] Sullivan BN, Fischer T. Age-associated neurological complications of COVID-19: A systematic review and meta-analysis. Frontiers in Aging Neuroscience. Aug 2021;**13**:374. DOI: 10.3389/fnagi.2021.653694

[94] Brown EE, Kumar S, Rajji TK, Pollock BG, Mulsant BH. Anticipating and mitigating the impact of COVID-19 pandemic on Alzheimer's disease and related dementias. The American Journal of Geriatric Psychiatry. 2020;**28**(7):712-721

[95] Iravani B, Arshamian A, Lundström JN. Loss of olfactory sensitivity is an early and reliable marker for COVID-19. Chemical Senses. 2022;**47**:bjac022. DOI: 10.1093/chemse/bjac022

[96] Guo P, Benito Ballesteros A, Yeung SP, Liu R, Saha A, Curtis L, et al. COVCOG 2: Cognitive and memory deficits in Long COVID: A second publication from the COVID and cognition study. Frontiers in Aging Neuroscience. Mar 2022;**14**. Article ID: 804937. DOI: 10.3389/fnagi.2022.804937

[97] Bougakov D, Podell K, Goldberg E. Multiple neuroinvasive pathways in COVID-19. Molecular Neurobiology. 2021;**58**:564-575

[98] Hampshire A, Trender W, Chamberlain SR, Jolly AE, Grant JE, Patrick F, et al. Cognitive deficits in people who have recovered from COVID-19. EClinicalMedicine. 2021;**39**:101044

[99] Hugon J, Msika E-F, Queneau M, Farid K, Paquet C. Long COVID: Cognitive complaints (brain fog) and dysfunction of the cingulate cortex. Journal of Neurology. 2022;**269**:44-46

[100] Kang YJ, Cho JH, Lee MH, Kim YJ, Park C-S. The diagnostic value of detecting sudden smell loss among asymptomatic COVID-19 patients in early stage: The possible early sign of COVID-19. Auris, Nasus, Larynx. 2020;**47**:565-573

[101] Bhattacharjee AS, Joshi SV, Naik S, Sangle S, Abraham NM. Quantitative assessment of olfactory dysfunction accurately detects asymptomatic COVID-19 carriers. EClinicalMedicine. 2020;**28**:100575

[102] Whitcroft KL, Hummel T. Olfactory dysfunction in COVID-19: Diagnosis and management. Journal of the American Medical Association. 2020;**323**:2512-2514

[103] Li J, Wang X, Zhu C, Lin Z, Xiong N. Affected olfaction in COVID-19: Re-defining "asymptomatic". EClinicalMedicine. Dec 2020;**29-30**:100628

[104] Doty RL, Shaman P, Dann M. Development of the University of Pennsylvania Smell Identification Test: A standardized microencapsulated test of olfactory function. Physiology & Behavior. 1984;**32**:489-502

[105] Ugurlu BN, Akdogan O, Yilmaz YA, Yapar D, Aktar Ugurlu G, Yerlikaya HS, et al. Quantitative evaluation and progress of olfactory dysfunction in COVID-19. European Archives of Oto-Rhino-Laryngology. 2021;**278**:2363-2369

[106] Moein ST, Hashemian SM, Mansourafshar B, Khorram-Tousi A, Tabarsi P, Doty RL. Smell dysfunction: A biomarker for COVID-19. International Forum of Allergy & Rhinology. (Chicago). 2020;**10**(8):944-950

[107] Hummel T, Pfetzing U, Lötsch J. A short olfactory test based on the identification of three odors. Journal of Neurology. 2010;**257**:1316-1321

[108] Bagnasco D, Passalacqua G, Braido F, Tagliabue E, Cosini F, Filauro M, et al. Quick olfactory Sniffin'Sticks test (Q-sticks) for the detection of smell disorders in COVID-19 patients. World Allergy Organization Journal. 2021;**14**:100497

[109] Parma V, Hannum ME, O'Leary M, Pellegrino R, Rawson NE, Reed DR, et al. SCENTinel 1.0: Development of a rapid test to screen for smell loss. Chemical Senses. 1 Jan 2021;**46**:bjab012. DOI: 10.1093/chemse/bjab012

[110] Said M, Davis P, Davis S, Smart K, Davis S, Yan CH. A rapid olfactory test as a potential screening tool for COVID-19. JAMA Otolaryngology—Head & Neck Surgery. 2021;**147**:828-831

[111] Albaharna HA, Alhajjaj AH, al Shabeb HA, Alghanim DA, Alkhabbaz FL, JM AJ. Screening for olfactory dysfunction in COVID-19 patients using quick smell identification test. Indian Journal of Otolaryngology and Head & Neck Surgery. 2021:1-7. DOI: 10.1007/s12070-021-02709-3

[112] Bhowmik R, Pardasani M, Mahajan S, Magar R, Joshi SV, Nair GA, et al. Persistent olfactory learning deficits during and post-COVID-19 infection. 2022. DOI: 10.2139/ssrn.4202478

[113] Abraham NM. Olfactory-action meter for precise quantification of olfactory dysfunctions and neurocognitive deficits. US Patent App. 17/443,527, 2022, Publication number: 20220054075, Feb 24, 2022

[114] Bhowmik R, Pardasani M, Mahajan S, Bhattacharjee AS, Konakamchi S, Phadnis S, et al. Uncertainty revealed by delayed responses during olfactory matching. BioRxiv. 2022. DOI: 10.1101/2022.09.11.507462

[115] Hummel T, Sekinger B, Wolf SR, Pauli E, Kobal G. "Sniffin'sticks": Olfactory performance assessed by the combined testing of odor identification, odor discrimination and olfactory threshold. Chemical Senses. 1997;**22**:39-52

[116] Hag-Ali M, AlShamsi AS, Boeijen L, Mahmmod Y, Manzoor R, Rutten H, et al. The detection dogs test is more sensitive than real-time PCR in screening for SARS-CoV-2. Communications Biology. 2021;**4**:1-7

[117] Grandjean D, Sarkis R, Lecoq-Julien C, Benard A, Roger V, Levesque E, et al. Can the detection dog alert on COVID-19 positive persons by sniffing axillary sweat samples? A proof-of-concept study. PLoS One. 2020;**15**:e0243122

[118] Snitz K, Andelman-Gur M, Pinchover L, Weissgross R, Weissbrod A, Mishor E, et al. Proof of concept for real-time detection of SARS CoV-2 infection with an electronic nose. PLoS One. 2021;**16**:e0252121

[119] Guest C, Dewhirst SY, Lindsay SW, Allen DJ, Aziz S, Baerenbold O, et al.

Using trained dogs and organic semi-conducting sensors to identify asymptomatic and mild SARS-CoV-2 infections: An observational study. Journal of Travel Medicine. 2022;**29**:taac043

[120] Galougahi MK, Ghorbani J, Bakhshayeshkaram M, Naeini AS, Haseli S. Olfactory bulb magnetic resonance imaging in SARS-CoV-2-induced anosmia: The first report. Academic Radiology. 2020;**27**:892

[121] Chan JF-W, Zhang AJ, Yuan S, Poon VK-M, Chan CC-S, Lee AC-Y, et al. Simulation of the clinical and pathological manifestations of coronavirus disease 2019 (COVID-19) in a golden Syrian hamster model: Implications for disease pathogenesis and transmissibility. Clinical Infectious Diseases. 2020;**71**:2428-2446

[122] Zazhytska M, Kodra A, Hoagland DA, Frere J, Fullard JF, Shayya H, et al. Non-cell-autonomous disruption of nuclear architecture as a potential cause of COVID-19-induced anosmia. Cell. 2022;**185**:1052-1064

[123] Sorek M, Meshorer E. Can't smell the virus: SARS-CoV-2, chromatin organization, and anosmia. Developmental Cell. 2022;**57**:1081-1082

[124] de Melo GD, Lazarini F, Levallois S, Hautefort C, Michel V, Larrous F, et al. COVID-19-related anosmia is associated with viral persistence and inflammation in human olfactory epithelium and brain infection in hamsters. Science Translational Medicine. 2021;**13**:eabf8396

Chapter 2

Neurological Effects of COVID-19 and Its Treatment/Management

John Teibo, Abolaji Olagunju, Festus Atiba, Olabode Omotoso, Titilade Teibo, Ahmad Babalghith and Gaber Batiha

Abstract

The impact of COVID-19 is significant in the body system, one of which is the central nervous system (CNS) involved in controlling all aspects of human behavior and coordination. This shows the need to assess from various studies in human and animal models the neurological effects of this virus. Some of the reported effects include loss of taste and smell, headaches, delirium, dizziness, ischemic stroke, and brain inflammation. It is essential to review the acute, chronic or transient neurological effects. This will enhance and/or improve treatment designs and management modalities for the COVID-19. We critically revise the literature and contribute to the body of knowledge in this line of research. Here in this chapter, we highlighted the various neurological disorders caused by COVID-19 and examined the relationship between the neurological systems and COVID-19. As well as evaluate current treatment/management modalities including vaccines and prospects for the future.

Keywords: COVID-19, SARS-CoV-2, neurological disorders, neurological symptoms, treatment/management modalities

1. Introduction

COVID-19 causative virus (SARS-CoV-2) affects many body organs and systems to induce its pathogenesis. The disease is severe in people with comorbidities such as obesity, diabetes, hypertension, chronic respiratory disease, cerebrovascular disease, and chronic kidney and liver disease [1].

In neural tissues, the mechanism of invasion is well-established. It involves the interaction of ACE2 (Angiotensin-converting enzyme 2) receptors and spike protein. SARS-CoV-2 enters the nervous system via neurotropism, hematological dissemination, vasculotropism, and cytokine storm [2, 3].

Some of the common neurological symptoms of SARS-CoV-2 include CNS symptoms; (dizziness, delirium, confusion, prominent agitation, and dizziness), acute cerebrovascular disease, and epilepsy; PNS symptoms; ageusia (loss of sense of taste), hypogeusia (reduction in the ability to taste), anosmia (inability to smell), hyposmia (reduction in the ability to smell), and neuralgia (painful sensation in the body) and skeletal muscular symptoms: myalgia/fatigue and muscle injury [3, 4].

Many bioactive compounds have been reviewed for their antiviral effects which may have both preventive and curative effects [5]. Mainstay pharmacological/non-pharmacological interventions for prevention, management, and treatment include COVID-19 vaccines, remdesivir [6], SARS-CoV-2 targeting monoclonal antibodies such as Casirivimab and Imdevimab, Immune modulators (Baricitinib), immunosuppressive therapy as well adherence to public health guidelines such as handwashing, use of alcohol gels and face masks, etc.

In this chapter, we highlighted various neurological disorders and symptoms caused by COVID-19 and examined the relationship between the neurological systems and COVID-19. Additionally, we evaluated current therapies including the administration of vaccines, anti-virals, and their prospects for future applications.

2. COVID-19

The novel coronavirus disease (COVID-19) has been a dire threat to public health, the global economy, and human co-existence since its first report in Wuhan, China in 2019 [7]. Globally, as of 2nd June 2022, there have been 6,293,414 deaths due to COVID-19 out of 528,275,339 confirmed cases. To curtail the menace of COVID-19, 11,947,644,522 vaccine doses have been reported administered globally [8]. Prior to the development and administration of vaccines, a number of preventive measures (hand-washing under running water, use of alcohol-based hand sanitizer, social distancing, wearing of face mask, etc.) were put in place by health regulatory bodies to manage the transmission of the disease [7]. These measures were evaluated to study compliance and effectiveness in curbing the spread of the virus [9–11]. Although the global incidence and mortality rate has declined, adherence to preventive measures and vaccination is still encouraged.

COVID-19 severity has been reported in elderly patients and those with comorbidities (obesity, diabetes, hypertension, chronic respiratory disease, cardiovascular disease, cerebrovascular disease, chronic kidney, and liver disease) [1, 12]. Due to the novelty of the disease, the possibility of other long-term effects is still unknown. However, those with severe cases of infection can develop acute or chronic effects (graphical abstract) such as chronic fatigue syndrome, complications of the heart, lung, and kidney, neurological defects (loss of taste and smell, delirium, headaches, brain inflammation, stroke, and Guillain-Barre syndrome) [12, 13]. This calls for a need for closer monitoring and more research into the aftermath effect of the COVID-19, even in well-managed patients.

3. Mechanism of neurological pathology

The SARS-CoV-2 respiratory indices are well known and reported. Recently, there has been a significant increase in evidence showing anosmia (complete loss of smell) as a SARS-CoV-2 symptom, indicating a high level of neurological involvement following the infection and also SARS-CoV-2 having neuro-invasive properties. Studies suggest that SARS-CoV-2 enters the central nervous system (CNS) in either of the two ways; through systemic vascular dissemination or across the cribriform plate of the ethmoid bone, which might have consequences concerning anosmia as experienced by the SARS-CoV-2 patients [14]. The virus invades the neural tissue once in the systemic circulation due to its neurotropism properties and then, binds and interacts with ACE2 (Angiotensin-converting enzyme 2) receptors in the endothelium capillary via the spike proteins [14, 15]. Previously, ACE2 has been shown to be expressed in the upper and lower epithelium of the airways together with the CNS endothelial capillary [16]. One of the studies conducted evaluating SARS-CoV-2 spike glycoprotein structural integrity showed an approximately 20- a fold affinity increases to ACE2 when compared to the spike protein of the sister virus SARS-CoV-2 [17]. However, using BLASTp, the spike proteins of the two sister viruses are structurally similar but not identical, explaining the differences in the neurological prevalence. Meanwhile, not all the human cell lines that express ACE2 are susceptible to the novel coronavirus infection. Nevertheless, several neurological manifestations of the SARS-CoV-2 infection should be given absolute attention together with its well-understood respiratory index.

3.1 Stroke

Stroke is now common, developing, and/or potentially devastating SARS-CoV-2 infection complication [18]; about 2–6% of hospitalized COVID-19 patients have developed an acute cerebrovascular event [19]. In 2020, a large vessel stroke was reported in five patients (< 50 years of age) infected with SARS-CoV-2 [20]. Studies on the thromboembolic complications rate in SARS-CoV-2 patients showed 1.6% [21] and 2.5% [22] reported ischemic stroke occurrences. Klok and Lodigiani showed that the thrombotic complications were significantly high for their respective institutions. However, there are other risk factors predisposing COVID-19 patients to thromboembolic stroke development beyond the usual metabolic and cardiovascular co-morbidities. At this moment, various mechanisms of SARS-CoV-2 induced stroke have been reported including myocardial damage with cerebral embolism, coagulopathy, or pre-existing atheroma plaque destabilization [23]. The viral invasion led to thrombosis by activating immune response involving platelets, endothelium, and coagulation. Furthermore, SARS-CoV-2 causes cytokine storms resulting in increased D-dimers, affecting coagulation, and inducing stroke. Also, viral invasion can lead to heart damage, resulting in viral myocarditis and finally cardioembolic stroke. Inflammation can destabilize the fibrous capsule surrounding the atheroma plaque, eventually, exposing the thrombogenic clotting material, initiating arteries clogging and thus, causing a stroke [23].

3.2 Guillain-Barré syndrome (GBS)

GBS is an acute acquired autoimmune disorder of the peripheral nerves that occurs as a result of infection [24]. Actually, GBS is symmetrical ascending paralysis, mostly due to bacteria or viral infection of the respiratory or gastrointestinal tract [25]. It is a rare disease of the peripheral nervous system (PNS) with approximately 1.11 in 100,000 incidences annually [26]. Since the COVID-19 outbreak, the number of GBS cases has increased significantly. There have been some confirmed cases and a potential report of GBS as significant SARS-CoV-2 neurological sequelae. Among the eleven cases published in the literature, there is substantial capriciousness in an indication of GBS onset, together with distinctive respiratory distress of SARS-CoV-2 [27]. GBS is related to recent inoculation from a possible range of pathogens, explaining the disease's clinical heterogeneity [28]. Despite the inconsistency in the symptom onset in relation to COVID-19 diagnosis, it is of note that most reports described constant clinical features of variable sensory abnormalities with deep tendon reflex loss and lower limb weakness over the upper limb. Various mechanisms the virus uses to trigger acute areflexic state in GBS have been reported. Possibly, antibodies against the surface glycoproteins are generated against the pathogen which also responds to the comparable native protein structures located on the neuronal surface leading to GBS clinical features [29]. Another probable mechanism is the macrophage activation syndrome (cytokine storm) and hyper-inflammation might be involved in GBS pathogenesis in SARS-CoV-2 individuals [30].

3.3 Neurocognitive disorder

Individuals with neurocognitive disorders have a high risk of being infected with COVID-19. APOE e4 increases the risk of Alzheimer's neurocognitive disorder. Previous studies revealed that the deformed blood–brain barrier (BBB) in Alzheimer's patients predisposes them to infections. Furthermore, memory impairment related to neurocognitive disorders could possibly affect the patient's capability to observe the COVID-19 preventive measures including the use of masks, hand-sanitizing, and social distancing [31]. Individuals with neurocognitive disorders are more liable to experience comorbidities including diabetes, pneumonia, or cardiovascular disease increasing their risk of severe morbidities or death if they contract COVID-19 [32]. Previous research has found a bidirectional association between viral infections and neurocognitive disorders. Patients with neurocognitive disorders have a higher chance of viral infection and patients with a poor immune response to the infection have a higher risk of neurocognitive disorders [31]. Further research is needed to understand if the molecular and socioeconomic interactions play role in the higher incidence of COVID-19 in patients with neurocognitive disorders patients, and to identify whether SARS-CoV-2 infection accelerates or triggers neurocognitive disorders [31].

3.4 Movement disorders

COVID-19 could potentially aggravate neurological symptoms in PD individuals [33]. The effect of COVID-19 on individuals with Parkinson's (PD) disease is multifaceted as SARS-CoV-2 can affect their health directly, with a downstream effect on the advancement of the disease and the quality of life. Several studies have reported the onset of deteriorating PD and motor symptoms (for example speech disturbance, fall, dystonic spasms) preceding COVID-19 diagnosis [34–36]. Motor symptom changes might be a result of a decrease in oral therapy absorption due to diarrhea -a COVID-19 symptom [37]. Worsening of the symptoms can be ascribed to the pandemic subordinate effects including changes in normal activities and stress. Fatigue, rigidity, pain, concentration, and tremor were recorded during neurological symptoms evaluation for individuals with PD a month before the pandemic began and beyond [38].

3.5 Hypoxia

Several COVID-19 patients appeared to have severely low blood oxygen saturation levels [39], leading to hypoxia which causes damage to the tissues [40]. Meanwhile, these patients do not get enough oxygenation via the blood, COVID-19 individuals with hypoxia often do not show much respiratory distress, but they feel alert, and can easily talk [39]. Hence, hypoxia in COVID-19 individuals is often known as "happy" or "silent" hypoxia due to its minimal additional effects [39]. In a study by Mortaz et al. COVID-19 participants' RBC had higher amounts of intracellular NO (nitric oxide). This is not due to hypoxia per se, but it could provide protection against the hypoxia reported in COVID-19 patients. Constitutive NO generation in RBCs is mostly dependent on NOS during health, although NO production in hypoxic settings may entail nitrite reduction by deoxyhemoglobin carbonic anhydrase and/or eNOS itself. Also, COVID-19 participants' RBC had higher amounts of intracellular NO [39].

4. Relationship and effects of COVID-19 on neurological systems

In the past, viruses such as arbovirus, measles virus, enterovirus, herpes simplex virus (HSV), Varicella-Zoster virus (VZV), Cytomegalovirus (CMV), Epstein -Barr virus (EBV), and Human JC virus (JCV) have been reported to invade the nervous systems of hosts with severe neurological effects [41]. Now, SARS CoV-2 (severe acute respiratory syndrome coronavirus 2), the virus that causes COVID-19 has joined that list with recently reported neurological manifestations of the disease. The mode of entry of these viruses including SARS CoV-2 has been thoroughly studied and classified into the several major routes: endocytosis (direct fusion with neurons), sensory nerve endings, synapses, and axons, circulating leukocytes, lymph nodes, the blood–brain barrier (BBB), the Central Nervous System (CNS) and the Peripheral Nervous System (PNS) [42].

4.1 SARS-CoV-2 and angiotensin-converting enzyme 2 (ACE2)

ACE2 has a high affinity for SARS-CoV-2 (**Figures 1** and **2**). SARS-CoV-2 interacts with ACE2 receptors to invade the cells in the body [45, 46] by receiving the spike (peplomer) glycoprotein of the virus. mRNA expression profile of ACE2 shows that the enzyme is organ-specific but expressed in almost every tissue in the body [46, 47]. ACE2 receptor is usually found in the pulmonary type II alveolar cells and respiratory epithelial at high levels because COVID-19 is primarily a respiratory disease [48, 49]. ACE2 is also found in other body tissues and cells such as myocardial and endothelial cells [50], kidney, stomach, colon, and ileum cells [51], oral mucosa cells [52], astrocytes, neuron and glial cells of the brain and spinal cord tissues (**Figure 1**) [14].

The ACE2 gene is located on chromosome Xp22.22 and contains 18 exons and 20 introns [53]. It produces an 805 amino acid, type I transmembrane glycoprotein which contains a 17-amino-acid N-terminal signal peptide and a 22-amino acid C-terminal membrane hydrophobic transmembrane region anchoring it in the cell membrane [46]. It also has a HEXXH zinc-binding metalloprotease motif, a C-terminal collecting domain, and an insulin-like domain [53]. ACE2 gene expression is also found in other respiratory disorders such as SARS, Middle East respiratory syndrome (MERS), and H1N1 influenza [54].

4.2 Relationship of COVID-19 with neurological systems

SARS-CoV-2 directly attacks neural cells and infects cerebrovascular endothelium and brain parenchyma (medial temporal lobe) causing early apoptosis and necrosis

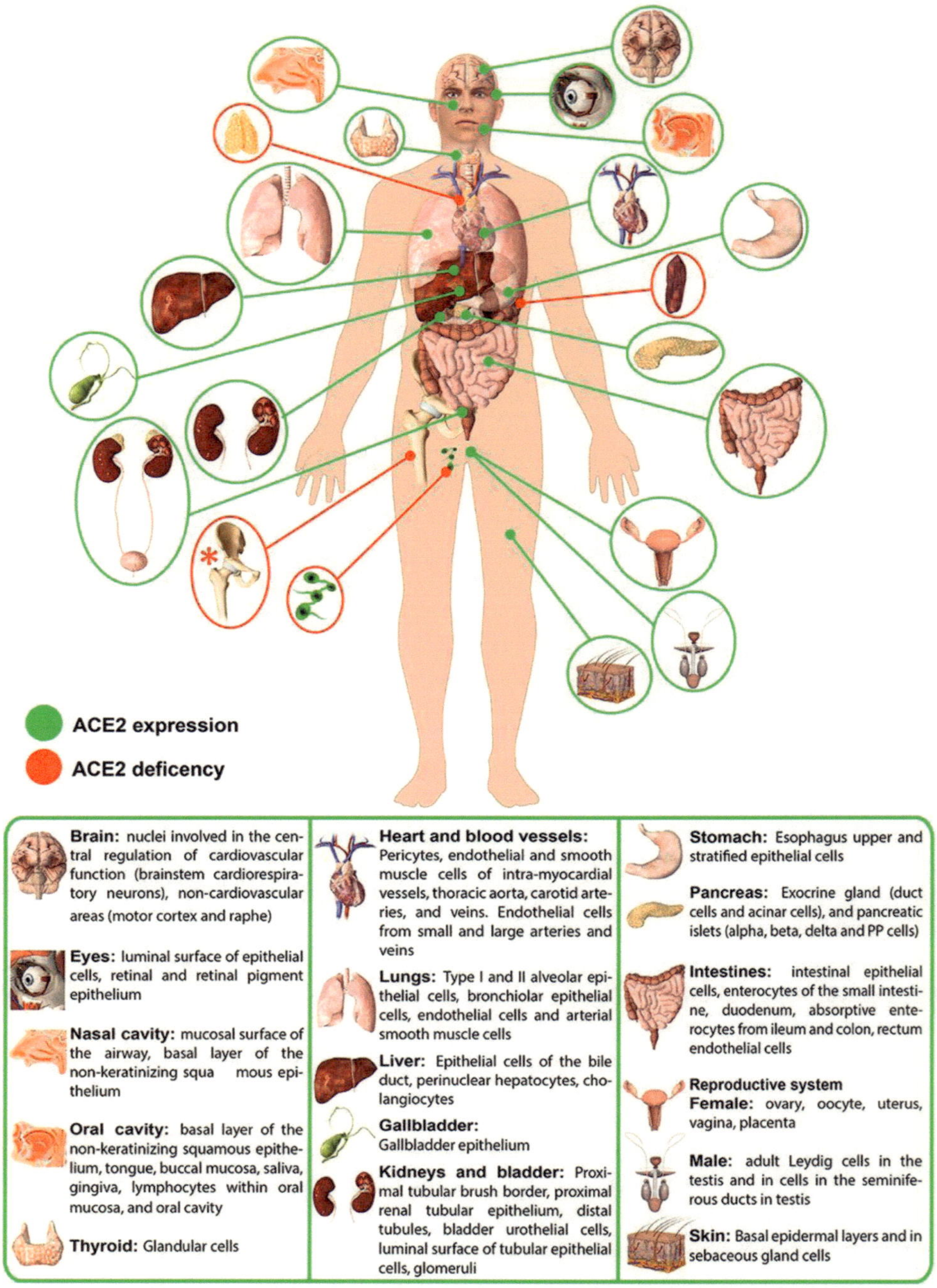

Figure 1.
Distribution of ACE 2 in the human body. (image adapted from [43]).

(**Figure 3**) [4, 44, 48]. This attack occurs through a series of mechanisms such as proteolysis, viral fusion with membrane, and entry mediated by ACE2 and transmembrane serine protease 2 (TMPRSS2) in some parts of the brain, CNS, PNS, and cerebrospinal fluid described through animal studies [see 55–58 for more details].

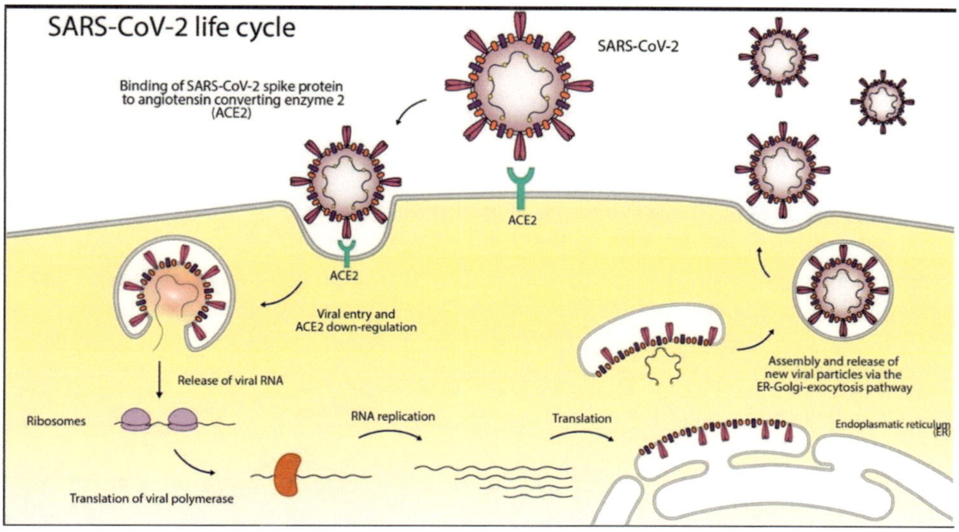

Figure 2.
SARS-CoV life cycle (image adapted from [44]).

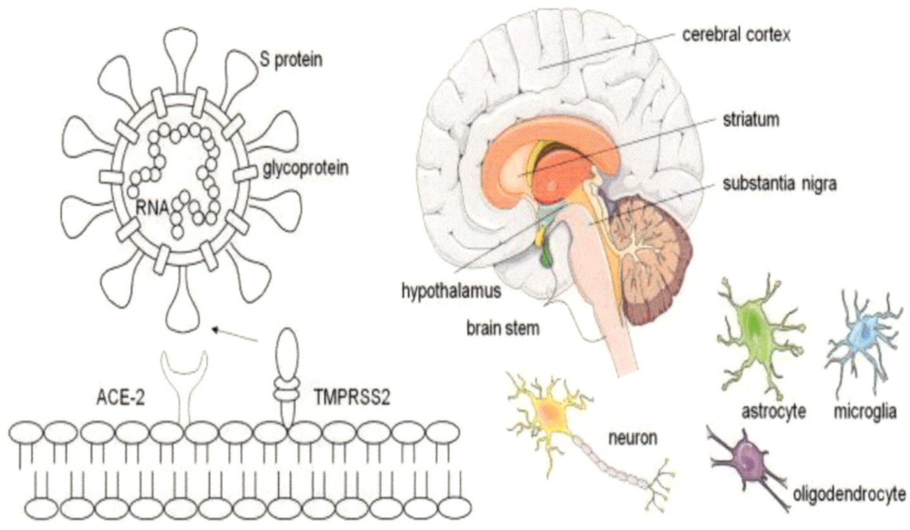

Figure 3.
Neurotropism of SARS-CoV-2. SARS-CoV-2 (image and description text and Servier medical art, https://smart.servier.com).

4.3 Proposed mechanisms of coronavirus entry into the nervous system

1. **Neurotropism:** retrograde transfer from the olfactory epithelium to the brain via cribriform plate (**Figure 4**) [3, 49].

2. **Hematological Dissemination:** damage to the blood–brain barrier during the viremia phase [3, 14]. Brain areas devoid of a blood–brain barrier such as the

circumventricular organs are particularly vulnerable to circulating inflammatory mediators.

3. **Vasculotropism:** Transfer from peripheral nerve terminal to CNS via synapse connected route [4, 13].

4. **Cytokine Storm:** increase in cytokine serum levels [4].

Spike (S) proteins bind the angiotensin-converting enzyme 2 (ACE-2) receptor of the target cell. Cleavage of the S protein by type II transmembrane serine protease (TMPRSS2), facilitates viral entry. ACE-2 mRNA expression and double-positive ACE-2 + TMPRSS2 + cells have been identified, among others, on neurons and glial

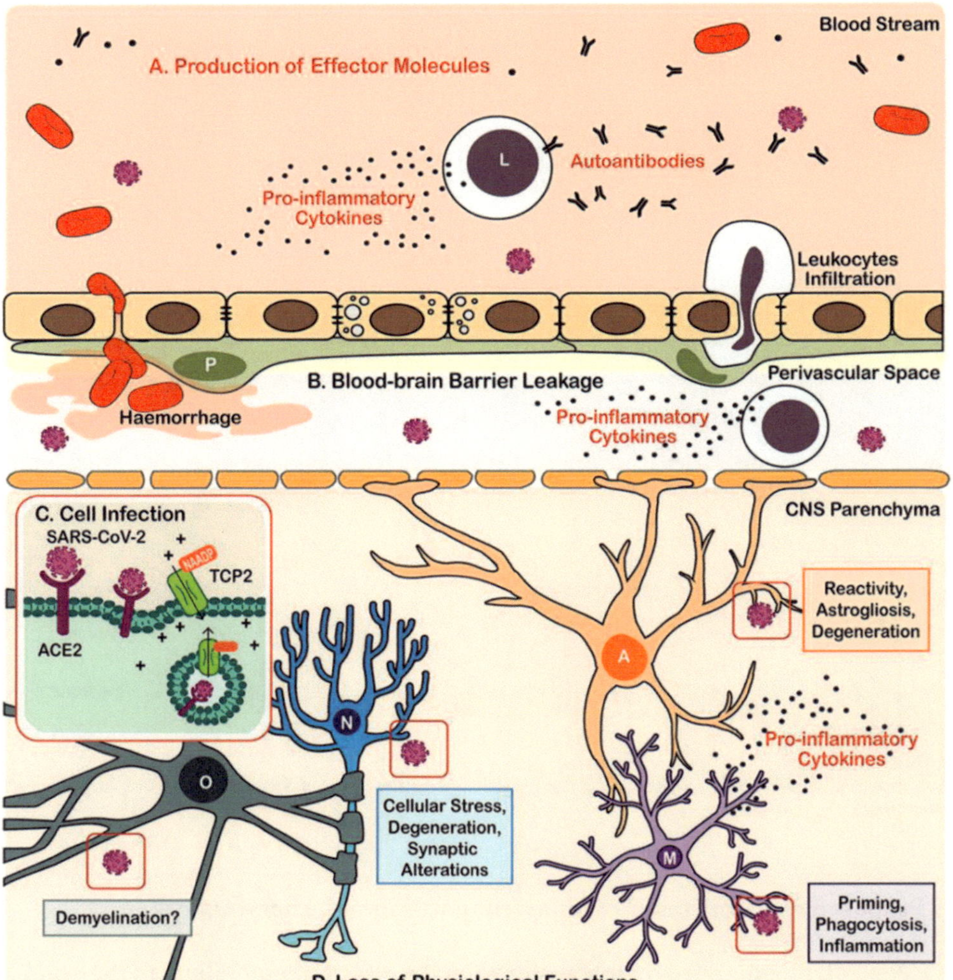

Figure 4.
Scheme illustration of the neurotropism, neuroinflammatory processes, and effects on brain cells triggered by COVID-19 in patients. Image and description text adapted from [59].

cells, in the cerebral cortex, striatum, hypothalamus, substantia nigra, and brain stem, making the CNS potential direct targets of SARS-CoV-2 infection.

Immune cells from the periphery and the central nervous system (CNS) (A) Produce effector molecules that include pro-inflammatory cytokines and autoantibodies. (B) SARS-CoV-2 infection also causes leakage of the blood–brain barrier leading in some cases to hemorrhage and cerebral infarct, as well as eliciting leukocyte infiltration. (C) In the parenchyma, the CNS cells become infected by SARS-CoV via angiotensin-converting enzyme 2 (ACE2) endocytosis mediated by the two-pore channel 2 (TCP2). (D) SARS-CoV-2 infection leads to loss of physiological functions of the brain cells, including neurons, astrocytes, microglia, and oligodendrocytes. Cell types are identified in the following manner; A, Astrocyte; L, Leukocyte; M, Microglia; N, Neurone; O, Oligodendrocyte.

4.4 Effects of COVID-19 on neurological systems

Several case reports of SARS-CoV-2 from hospitals, clinical settings, and study groups indicate different manifestations of neurological symptoms and effects [43, 60]. These studies report these common neurological manifestations to occur in the brain, olfactory areas, and central nervous system. A report from the treatment of a COVID-19 patient carried out by [61] described encephalitis (inflammation of the brain) detected through CT scans as a clinical manifestation of SARS-CoV-2 infection. One study in China. Another study in the UK reported that patients developed unexplained encephalopathic features (detected through MRI) and showed a cognitive decline [62]. Additionally, an autopsy of human brain samples from neurologically diseased patients showed the presence of the virus in the cortical neurons of the brain [55, 63]. This presence is attributed to inter-neuronal propagation and axonal transport of the virus into the CNS. These reports constitute evidence that SARS-CoV-2 has neuro-invasive potential. It also stresses the need for further research to ascertain the level of damage it can cause in neurological systems as the exact mechanism of invasion is still unclear.

4.5 Neurological symptoms are classified into three categories

1. **CNS symptoms or diseases:** headache, ataxia, corticospinal tract signs, impaired consciousness (confusion, prominent agitation, and dizziness), acute cerebrovascular disease, and epilepsy [2, 3, 14, 59, 64].

2. **PNS symptoms**: ageusia (loss of sense of taste), hypogeusia (reduction in the ability to taste), anosmia (inability to smell), hyposmia (reduction in the ability to smell), and neuralgia (painful sensation in the body).

3. **Skeletal muscular symptoms**: myalgia/fatigue and muscle injury.

Similarly, clinical manifestations such as stroke, acute necrotizing hemorrhagic encephalopathy, acute Guillain–Barré syndrome, and meningitis usually accompany the neurological effects of COVID-19. But they are frequent in individuals who are critically ill, adults who are old, and people who have suffered from previous infections of embolism or cardiovascular diseases [20, 65, 66].

5. Possible therapies for COVID-19

Numerous probable therapies for COVID-19 are being studied and tested, but, fortuitously, some medications have been approved by the FDA and made available for infected individuals [6]. Some pharmaceutical medications are being evaluated as possible therapies with different degrees of success [67]. Hydroxychloroquine, an antimalarial and anti-inflammatory drug, was first suggested to have potential against COVID-19 [6], but was later shown to be ineffective [68]; Ribavirin inhibits viral fusion and entry into host cells [6]. The use of Remdesivir for COVID-19 treatment prevented SARS-CoV-2 replication, while tocilizumab, an antagonist drug, also prevents the virus entry into the host cells [6].

ATN-161 has been shown to affect as an anti-cancer and ischemic stroke agent and has successfully completed phase I clinical trial for cancer showing to be well-tolerated without any toxicity. In an ischemic stroke study, increased expression of α5β1 integrin in post-stroke brain endothelial cells was linked to BB breakdown and then increased neuroinflammation and edema. These conditions can be inhibited by ATN-161 [71]. ATN-161 has been shown to be a potential antiviral therapy following a study that reported ATN-161 blocking viral replication of the beta-coronavirus porcine hemagglutinating encephalomyelitis virus (PHEV) in mice through the α5β1-FAK signaling mechanism [69]. In the study, it was found that SARS-CoV-2 spike protein was attached to α5β1 and α5β1/hACE2 which was inhibited by ATN-161 in VeroE6 cells in vitro. This study, therefore, recommends further studies on the ATN-161 as a possible COVID-19 therapy against COVID-19 related neurological disorders. The last possibility for a possible treatment is convalescent plasma, in which the infected individual receives plasma from a recovered COVID-19 individual. This was done in optimisms that the antibodies in the plasma of the improved individuals could help fight the virus in infected ones [67].

Managing prior neurological diseases such as stroke might remain similar to the pre-COVID-19 era. Continuing immunomodulation should continue as well as constant for drug-related adverse effects observation, since withdrawal may initiate a reversion [70]. Individuals involved must consciously observe hand hygiene and social distancing to avoid being infected with SARS CoV-2 [71, 72].

6. Conclusion

The COVID-19 pandemic has impacted our lives beyond health. Today, we have learned new ways of dealing with a pandemic and our understanding of viruses has expanded to newer dimensions. In this chapter, we reviewed the specific effects of COVID-19 on the neurological system and the various symptoms in the CNS, PNS, and skeletomuscular systems. Studies done so far emphasize the need for further research to ascertain the level of damage SARS-CoV-2 can cause in neurological systems as the exact mechanism of invasion remains unclear. Once clearly defined, existing drugs can be repurposed, new pharmacological interventions can be developed, and combination therapies can be designed to relieve neurological symptoms and the effects of SARS-CoV-2 on neurological systems.

Conflict of interest

The authors declare no conflict of interest.

Author details

John Teibo[1*], Abolaji Olagunju[2], Festus Atiba[1], Olabode Omotoso[3], Titilade Teibo[4]
Ahmad Babalghith[5] and Gaber Batiha[6]

1 Department of Biochemistry and Immunology, Ribeirão Preto Medical School, University of São Paulo, Ribeirão Preto, São Paulo, Brazil

2 Department of Immunology, Institute of Biomedical Sciences, University of São Paulo, Brazil

3 Department of Biochemistry, Faculty of Basic Medical Sciences, University of Ibadan, Ibadan, Nigeria

4 Department of Maternal-Infant and Public Health Nursing, College of Nursing, Ribeirão Preto, University of São Paulo, Ribeirão Preto, São Paulo, Brazil

5 Medical Genetics Department, College of Medicine, Umm alqura University, Makkah, Saudi Arabia

6 Department of Pharmacology and Therapeutics, Faculty of Veterinary Medicine, Damanhour University, AlBeheira, Egypt

*Address all correspondence to: johnteibo@usp.br

References

[1] Zhou Y, Yang Q, Chi J, Dong B, Lv W, Shen L, et al. Comorbidities and the risk of severe or fatal outcomes associated with coronavirus disease 2019: A systematic review and meta-analysis. International Journal of Infectious Diseases. 2020;**99**:47-56. DOI: 10.1016/j.ijid.2020.07.029

[2] Altunisik E, Sayiner HS, Aksoz S, Cil E, Ozgenc G. Neurological symptoms in COVID-19 patients. Bratislavské Lekárske Listy. 2021;**122**(1):39-44. DOI: 10.4149/BLL_2021_004

[3] Haider A, Siddiqa A, Ali N, Dhallu M. COVID-19 and the brain: Acute encephalitis as a clinical manifestation. Cureus. 2020;**12**(10):e10784. DOI: 10.7759/cureus.10784

[4] Aghagoli G, Gallo Marin B, Katchur NJ, Chaves-Sell F, Asaad WF, Murphy SA. Neurological involvement in COVID-19 and potential mechanisms: A review. Neurocritical Care. 2021;**34**(3):1062-1071. DOI: 10.1007/s12028-020-01049-4

[5] Teibo J, Olorunfemi F, Ajayi J, Adewolu M. Frugal chemo-prophylaxis against COVID19: Possible preventive benefits for the populace. International Journal Advanced Research in Biological Sciences. 2020;**7**:44-64

[6] Jean SS, Lee PI, Hsueh PR. Treatment options for COVID-19: The reality and challenges. Journal of Microbiology, Immunology, and Infection. 2020;**53**(3):436-443

[7] Omotoso OE. Contributory role of SARS-CoV-2 genomic variations and life expectancy in COVID-19 transmission and low fatality rate in Africa. Egyptian Journal of Medical Human Genetics. 2020;**21**:72. DOI: 10.1186/s43042-020-00116-x

[8] WHO, 2022 Available from: https://covid19.who.int/

[9] Omotoso OE, Awoyemi P-P, Wahab VJ, Ragab M, Teibo JO, Akinfe O, et al. Knowledge and level of adherence to COVID-19 preventive measures: A Bi-national web-based survey in Africa December. Saudi Journal of Health Sciences. 2021;**10**:80-87

[10] Teibo JO, Teibo TKA, Omotoso OE, Olagunju AS, Omotoso E. A Bi-continental review of the knowledge and adherence to COVID-19 public health guidelines in north and South America. Infectious Diseases and Tropical Medicine. 2021;**7**:e728

[11] Omotoso OE, Omotoso EF, Paimo KO, Teibo JO, Olagunju AO. Knowledge and adherence to COVID-19 preventive measures: A continental review. Sudan Journal of Medical Sciences. 2021b;**16**(3):371-385

[12] https://www.nih.gov/news-events/news-releases/researchers-highlight-covid-19-neurological-symptoms-need-rigorous-studies#:~:text=Neurological%20symptoms%20that%20have%20been,%2C%20delirium%2C%20and%20brain%20inflammation.

[13] https://www.mayoclinic.org/diseases-conditions/coronavirus/in-depth/coronavirus-long-term-effects/art-20490351

[14] Baig A, Khaleeq A, Ali U, Syeda H. Evidence of the COVID-19 virus targeting the CNS: Tissue distribution,

host-virus interaction, and proposed neurotropic mechanisms. ACS Chemical Neuroscience. 2020;**11**:995-998

[15] Olagunju AS, Oladapo IP, Kosemani SO, Olorunfemi FG, Adeyemo AS. Pathogenesis of severe acute respiratory syndrome coronavirus-2 (SARS-CoV-2) respiratory infection. International Journal of Travel Medical Global Health. 2020;**8**(4):137-145. DOI: 10.34172/ijtmgh.2020.24

[16] Li YC, Bai WZ, Hashikawa T. The neuroinvasive potential of SARSCoV2 may be at least partially responsible for the respiratory failure of COVID-19 patients. Journal of Medical Virology. 2020;**92**:552-555

[17] Wrapp D, Wang N, Corbett K, et al. Cryo-EM structure of the 2019-nCoV spike in the prefusion conformation. Science. 2020;**367**:1260-1263

[18] Amruta N, Chastain WH, Paz M, Solch RJ, Murray-Brown IC, Befeler JB, et al. SARS-CoV-2 mediated neuroinflammation and the impact of COVID-19 in neurological disorders. Cytokine & Growth Factor Reviews. 2021;**58**:1-15. DOI: 10.1016/j.cytogfr.2021.02.002

[19] Ellul MA, Benjamin L, Singh B, Lant S, Michael BD, Easton A, et al. Neurological associations of COVID-19. Lancet Neurology. 2020;**19**(9):767-783

[20] Oxley T, Mocco J, Majidi S, et al. Large-vessel stroke as a presenting feature of Covid-19 in the young. The New England Journal of Medicine. 2020;**382**(20):e60

[21] Klok F, Kruip M, van der Meer N, Arbuos M, Gommers D, Kant K. Incidence of thrombotic complications in critically ill ICU patients with COVID-19. Thrombosis Research. 2020;**S0049-3848**(20):30120-30121

[22] Lodigiani C, Lapichino G, Carenzo L, Cecconi M, Ferrazzi P, Sebastian T. Venous and arterial thromboembolic complications in COVID 19 patients admitted to an academic hospital in Milan, Italy. Thrombosis Research. 2020;**191**:9-14

[23] Trejo-Gabriel-Galan JM. Stroke as a complication and prognostic factor of COVID-19. Neurología. 2020;**35**(5):318-322

[24] Yamana M, Kuwahara M, Fukumoto Y, Yoshikawa K, Takada K, Kusunoki S. Guillain-Barré syndrome and related diseases after influenza virus infection. Neurology: Neuroimmunology, Neuroinflammation. 2019;**6**:1-7. DOI: 10.1212/NXI.0000000000000575

[25] Bridwell R, Long B, Gottlieb M. Neurologic complications of COVID-19. The American Journal of Emergency Medicine. 2020;**38**(1549):e3-e7. DOI: 10.1016/j.ajem.2020.05.024

[26] Asiri S, Altwaijri WA, Ba-Armah D, Alrifai AARMT, Salam M, Almutairi AF. Prevalence and outcomes of Guillain-Barré syndrome among pediatrics in Saudi Arabia: A 10-year retrospective study. Neuropsychiatric Disease and Treatment. 2019;**15**:627-635. DOI: 10.2147/NDT.S187994

[27] Whittaker A, Anson M, Harky A. Neurological manifestations of COVID-19: A review. Acta Neurologica Scandinavica. 2020;**142**:14-22. DOI: 10.1111/ane.13266

[28] Jacobs B, Rothbarth P, van der Meche F, et al. The spectrum of antecedent infections in Guillain-Barre syndrome: A case-control study. Neurology. 1998;**51**:1110-1115

[29] Virani A, Rabold E, Hanson T, Haag A, Elrufay R, Cheema T. Guillain-Barré syndrome associated with SARS-CoV-2 infection. IDCases. 2020;**20**:e00771

[30] McGonagle D, Sharif K, O'Regan A, Bridgewood C. The role of cytokines including Interleukin-6 in COVID-19 induced pneumonia and macrophage activation syndrome-like disease. Autoimmunity Reviews. 2020;**19**(6):102537

[31] Wood H. Elevated risk of COVID-19 in people with dementia nature reviews. Neurology. 2021;**17**:194. DOI: 10.1038/s41582-021-00473-0

[32] Brown EE, Kumar S, Rajji TK, Pollock BG, Mulsant BH. Anticipating and mitigating the impact of the COVID-19 pandemic on Alzheimer's disease and related dementias. The American Journal of Geriatric Psychiatry. 2020;**28**(7):712-721

[33] Kubota T, Kuroda N. Exacerbation of neurological symptoms and COVID-19 severity in patients with preexisting neurological disorders and COVID-19: A systematic review. Clinical Neurology and Neurosurgery. 2021;**200**:106349

[34] Antonini A, Leta V, Teo J, Chaudhuri KR. Outcome of parkinson's disease patients affected by COVID-19. Movement Disorders. 2020;**35**(6):905-908

[35] Hainque E, Grabli D. Rapid worsening in parkinson's disease may hide COVID-19 infection. Parkinson Related Disordered. 2020;**75**:126-127

[36] Lo Monaco MR, Bentivoglio AR, Fusco D, Calabresi P, Piano C. Subacute onset dystonia in a woman affected by parkinson's disease following SARS-COV-2 infection. Clinical Parkinsonism Related Disordered. 2021;**4**:100082-100082

[37] Cilia R, Bonvegna S, Straccia G, Andreasi NG, Elia AE, Romito LM, et al. Effects of COVID-19 on parkinson's disease clinical features: A community-based case-control study. Movement Disorders. 2020;**35**(8):1287-1292

[38] Van der Heide A, Meinders MJ, Bloem BR, Helmich RC. The impact of the COVID-19 pandemic on psychological distress, physical activity, and symptom severity in parkinson's disease. Journal of Parkinson's Disease. 2020;**10**(4):1355-1364

[39] Mortaz E, Malkmohammad M, Jamaati H, Naghan PA, Hashemian SM, Tabarsi P, et al. Silent hypoxia: Higher NO in red blood cells of COVID-19 patients. BMC Pulmonary Medicine. 2020;**20**(1):269

[40] Cafaro RP. Hypoxia: Its causes and symptoms. Journal of the American Dental Society of Anesthesiology. 1960;**7**(4):4-8

[41] Kennedy PGE. An overview of viral infections of the nervous system in the immunosuppressed. Journal of Neurology. 2021;**268**(8):3026-3030. DOI: 10.1007/s00415-020-10265-z

[42] Koyuncu OO, Hogue IB, Enquist LW. Virus infections in the nervous system. Cell Host & Microbe. 2013;**13**(4):379-393. DOI: 10.1016/j.chom.2013.03.010

[43] Lan J, Ge J, Yu J, Shan S, Zhou H, Fan S, et al. Structure of the SARS-CoV-2 spike receptor-binding domain bound to the ACE2 receptor. Nature. 2020;**581**(7807):215-220. DOI: 10.1038/s41586-020-2180-5

[44] Fu J, Zhou B, Zhang L, Balaji KS, Wei C, Liu X, et al. Expressions and

significances of the angiotensin-converting enzyme 2 gene, the receptor of SARS-CoV-2 for COVID-19. Molecular Biology Reports. 2020;**47**(6):4383-4392. DOI: 10.1007/s11033-020-05478-4

[45] Abdel Hafez SMN. Can Covid-19 attack our nervous system? Journal of Chemical Neuroanatomy. 2021;**117**:102006. DOI: 10.1016/j.jchemneu.2021.102006

[46] Beyerstedt S, Casaro EB, Rangel ÉB. COVID-19: Angiotensin-converting enzyme 2 (ACE2) expression and tissue susceptibility to SARS-CoV-2 infection. European Journal of Clinical Microbiology & Infectious Diseases. 2021;**40**:905-919. DOI: 10.1007/s10096-020-04138-6

[47] Zou X, Chen K, Zou J, Han P, Hao J, Han Z. Single-cell RNA-seq data analysis on the receptor ACE2 expression reveals the potential risk of different human organs vulnerable to 2019-nCoV infection. Frontiers of Medicine. 2020;**14**:185-192

[48] Qi F, Qian S, Zhang S, Zhang Z. Single cell RNA sequencing of 13 human tissues identify cell types and receptors of human coronaviruses. Biochemical and Biophysical Research Communications. 2020;**526**(1):135-140. DOI: 10.1016/j.bbrc.2020.03.044

[49] Xu H, Zhong L, Deng J, Peng J, Dan H, Zeng X, et al. High expression of ACE2 receptor of 2019-nCoV on the epithelial cells of oral mucosa. International Journal of Oral Science. 2020;**12**(1):8. DOI: 10.1038/s41368-020-0074-x

[50] Harmer D, Gilbert M, Borman R, Clark KL. Quantitative mRNA expression profiling of ACE 2, a novel homologue of angiotensin converting enzyme. FEBS Letters. 2002;**532**(1-2):107-110. DOI: 10.1016/s0014-5793(02)03640-2

[51] Devaux CA, Rolain J-M, Raoult D. ACE2 receptor polymorphism: Susceptibility to SARS-CoV-2, hypertension, multi-organ failure, and COVID-19 disease outcome. Journal of Microbiology, Immunology, and Infection. 2020;**53**:425-435. DOI: 10.1016/j.jmii.2020.04.015

[52] Kochi AN, Tagliari AP, Forleo GB, Fassini GM, Tondo C. Cardiac and arrhythmic complications in patients with COVID-19. Journal of Cardiovascular Electrophysiology. 2020;**31**(5):1003-1008. DOI: 10.1111/jce.14479

[53] Hamming I, Timens W, Bulthuis ML, Lely AT, Navis G, van Goor H. Tissue distribution of ACE2 protein, the functional receptor for SARS coronavirus. A first step in understanding SARS pathogenesis. The Journal of Pathology. 2004;**203**:631-637. DOI: 10.1002/path.1570

[54] Song E, Zhang C, Israelow B, Lu-Culligan A, Prado AV, Skriabine S, et al. Neuroinvasion of SARS-CoV-2 in human and mouse brain. The Journal of experimental medicine, 2021;**218**(3):e20202135. DOI: 10.1084/jem.20202135

[55] Zhao Y, Zhao Z, Wang Y, Zhou Y, Ma Y, Zuo W. Single-cell RNA expression profiling of ACE2, the receptor of SARS-CoV-2. American Journal of Respiratory and Critical Care Medicine. 2020;**202**(5):756-759. DOI: 10.1164/rccm.202001-0179LE Erratum in: Am J Respir Crit Care Med. 2021 Mar 15;203(6):782

[56] Gemmati D, Bramanti B, Serino ML, Secchiero P, Zauli G, Tisato V. COVID-19 and individual genetic susceptibility/

receptivity: Role of ACE1/ACE2 genes, immunity, inflammation and coagulation. Might the double X-chromosome in females Be protective against SARS-CoV-2 compared to the single X-chromosome in males? International Journal of Molecular Sciences. 2020;**21**(10):3474. DOI: 10.3390/ijms21103474

[57] Reza-Zaldívar EE, Hernández-Sapiéns MA, Minjarez B, Gómez-Pinedo U, Márquez-Aguirre AL, Mateos-Díaz JC, et al. Infection Mechanism of SARS-COV-2 and Its Implication on the Nervous System. Frontiers in immunology, 2021;**11**:621735. DOI: 10.3389/fimmu.2020.621735

[58] Bolay H, Gül A, Baykan B. COVID-19 is a real headache! Headache. 2020;**60**(7):1415-1421. DOI: 10.1111/head.13856

[59] Mao L, Jin H, Wang M, Hu Y, Chen S, He Q, et al. Neurologic manifestations of hospitalized patients with coronavirus disease 2019 in Wuhan, China. JAMA Neurology. 2020;**77**(6):683-690. DOI: 10.1001/jamaneurol.2020.1127

[60] Ye M, Ren Y, Lv T. Encephalitis as a clinical manifestation of COVID-19. Brain, Behavior, and Immunity. 2020;**88**:945-946. DOI: 10.1016/j.bbi.2020.04.017

[61] Douaud G, Lee S, Alfaro-Almagro F, Arthofer C, Wang C, McCarthy P, et al. SARS-CoV-2 is associated with changes in brain structure in UK Biobank. Nature, 2022;**604**(7907):697-707. DOI: 10.1038/s41586-022-04569-5

[62] Matschke J, Lütgehetmann M, Hagel C, Sperhake JP, Schröder AS, Edler C, et al. Neuropathology of patients with COVID-19 in Germany: A post-mortem case series. Lancet Neurology. 2020;**19**(11):919-929. DOI: 10.1016/S1474-4422(20)30308-2

[63] Chen X, Laurent S, Onur OA, Kleineberg NN, Fink GR, Schweitzer F, et al. A systematic review of neurological symptoms and complications of COVID-19. Journal of Neurology. 2021;**268**(2):392-402. DOI: 10.1007/s00415-020-10067-3

[64] Helms J, Kremer S, Merdji H, Clere-Jehl R, Schenck M, Kummerlen C, et al. Neurologic features in severe SARS-CoV-2 infection. The New England Journal of Medicine. 2020;**382**(23):2268-2270. DOI: 10.1056/NEJMc2008597

[65] Nannoni S, de Groot R, Bell S, Markus HS. Stroke in COVID-19: A systematic review and meta-analysis. International Journal of Stroke. 2021;**16**(2):137-149. DOI: 10.1177/1747493020972922

[66] Majidi S, Fifi JT, Ladner TR, Lara-Reyna J, Yaeger KA, Yim B, et al. Emergent large vessel occlusion stroke during new York City's COVID-19 outbreak: Clinical characteristics and Paraclinical findings. Stroke. 2020;**51**(9):2656-2663. DOI: 10.1161/STROKEAHA.120.030397

[67] Barati F, Pouresmaieli M, Ekrami E, Asghari S, Ziarani FR, Mamoudifard M. Potential drugs and remedies for the treatment of COVID-19: A critical review. Biological Proceedings. 2020;**22**:15

[68] Smit M, Marinosci A, Agoritsas T, Calmy A. Prophylaxis for COVID-19: a systematic review. Clinical microbiology and infection: the official publication of the European Society of Clinical Microbiology and Infectious Diseases, 2021;**27**(4):532-537. DOI: 10.1016/j.cmi.2021.01.013

[69] Lv X, Li Z, Guan J, Zhang J, Xu B, He W, et al. ATN-161 reduces virus proliferation in PHEV-infected mice

by inhibiting the integrin alpha5beta1-FAK signaling pathway. Veterinary Microbiology. 2019;**233**:147-153

[70] Sanders JM, Monogue ML, Jodlowski TZ, Cutrell JB. Pharmacologic treatments for coronavirus disease 2019 (COVID-19): A review. JAMA. 2020;**323**(18):1824-1836

[71] Zubair AS, McAlpine LS, Gardin T, Farhadian S, Kuruvilla DE, Spudich S. Neuropathogenesis and neurologic manifestations of the coronaviruses in the age of coronavirus disease 2019: A review. JAMA Neurology. 2020;**77**(8):1018-1027

[72] Manji H, Carr AS, Brownlee WJ, Lunn MP. Neurology in the time of COVID-19. Journal of Neurology, Neurosurgery, and Psychiatry. 2020;**91**(6):568-570

Chapter 3

COVID-19 and Its Impact on Onset and Progression of Parkinson's and Cognitive Dysfunction

Swapan Kumar Chatterjee, Snigdha Saha and Shahin Muhammed T.K.

Abstract

In the COVID-19 pandemic, neurological complications have emerged as a significant cause of morbidity and mortality. A wide range of neurological manifestations ranging from cognitive or memory disturbances, headache, loss of smell or taste, confusion, and disabling strokes have been reported during and post COVID conditions. The COVID-19 virus can utilize two possible pathways for invasion into the brain, either through retrograde axonal transport (olfactory route) or by crossing the blood-brain barrier (BBB). Furthermore, the production of SARS-CoV-2-associated cytokines, such as interleukin (IL)-6, IL-17, IL-1b, and tumor necrosis factor (TNF), is able to disrupt the BBB. The neuroinvasive nature of SARS-CoV-2 has a more severe impact on patients with preexisting neurological manifestations such as Parkinson's disease (PD). Pathological features of PD include selective loss of dopaminergic neurons in the substantia nigra pars compacta and aggregation of α-syn proteins present in neurons. Interaction between SARS-COV-2 infection and α-synuclein might have long-term implications on the onset of Parkinsonism by the formation of toxic protein clumps called amyloid fibrils—a hallmark of Parkinson's. Molecular modeling is an emerging tool to predict potential inhibitors against the enzyme α-synuclein in neurodegenerative diseases by using plant bioactive molecules.

Keywords: neurotropism, neuroinflammation, cytokine storm, ACE-2, Parkinson's, α-synuclein amyloid fibrils, molecular modeling, COVID-19

1. Introduction

Since the onset of pandemics, our world has witnessed over 500 million confirmed cases of COVID-19 and over 15 million related (direct and indirect) deaths till date [1]. With the progression of the disease, severe and more complex processes like acute respiratory distress syndrome, cytokine storm, and NETosis may develop [2, 3]. This is the tip of the iceberg. Our knowledge about the disease manifestation is increasing day by day. A wide spectrum of illnesses vary from a simple cold and fever to multisystemic diseases. It has been reported that a hypercoagulable state, damage of renal tubule cells, and heart muscles are also associated with the development of COVID 19 [4–6].

IntechOpen

Besides respiratory insufficiency, neurological complications like seizures, loss of consciousness, encephalitis, Guillain-Barre syndrome, acute necrotizing, hemophagocytic lymphohistiocytosis, acute ischemic cerebrovascular syndrome, anosmia, or ageusia as well as neuropsychiatric symptoms like headaches, nausea, dizziness, hallucinations, and depression have emerged as a significant cause for COVID-related morbidity and mortality [6–8]. Of note, these damages may significantly increase the incidence rate of other neurodegenerative diseases and foster dementia (**Figure 1**) [8].

Over the past few decades, different novel viral epidemics, such as influenza, Middle Eastern respiratory syndrome (MERS), and severe acute respiratory syndrome (SARS) have appeared, with the aid of zoonosis [9]. So far, various studies have been done to establish the link between viral infections and neurodegeneration disease. The most eminent of them is the 1918 influenza pandemic (Spanish flu) which coexisted with an increased rate of encephalitis lethargica, followed by postencephalitic Parkinsonism [10]. In recent times, multiple studies have indicated a possible relation between onset and/or worsening progression of PD and viral infections. Although the detailed mechanism of viral infections–induced neurodegeneration is still unclear, the role of the immune system or the direct effect of zoonosis cannot be overruled. Neurodegenerative diseases like PD and Alzheimer's disease (AD) are

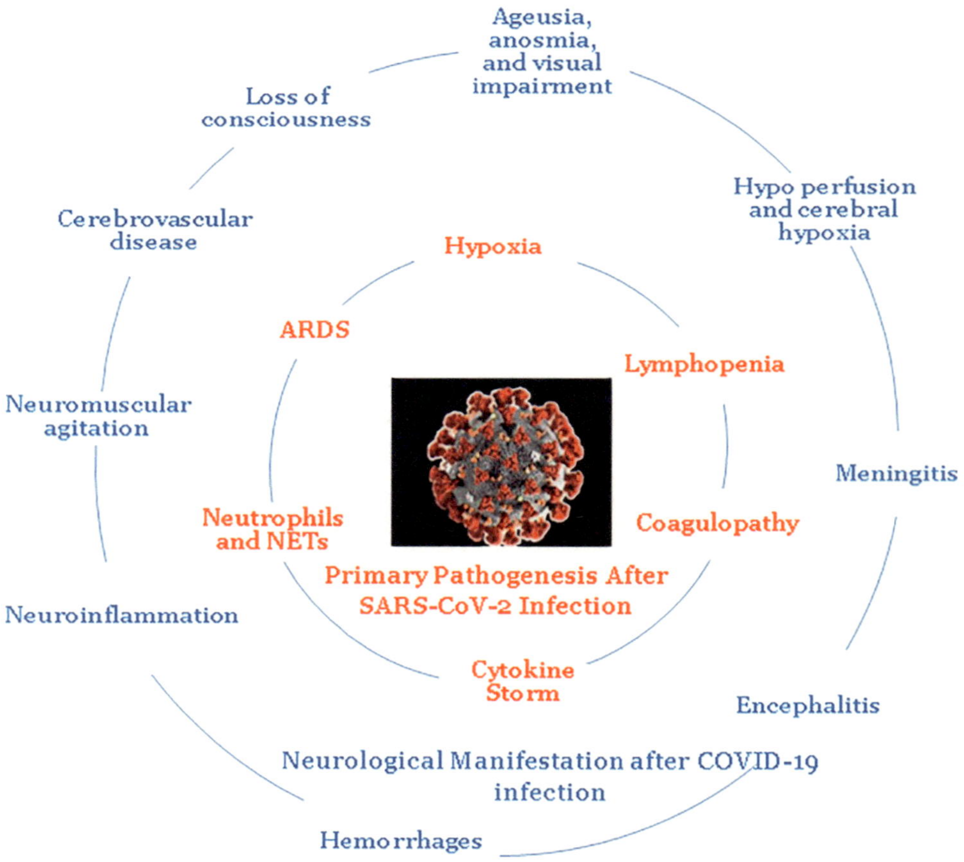

Figure 1.
Schematic representation of COVID-19-related symptoms. Primary pathogenesis associated with COVID-19 are shown in inner circle (in red). The outer circle (in blue) depicts the neurological manifestation related to COVID-19.

mainly protein aggregation diseases in which specific proteins, such as α-synuclein (α-Syn) in PD and tau and Aβ peptide in AD aggregate together to form amyloids. Once triggered, the aggregation process begins to spread from cell to cell and continues to form and deposit amyloids that in turn hamper the brain function [9–11]. A detailed study on molecular pathogenesis of the acute and delayed neurological manifestations and establishment of the link between SARS-CoV-2 infections and the development of PD will be helpful to design the new therapeutic approach.

2. Brain expression of SARS-CoV-2 receptor and molecular pathogenesis

The beta-coronaviruses are large enveloped non-segmented positive-sense RNA viruses. Like its related family members MERS-CoV (exploits dipeptidyl peptidase 4), and SARS-CoV-1, SARS-CoV-2 utilizes its specific proteins, in particular, Spike (S) protein, to bind to a number of host proteins (virus receptors) that assist in its entry [12]. Distributions of host receptors on various tissues are generally believed to decide the virus tropisms within the host cell. For an efficient host cell entry similar to SARS-CoV-1, SARS-CoV-2 uses angiotensin converting enzyme-2 (ACE2) type 1 transmembrane receptors as the major docking receptor followed by proteolytic processing of the spike protein by transmembrane protease serine 2 (TMPRSS2) [13]. Targeting of different cell types by the viral protein has been partially attributed to the distribution ACE2 receptors on the endothelial and epithelial cells of the respiratory system, as well as on immune cells. Along with that, expression of ACE2 is widely found in lung parenchyma, vasculature, heart, kidney, and the gastrointestinal tract [14, 15]. Expression of ACE2 receptors is widespread within brain structures, such as the central nervous system, in human brain vessels, pericytes and smooth muscle cells in the vascular wall, hypothalamus, and visual tracts, which are associated with the various neurological symptoms in coronavirus disease 2019 (COVID-19) infection [10, 11, 14]. However, data mining study of human brain single-nuclear RNA sequencing (RNA-seq) data has also found the expression of ACE2 receptors in the choroid plexus and neocortical neurons, in less amount [16]. Even presence of non-canonical SARS-CoV-2 receptors in other brain cell types makes them vulnerable to the virus.

Interaction with viral S protein and ACE2 receptors on the vascular endothelial cells leads to disruption of the blood-brain barrier, resulting in consequent cerebral edema and microhemorrhages. In addition to this, SARS-CoV-2 may expend direct neuronal damage due to the affinity of the spike S1 protein toward ACE2 receptors expressed on neurons. In short, the virus can utilize two possible pathways for invasion into the brain, either through retrograde axonal transport (olfactory route) or by crossing the blood-brain barrier [17]. Furthermore, production of SARS-CoV-2-associated cytokines, such as interleukin (IL)-6, IL-17, IL-1b, and tumor necrosis factor (TNF), are able to disrupt the BBB [18] and could facilitate the viral entry. Even in some studies SARS-CoV-2 has been predicted to induce infection in cerebral endothelial cells as well as inflammation in peripheral vessels [19], but direct evidence has not been far provided. Co-morbidity factors like cardiovascular risk factors and/or pre-existing neurological diseases could alone or in combination with cytokines intensify the rate of BBB permeability [18]. Nonetheless, viruses are able to enter the brain by carried by infected immune cells that also act as a reservoir [20]. Neutrophils T cells and Monocytes, may traffic into the brain through the vasculature, whereas the meninges and the choroid plexus [21], could be considered as entry points for infected immune cells. In COVID-19 loss of smell is considered a frequent neurological manifestation that is consistent with infection of the olfactory system. The internalization of the virus in nerve terminals by endocytosis, transportation retrogradely, and spread trans-synaptically to other regions of brain, has been studied in other coronaviruses [22]. Detection of ACE2and TMPRSS2 in the nasal mucosa at both RNA and protein levels increases the chance of involvement of olfactory neurons in viral transmission. The hypothalamus could contribute to the dysregulation of the immune cells. In COVID-19, upregulation of cytokines like IL-6, IL-1b, and TNF act as the activators of the hypothalamic-pituitary-adrenocortical (HPA) axis. This HPA axis acts as the center of the systemic immune activity regulation and is activated by BBB dysfunction and neurovascular inflammation [23].

However, apart from ACE2, SARS-CoV-2 can utilize neuropilin-1 (NRP1) and basigin (BSG; CD147) as docking receptors, whereas a variety of proteases such as cathepsin B and L,TMPRSS11A/B, and furin (FURIN) have been shown to promote viral cell entry as well as replication within the host cell [24–26]. Exposure of brain tissue to COVID-19-related injuries like hypercoagulable states, inflammation, hypoxia, immune response (cytokine storm), or dyselectrolytemia is thought to play the main role in the cerebral pathomechanism of viral damage and cause all the neurodegenerative conditions like AD and PD [27].

3. Molecular link between COVID-19 and Parkinson's

Parkinson's disease (PD) is a neurodegenerative disorder, defined as α-synucleinopathy that affects 1% of the population aged above 60 years with an annual incidence of 15 per 100,000 populations. It is a disorder of the central nervous system (progressive loss of dopamine neurons) that mainly affects the motor system, particularly, the nigrostriatal pathway. Therefore, the major PD symptoms include tremor, bradykinesia/akinesia, rigidity, and postural instability. The clinical manifestations of PD also include non-motor symptoms (NMS) such as dementia, anxiety, depression, fatigue, and others [28]. The major pathological features of PD include selective loss of dopaminergic neurons in the substantia nigra pars compacta and aggregation of protein (called Lewy neurites and Lewy bodies) consisting mainly of α-syn proteins present in neurons [29, 30].

Alpha-synuclein (α-syn), is a small protein (forms an α-helix-rich tetramer) that comprises of 140 amino acids, and the human *SNCA* gene encodes them. Expression of α-syn takes place in the central nervous system (CNS) and is mainly localized in synapses and nuclei. Although the exact function of α-syn is not clearly explained yet, various studies have shown that maintaining synaptic plasticity, vesicle trafficking, and interaction with synaptic vesicles as well as physiological regulation of vesicle recycling is regulated by α-syn [30–32]. The major biological function of α-syn is employed through the non-amyloid-beta component (NAC), N-terminal, and C-terminal domains. The KTKEGV motif is present in the N-terminus that maintains tetramerization of α-syn, and mutations in this motif lead to neurotoxicity. NAC is a highly hydrophobic domain and was first identified in patients with AD. It forms a β-sheet structure for α-syn aggregation. The C-terminus of α-syn is a proline-rich region domain that helps in interaction with other proteins [30, 33]. Misfolded or unfolded α-syn protein forms fibrillar aggregates that generate insoluble inclusions in the affected neurons and glial cells. Aggregated α-syn can induce other pathological features, such as mitochondrial dysfunction, dysregulation of calcium homeostasis, endoplasmic reticulum (ER) stress, neuroinflammation, Golgi fragmentation, lysosomal dysfunction, and impaired protein quality control that lead to neuronal toxicity [30, 33–35]. The non-neuronal cells present in the brain are called Gila cells that play a critical role in maintenance of the neuronal system. Glia cells are comprised of microglia, astrocytes, and oligodendrocytes in the CNS. The glial cells comprise a majority of brain cells, and they regulate neurogenesis and synaptogenesis. Furthermore, glial cells influence the development and function of brain-blood barrier (BBB) by interactions with endothelial cells and neurons to protect the brain from pathogenic attacks [30, 33]. Although the major function of astrocytes and microglia involves the immune response but under pathological conditions, they seem to be activated by specific stimuli. Upon activation, microglia and astrocytes can release pro-inflammatory cytokines like tumor necrosis factor-alpha (TNF-α), interleukin-1 (IL-1), IL-2, IL-4, interleukin-6 (IL-6), and also causes reduced levels of neurotrophins, like nerve growth factor and brain-derived neurotrophic factor (BDNF) that lead to the reactive oxidative stress (ROS) production followed by BBB dysfunction. Intercellular crosstalk between these factors induces neuronal cell death and engenders neurodegenerative diseases such as AD or PD [30, 33, 36].

In patients with PD/parkinsonism, the COVID-19 pandemic has had an indirect and negative impact that might be explained by the dopamine-dependent adaptation hypothesis. Due to the pandemic, there is a change in daily life and routine; therefore, flexibility in cognitive (and motor) functions is required to adapt to such changes. Even pharmacodynamic effects, social isolation, stress, and anxiety as well as prolonged immobility have detrimental effects on motor and non-motor symptoms and quality of life in PD. In patients with PD, damage to nigrostriatal dopamine neurons results in lower cognitive as well as motor neuron flexibility. Such patients often experience confusion and increased psychological stress, which can lead to the worsening of parkinsonism symptoms as well as mental illnesses such as anxiety and depression [37]. The development of permanent or transient Parkinsonism followed by a viral might occur through different mechanisms:

1. Damage to structural and functional basal ganglia mainly involving the substantia nigra pars compacta and nigrostriatal dopaminergic projection;

2. Extensive inflammation including hypoxic brain injury within the context of an encephalopathy;

3. Unmasking hidden non-symptomatic Parkinson's disease; or

4. A series of processes that might be triggered by a viral infection that result in Parkinson's disease development over the long term in individuals with genetic susceptibility.

There are fundamental clinical and anatomopathological differences present in each of these instances [37, 38].

The onset of transient parkinsonism has been associated with many viral infections including West Nile Virus, Japanese Encephalitis, Western Equine virus, Coxsackie virus, Epstein Barr virus, HIV, and currently SARS- CoV-2. Expression of high level ACE2 receptor on the midbrain dopamine neurons could facilitate entry of SARS-CoV-2 that can alter the expression of alpha-synuclein [39–41]. Since elevated alpha-synuclein levels can promote aggregation of the protein, this could predispose an infected patient to PD down the line. Various experimental models also suggest that SARS-CoV-2 may interact with different proteins in age-related pathways (lipid metabolism, proteostasis, mitochondrial function, and stress responses) [37, 40]. Dysfunction of these pathways could lead to alpha-synuclein aggregation and selective neurodegeneration. Even elevated cytokines (the primary mediators of inflammation in SARS-CoV-2) can accelerate the neurodegeneration in PD [41]. Studies revealed that the release of cytokines may activate the resident immune cells in the CNS. Activation of immune cells leads to their infiltration including activated T cells and microglia from the periphery that may kill neurons, astrocytes, and vascular cell types. Elevated levels of pro-inflammatory cytokines, such as TNF and IL-1beta, are also associated with increased risk of PD [41].

A current study has established the possible mechanism of triggering PD followed by COVID-19 infection. Virus-initiated amyloid-formation of α-synuclein acts as the main cell-toxic agent in the death of dopamine-producing neurons in the brain. By interacting with amyloidogenic regions with nucleocapsid protein (that encapsulates the RNA genome inside the virus), SARS-COV-2 speeds up the formation of amyloid fibrils. In the context of Alzheimer's disease, it has been speculated that amyloid fibrils are formed as an immune response to an infection, and neutralizing pathogens. A similar mechanism may play a role in progression of PD. In a current study, test tube experiments have shown that SARS-CoV-2 spike protein (S-protein) has no effect on α-synuclein aggregation, whereas SARS-CoV-2 nucleocapsid protein (N-protein) considerably speeds up the aggregation process That results in formation of multiprotein complexes and eventually amyloid fibrils that disturb the α-synuclein proteostasis and increase the rate of cell death (**Figure 2**) [42, 43].

As the cases of PD rises sharply in the older age group, particularly in those over the age of 80 years, a personalized approach to the clinical management of PD patients affected by COVID-19 is need of the hour. In addition, disturbance of α-synuclein proteostasis might be considered the first step toward nucleation of fibrils. Direct

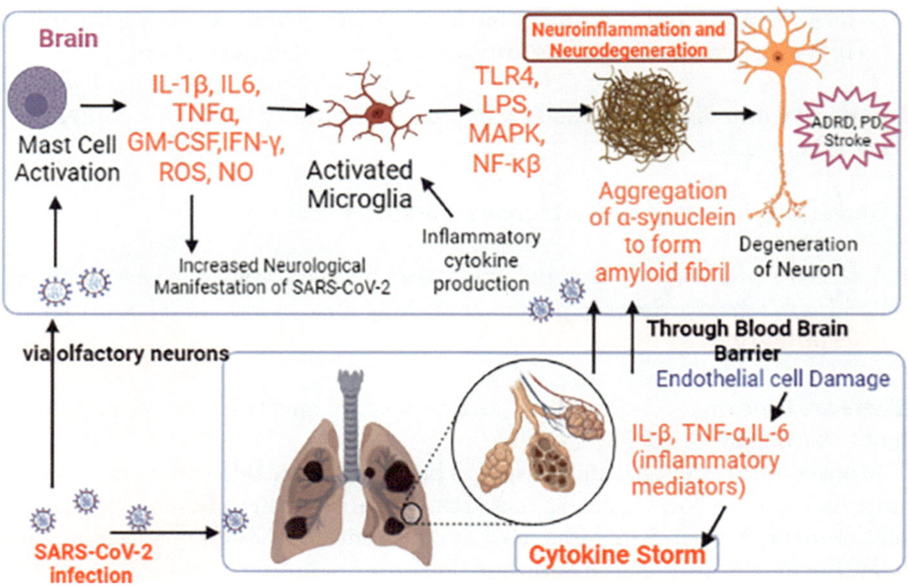

Figure 2.
Schematic representation of neuroinflammation and neurodegeneration due to SARS-CoV-2 infection. A immunological crosstalk between different organs. Created with BioRender.com.

interaction between the N-protein of SARS-CoV-2 and α-synuclein establishes a molecular link between virus infections and Parkinsonism. This piece of puzzle thus suggests that SARS-CoV-2 infections may have prolonged implications and consider N-protein as an attractive alternative target in designing novel vaccination strategies.

4. Targeted therapies for Parkinson's disease

Till date, no specific curative therapy is available for PD. There are two main approaches such as protective therapy and symptomatic therapy that have been practiced for the treatment of PD. Under symptomatic therapy, anticholinergic agents and some dopamine analogs help to restore the dopamine levels and result in improvement of the movement disabilities. Though, anticholinergic agents cause some serious effects on central nervous system such as cognitive impairment and hallucination along with constipation and dryness of mouth. In the field of PD management Levodopa brought a revolution by improving quality of life, parkinsonian symptoms, and normalizing life expectancy [44]. Other recent dopaminergic therapies, such as monoamine oxidase B inhibitors, dopamine agonists, catechol-O-methyltransferase inhibitors, and other unique formulations of levodopa, have also been developed to address parkinsonian symptoms [44, 45]. Continuous duodenal infusion of levodopa/carbidopa intestinal gel and apomorphine subcutaneous pumps are used to overcome the levodopa shortcomings. On the other hand, as PD pathogenesis mainly deals with oxidative damage, protective therapy that has free radical scavenging properties helps to reduce the side effects of drugs. Selegiline, bromocriptine, ropinirole, pramipexole, and vitamin E fall under this category [46].

Moreover, deep brain stimulation (DBS) is considered a very useful approach for patients with motor complications [47]. All these therapies have been of great value in the PD symptoms management in patients who are not responsive to medication. Currently, development of PD treatments majorly depends upon development and application of biomarkers that will help to improve the target engagement, disease state, safety, and disease outcome [48]. The development of new genetic editing technologies can open the possibility to correct mutated genes and regulatory DNA in the monogenic forms of PD [49–51]. Several methods of gene delivery that include use of viral vectors and CRISPR as well as the process of genome editing have been developed to manage PD symptoms. Currently, clinical trials of Gene therapy in PD have tried to focus on 4 main targeted approaches such as restoring dopamine synthesis, neuroprotection, genetic neuromodulation, and addressing disease-specific pathogenic variants [52].

To prevent the neurodegeneration of dopaminergic neurons by the overexpression of neurotrophic factors (NTF) is considered as a powerful strategy in PD management. The delivery of these factors, such as the glial cell line-derived neurotrophic factor (GDNF), neurotrophic factor (NF), cerebral dopamine neurotrophic factor (CDNF), neurturin (NRTN), and growth/differentiation factor 5 (GDF5) by the use of recombinant viral vectors to enable long-term expression might open a new way in PD management [53].

Even experimental studies have shown that down-regulation of α-syn levels by gene silencing with RNA interference (RNAi) can be beneficial in the normalizing expression of α-syn and improving motor function, though balance is important to avoid nigrostriatal neurotoxicity caused by excess downregulation. At epigenetic level, DNA methylation at SNCA intron1 acts as a regulator of the α-syn transcription, and thus it can consider a target for tight control of α-syn expression. In recent times, active immunization approaches are involved to develop vaccines targeting either the N or C-terminal of α-syn or its aggregation forms. Extensive clinical trials on these advanced techniques are required to prove their efficacy against PD symptoms [54].

4.1 In silico studies and prediction of therapeutic drug

In the absence of extensive experimental and pharmacological studies, none of the drug candidates are recommended for human use. Molecular docking or in silico studies is the answer to the problem with good potential tool in drug development. Molecular docking is an early guidance tool in contemporary drug discovery that minimizes not only time but also resource. In some cases, scientific data shows that the prediction results based on in silico studies are comparable with in vitro and in vivo results [55]. Molecular docking studies depend upon on joining of a particular ligand to a receptor region, providing information about orientation, conformation, and organization at the receptor site [55]. Nowadays, studies using computational chemistry have been done to predict potential inhibitors for neurodegenerative diseases from flavonoid derivatives [39]. During the pandemics or for the disease like PD or AD alternative food-based medicine or the flavonoids or bioactive compounds from the plant can be considered as the good alternatives. Development of the drug from the plant bioactive compound depends upon a great deal of in silico molecular docking investigation.

In silico studies, involving Parkinson's disease and anti-inflammatory activity of novel bioactive compounds such as quercetin, epigallocatechin gallate (EGCG), and acacetin have been done to predict inhibitory activities against the enzyme α-synuclein. According to other studies involving flavonoids including morin, naringenin, taxifolin, esculatin, daidzein, genistein, scopoletin, galangin, and silbinin have proven their inhibitory effect against lipoxygenase enzyme. Moreover, data using karanjin against several protein targets in relation to AD and PD have shown their efficiency in management of PD. Ligand-based-virtual screening together with structure-based virtual screening (docking) can be done to prove the efficiency of plant-based bioactive compounds, like alkaloids or flavonoids as inhibitors of PD- or AD-related proteins [56–58].

4.2 Treatment of Parkinson's disease and its impact on SARS-CoV-2 infection

Till now, no specific medicine is available to treat the SARS-CoV-2 infection. Nowadays, drug repurposing by the in silico studies is an essential technique for quick identification of frontline weapons to combat COVID-19. Antiviral and other life-saving drugs are trying to repurpose for the treatment of COVID-19 as SARS-CoV-2 replication shows a variety of clinical symptoms. Some of them are investigated to block different steps of host tropism such as transmembrane serine protease 2 (TMPRSS2), and/or viral entrance through the ACE2 receptor, viral membrane fusion, endocytosis, the activity of the SARS-CoV-2-3-chymotrypsin-like protease, etc. Treatment options for various diseases linked with COVID-19 such as obesity, sleep apnea, Parkinson's disease, and Alzheimer's disease have markedly changed during the pandemic. FDA-approved drug levodopa is mainly involved in alteration in dopamine synthetic pathways but studies have shown its involvement in the pathophysiology of SARS-CoV-2. DDC inhibitors act upon *DDC* and also *ACE2*, the gene encoding, the main receptor to SARS-CoV2. On the other hand, dopamine agonists are found to have detrimental effects on patients with PD symptoms and positive for the COVID-19. As per a study, a small number of COVID-19-positive PD patients were prescribed to take amantadine but did not manifest symptoms of the disease. Furthermore, COMT inhibitors like entacapone have shown potential effects against the virus SARS-CoV-2, when interactome analysis of potential drug repurposing studies was done [59, 60].

5. Conclusion

Since the beginning of the pandemics, SARS-CoV-2 has become one of the main research interests, especially due to high mortality rates among different populations and its catastrophic impact on global healthcare as well as socio-economic condition. Like other members of the Coronaviridae family, SARS-CoV-2 also has neurotropic properties. The harmful effects of the virus seem to exert either in a direct manner—by spreading through gastrointestinal nervous and/or olfactory pathways, or by evoking an inflammatory response. Along with the inflammatory response, the pathophysiology of COVID-19 also involves the complement and the coagulation systems. These triad systems interact with each other and show detrimental effects like appearance of the cytokine storm in ARDS. This leads to multisystem failure, especially in the case of disseminated intravascular coagulation disorders. In both cases – prodromal PD and COVID-19 induced PD. Parkinsonism is majorly associated with motor dysfunction, the hyposmia and hypogeusia. The cytoplasmic alpha-synuclein accumulation is associated with neurodegeneration in the nigrostriatal system of PD-affected patients [6, 8].

As SARS-CoV-2 may have a trigger for blood-brain barrier impairment and gain direct access to brain regions, the N-protein of the virus may play a major role in PD pathogenesis. Interaction between viral N-protein and alpha-synuclein promotes formation of amyloid fibril and hallmark of Parkinson's. There is a broad spectrum of COVID-19-related symptoms, perhaps associated with either pre-existing conditions or the presence of T cells that are reactive to previous coronavirus infections or in part of viral entry points. The neurological manifestations may be involved with capillaries inflammation, hypoxemia, the blood-brain barrier, and thrombosis that act as triggers for seizures or ischemic or hemorrhagic strokes. Production of pro-inflammatory cytokines and chemokines by activated microglia, astrocytes, or mitochondrial dysfunction in glial cells is considered as a major contributor to neuroinflammation. The crosstalk between these contributors may induce α-syn accumulation mediated neurodegeneration in α-synucleinopathies. This crosstalk mechanism may be considered a favorable target for α-synucleinopathy-associated neurodegenerative disease treatment [17, 18, 24]. Due to various impeding factors, such as limited understanding of the neurodegeneration mechanisms in PD, the heterogeneity of the pathology, absence of reliable biomarkers to diagnose the pathology, and the lack of adequate animal models, the development of effective preventive or curative therapies for PD has become extremely challenging. Though some medicine and therapy are available for the management of PD, they have severe detrimental effects on the central nervous system. Molecular docking or in silico studies are good potential tools in drug development for repurposing the drug or identification of new plant-based bioactive with potential neuroprotective activity. Shortly, by using this technology it will be possible to develop broad-spectrum, novel drugs active against not only a larger array of coronavirus but also will be the ultimate treatment strategy for circulating and emerging COVID-related neurological manifestations.

Author details

Swapan Kumar Chatterjee[1*], Snigdha Saha[1] and Shahin Muhammed T.K.[2]

1 Molecular Pharma Pvt. Ltd, Kolkata, West Bengal, India

2 College of Pharmaceutical Sciences, Government Medical College, Kannur, Kerala, India

*Address all correspondence to: swapan1chatterjee@gmail.com

References

[1] World Health Organization. Weekly Epidemiological Update. 2022. Available from: https://www.who.int/publications/m/item/weekly-epidemiological-update-on-covid-19---11-may-2022 [Accessed: May 15, 2022]

[2] Gillot C, Favresse J, Mullier F, LecompteT, DognéJM, DouxfilsJ. NETosis and the immune system in COVID-19: Mechanisms and potential treatments. Frontiers in Pharmacology. 2021;**12**:708302

[3] Iadecola C, Anrather J, Kamel H. Effects of COVID-19 on the nervous system. Cell. 2020;**183**(1):16-27. DOI: 10.1016/j.cell.2020.08.028

[4] Jain U. Effects of COVID-19 on the organs. Cureus. 2020;**12**(8):e9540

[5] Nadim MK, Forni LG, Mehta RL, et al. COVID-19-associated acute kidney injury: Consensus report of the 25th Acute Disease Quality Initiative (ADQI) Workgroup. Nature Review in Nephrology. 2020;**16**:747-764. DOI: 10.1038/s41581-020-00356-5

[6] Abou-Ismail MY, Diamond A, Kapoor S, Arafah Y, Nayak L. The hypercoagulable state in COVID-19: Incidence, pathophysiology, and management. Thrombotic Research. 2020;**194**:101-115

[7] Tiet MY, AlShaikh N. Guillain-Barré syndrome associated with COVID-19 infection: A case from the UK. BMJ Case Reports. 2020;**13**:e236563

[8] Guerrero JI, Barragán LA, Martínez JD, et al. Central and peripheral nervous system involvement by COVID-19: A systematic review of the pathophysiology, clinical manifestations, neuropathology, neuroimaging, electrophysiology, and cerebrospinal fluid findings. BMC Infectious Diseases. 2021;**21**(1):515

[9] Ye ZW, Yuan S, Yuen KS, Fung SY, Chan CP, Jin DY. Zoonotic origins of human coronaviruses. International Journal of Biological Science. 2020;**16**(10):1686-1697

[10] Henry J, Smeyne RJ, Jang H, Miller B, Okun MS. Parkinsonism and neurological manifestations of influenza throughout the 20th and 21st centuries. Parkinsonism Related Disorders. 2010;**16**(9):566-571. DOI: 10.1016/j.parkreldis.2010.06.012

[11] Vasili E, Dominguez-Meijide A, Outeiro TF. Spreading of α-synuclein and Tau: A systematic comparison of the mechanisms involved. Frontiers in Molecular Neuroscience. 2019;**12**:107

[12] Gerges Harb J, Noureldine HA, Chedid G, et al. SARS, MERS and COVID-19: Clinical manifestations and organ-system complications: A mini review. Pathogenesis Diseases. 2020;**78**(4):ftaa033

[13] Hoffmann M, Kleine-Weber H, Schroeder S, et al. SARS-CoV-2 cell entry depends on ACE2 and TMPRSS2 and is blocked by a clinically proven protease inhibitor. Cell. 2020;**181**(2):271-280. DOI: 10.1016/j.cell.2020.02.052

[14] Salamanna F, Maglio M, Landini MP, Fini M. Body localization of ACE-2: On the trail of the keyhole of SARS-CoV-2. Frontiers in Medicine. 2020;**7**:594495

[15] Song E, Zhang C, Israelow B, et al. Neuroinvasion of SARS-CoV-2 in human and mouse brain. J Exp Med. 2021;**218**(3):e20202135. DOI: 10.1084/jem.20202135

[16] Chen R, Wang K, Yu J, et al. The spatial and cell-type distribution of SARS-CoV-2 receptor ACE2 in the human and mouse brains. Front Neurol. 2021;**11**:573095. Published 2021 Jan 20. DOI: 10.3389/fneur.2020.573095

[17] Zhang L, Zhou L, Bao L, et al. SARS-CoV-2 crosses the blood–brain barrier accompanied with basement membrane disruption without tight junctions alteration. Signal Transduction and Target Therapy. 2021;**6**:337. DOI: 10.1038/s41392-021-00719-9

[18] Erickson MA, Banks WA. Neuroimmune axes of the blood-brain barriers and blood-brain interfaces: Bases for physiological regulation, disease states, and pharmacological interventions. Pharmacological Review. 2018;**70**(2):278-314

[19] Teuwen LA, Geldhof V, Pasut A, Carmeliet P. COVID-19: The vasculature unleashed. Nature Reviews in Immunology. 2020;**20**(7):389-391. DOI: 10.1038/s41577-020-0343-0

[20] Bergmann CC, Lane TE, Stohlman SA. Coronavirus infection of the central nervous system: Host-virus stand-off. Nature Review in Microbiology. 2006;**4**(2):121-132. DOI: 10.1038/nrmicro1343

[21] Engelhardt B, Vajkoczy P, Weller RO. The movers and shapers in immune privilege of the CNS. Nature Immunology. 2017;**18**(2):123-131. DOI: 10.1038/ni.3666

[22] Dubé M, Le Coupanec A, Wong AHM, Rini JM, Desforges M, Talbot PJ. Axonal transport enables neuron-to-neuron propagation of human coronavirus OC43. Journal of Virology. 2018;**92**(17):e00404

[23] Dantzer R. Neuroimmune interactions: From the brain to the immune system and vice versa. Physiological Review. 2018;**98**(1):477-504. DOI: 10.1152/physrev.00039.2016

[24] Cantuti-Castelvetri L, Ojha R, Pedro LD, et al. Neuropilin-1 facilitates SARS-CoV-2 cell entry and infectivity. Science. 2020;**370**(6518):856-860. DOI: 10.1126/science.abd2985

[25] Wang K, Chen W, Zhang Z, et al. CD147-spike protein is a novel route for SARS-CoV-2 infection to host cells. Signal Transduct Target Ther. 2020;**5**(1):283. Published 2020 Dec 4. DOI: 10.1038/s41392-020-00426-x

[26] Shang J, Wan Y, Luo C, et al. Cell entry mechanisms of SARS-CoV-2. Proceedings of the National Academy of Science USA. 2020;**117**(21):11727-11734. DOI: 10.1073/pnas.2003138117

[27] Estrada E. Cascading from SARS-CoV-2 to Parkinson's disease through protein-protein interactions. Viruses. 2021;**13**(5):897

[28] Rodriguez-Oroz MC, Jahanshahi M, Krack P, et al. Initial clinical manifestations of Parkinson's disease: Features and pathophysiological mechanisms. Lancet Neurology. 2009;**8**(12):1128-1139. DOI: 10.1016/S1474-4422(09)70293-5

[29] Mahul-Mellier AL, Burtscher J, Maharjan N, et al. The process of Lewy body formation, rather than simply α-synuclein fibrillization, is one of the major drivers of neurodegeneration. Proceedings of the National Academy of Science USA. 2020;**117**(9):4971-4982. DOI: 10.1073/pnas.1913904117

[30] Gómez-Benito M, Granado N, García-Sanz P, Michel A, Dumoulin M, Moratalla R. Modeling Parkinson's disease with the alpha-synuclein protein. Frontiers in Pharmacology. 2020;**11**:356

[31] Bridi JC, Hirth F. Mechanisms of α-synuclein induced synaptopathy in Parkinson's disease. Frontiers in Neuroscience. 2018;**12**:80

[32] Cardinale A, Calabrese V, de Iure A, Picconi B. Alpha-Synuclein as a prominent actor in the inflammatory synaptopathy of Parkinson's disease. International Journal of Molecular Science. 2021;**22**(12):6517

[33] Jeon YM, Kwon Y, Jo M, Lee S, Kim S, Kim HJ. The role of glial mitochondria in α-synuclein toxicity. Frontiers in Cell Development Biology. 2020;**8**:548283

[34] Al-Mansoori KM, Hasan MY, Al-Hayani A, El-Agnaf OM. The role of α-synuclein in neurodegenerative diseases: From molecular pathways in disease to therapeutic approaches. Current Alzheimer Research. 2013;**10**(6):559-568. DOI: 10.2174/1567205011310060002

[35] Allen NJ, Lyons DA. Glia as architects of central nervous system formation and function. Science. 2018;**362**(6411):181-185. DOI: 10.1126/science.aat0473

[36] Kwon HS, Koh SH. Neuroinflammation in neurodegenerative disorders: The roles of microglia and astrocytes. Translational Neurodegeneration. 2020;**9**(1):42

[37] Domingues AV, Pereira IM, Vilaça-Faria H, Salgado AJ, Rodrigues AJ, Teixeira FG. Glial cells in Parkinson's disease: Protective or deleterious? Cell Molecular Life Sciences. 2020;**77**(24):5171-5188. DOI: 10.1007/s00018-020-03584-x

[38] Sulzer D, Antonini A, Leta V, et al. COVID-19 and possible links with Parkinson's disease and parkinsonism: From bench to bedside. NPJ Parkinsons Diseases. 2020;**6**:18

[39] Limphaibool N, Iwanowski P, Holstad MJV, Kobylarek D, Kozubski W. Infectious etiologies of Parkinsonism: Pathomechanisms and clinical implications. Frontiers in Neurology. 2019;**10**:652

[40] Toscano G, Palmerini F, Ravaglia S, et al. Guillain-Barré syndrome associated with SARS-CoV-2. New England Journal of Medicine. 2020;**382**(26):2574-2576. DOI: 10.1056/NEJMc2009191

[41] Schetters STT, Gomez-Nicola D, Garcia-Vallejo JJ, Van Kooyk Y. Neuroinflammation: Microglia and T cells get ready to Tango. Frontiers in Immunology. 2018;**8**:1905

[42] Semerdzhiev SA, Fakhree MAA, Segers-Nolten I, Blum C, Claessens MMAE. Interactions between SARS-CoV-2 N-protein and α-synuclein accelerate amyloid formation. ACS Chemical Neuroscience. 2022;**13**(1):143-150. DOI: 10.1021/acschemneuro.1c00666

[43] Jana AK, Greenwood AB, Hansmann UHE. Presence of a SARS-CoV-2 protein enhances amyloid formation of serum Amyloid A. J Phys Chem B. 2021;**125**(32):9155-9167. DOI: 10.1021/acs.jpcb.1c04871

[44] Tambasco N, Romoli M, Calabresi P. Levodopa in Parkinson's disease: Current status and future developments. Current Neuropharmacology. 2018;**16**(8):1239-1252. DOI: 10.2174/1570159X15666170510143821

[45] Armstrong MJ, Okun MS. Diagnosis and treatment of Parkinson disease: A review. JAMA. 2020;**323**(6):548-560. DOI: 10.1001/jama.2019.22360

[46] DeMaagd G, Philip A. Parkinson's disease and its management: Part 3: Nondopaminergic and nonpharmacological treatment options. P T. 2015;**40**(10):668-679

[47] Zhang C, Zhang J, Qiu X, et al. Deep brain stimulation for Parkinson's disease during the COVID-19 pandemic: Patient perspective. Frontiers in Human Neuroscience. 2021;**15**:628105

[48] Matthews DC, Lerman H, Lukic A, et al. FDG PET Parkinson's disease-related pattern as a biomarker for clinical trials in early stage disease. Neuroimage Clinic. 2018;**20**:572-579

[49] Iarkov A, Barreto GE, Grizzell JA, Echeverria V. Strategies for the treatment of Parkinson's disease: Beyond dopamine. Frontiers in Aging Neuroscience. 2020;**12**:4

[50] Kabra A, Sharma R, Kabra R, Baghel US. Emerging and alternative therapies for Parkinson disease: An updated review. Current Pharmaceutical Research. 2018;**24**(22):2573-2582. DOI: 10.2174/1381612824666180820150150

[51] Lu X, Cui Z, Liu S, Yin F. MiRNAs participate in the diagnosis, pathogenesis and therapy of Parkinson's disease. Histological and Histopathological. 2018;**33**(5):447-453. DOI: 10.14670/HH-11-944

[52] Merola A, Romagnolo A, Dwivedi AK, et al. Benign versus malignant Parkinson disease: The unexpected silver lining of motor complications. Journal of Neurology. 2020;**267**(10):2949-2960. DOI: 10.1007/s00415-020-09954-6

[53] Tenenbaum L, Humbert-Claude M. Glial cell line-derived neurotrophic factor gene delivery in Parkinson's disease: A delicate balance between neuroprotection, trophic effects, and unwanted compensatory mechanisms. Frontiers in Neuronanotechnology. 2017;**11**:29

[54] Ntetsika T, Papathoma PE, Markaki I. Novel targeted therapies for Parkinson's disease. Molecular Medicine. 2021;**27**:17

[55] Torres PHM, Sodero ACR, Jofily P, Silva-Jr FP. Key topics in molecular docking for drug design. International Journal of Molecular Science. 2019;**20**:4574

[56] Monteiro AFM, Viana JO, Nayarisseri A, et al. Computational studies applied to flavonoids against Alzheimer's and Parkinson's diseases. Oxidative Medical Cell Longevity. 2018;**2018**:7912765

[57] Madeswaran A, Umamaheswari M, Asokkumar K, Sivashanmugam T, Subhadradevi V, Jagannath P. Docking studies: In silico lipoxygenase inhibitory activity of some commercially available flavonoids. Bangladesh Journal of Pharmacology. 2011;**6**(2). DOI: 10.3329/bjp.v6i2.9408

[58] Garg S, Roy A. In silico analysis of selected alkaloids against main protease (M^{pro}) of SARS-CoV-2. Chemical Biological Interaction. 2020;**332**:109309. DOI: 10.1016/j.cbi.2020.109309

[59] Kaakkola S. Clinical pharmacology, therapeutic use and potential of COMT inhibitors in Parkinson's disease. Drugs. 2000;**59**(6):1233-1250. DOI: 10.2165/00003495-200059060-00004

[60] Fakhri S, Piri S, Majnooni MB, Farzaei MH, Echeverría J. Targeting neurological manifestations of coronaviruses by candidate phytochemicals: A mechanistic approach. Frontiers in Pharmacology. 2021;**11**:621099

Chapter 4

COVID-19 Pandemic and Neurocognitive Process: New Scenarios for Understanding and Treatment

Serefnur Ozturk and Fettah Eren

Abstract

COVID-19 disease was defined as a disease of primary respiratory system. However, symptoms associated with central nervous system were detected in approximately 2/3 of the hospitalized patients. The rate of ischemic cerebrovascular diseases is higher in central nervous system. In addition, hemorrhagic cerebrovascular diseases, encephalitis and/or encephalopathy are the other diseases. Complex pathogenesis was demonstrated in the central nervous system diseases associated with SARS-CoV-2. It was reported that SARS-CoV-2 virus could directly invade the central nervous system, especially via the olfactory nerves or the haematological pathway. As a result, endothelial cells, pericytes and/or neurons can be infected (direct pathway). Another mechanism is central nervous system deficit resulting from peripheral immune reactivation (indirect pathway). All these etiopathogenetic results support that COVID-19 disease is associated with cognitive dysfunction. Cerebral hypoperfusion associated with vascular endothelial structures is the main factor in the etiopathogenesis. It was reported that COVID-19 disease induced amyloid-β (Aβ) and α-synuclein phosphorylation. Besides, it was detected that this process was associated with tau and TDP-43 pathology. "Cognitive COVID-19" is a term that describes acute and long-term cognitive changes in people infected with SARS-CoV-2. Encephalopathy, delirium and cognitive disorders are most frequently detected. In this chapter, the clinical and etiopathogenetic processes of cognitive dysfunction after COVID-19 disease were evaluated. In addition, the disease, disease process and treatment were evaluated in general.

Keywords: COVID-19 disease, SARS-CoV-2 infection, pandemic, cognitive function, neurocognitive disorder

1. Introduction

Coronavirus disease 2019 (COVID-19) was initially defined as a disease that only causes respiratory system infiltration. However, in addition to major respiratory system symptoms, some systemic and neurocognitive symptoms were also detected in the acute or subacute/chronic period [1]. In these studies, the sample size and clinical and sociodemographic characteristics of the patients were heterogeneous. Therefore, the relationship between COVID-19 disease and neurocognitive dysfunction could not be determined definitively. Recent studies confirmed this relationship. Based on these results, the disease was named "infectious disease-associated encephalopathy" or "Cognitive COVID [2]." Neurological deficits associated with COVID-19 disease were investigated in the several studies. Cognitive deficits were detected more frequently in the post-hospitalization period associated with COVID-19 disease [2–4]. In addition, severe cognitive impairment was observed in some patients with COVID-19 [5, 6].

Nonspecific encephalopathy symptoms (headache, confusion, delirium, disorientation, etc.) were detected in 25% (53/214) of hospitalized patients [7]. This rate is higher in studies reported from Europe. Neurocognitive disorders and psychosis were detected 69% in studies from France and 31% from the United Kingdom (UK) [8, 9]. In a recent study, inattention and disorientation were detected at a frequency of 33% after hospitalization in patients with COVID-19 disease [8]. Micro-structural changes and functional disorders were reported during 3-month follow-up of COVID-19 patients [10]. These results demonstrate that COVID-19 disease causes structural and functional changes in the brain over a long period.

Previous studies have emphasized that the pathogenesis of encephalopathy associated with infection is different from non-infectious encephalopathy. In the literature, there are some studies on the effects of influenza A virus subtype H1N1 (A/H1N1) virus and severe acute respiratory syndrome coronavirus (SARS-CoV) virus on the central nervous system. However, scientific data regarding the etiopathogenesis of cognitive impairment are insufficient [2, 3]. Many mechanisms were reported about the acute, subacute and chronic effects of the SARS-CoV-2 virus. The first mechanism is viral neurotropism. The second mechanism is the general systemic inflammation and secondary effects of cytokine storm. The rates of acute and chronic cognitive dysfunction are higher in patients with acute respiratory distress syndrome (ARDS) and mechanical ventilation [4]. The third mechanism is neurocognitive dysfunction associated with psychosocial isolation. Pandemic-related social isolation and increasing death rates have revealed neurocognitive and neuropsychiatric symptoms over a long period [3, 11]. Evaluating the mechanisms and results of this process is important for the disease and possible treatment strategies.

COVID-19 disease affects the central nervous system with vascular and parenchymal deficits. Many cases of encephalopathy associated with COVID-19 have been reported without cerebral lesions [12]. Patients with neurological clinical symptoms are older and have more severe respiratory symptoms [7]. It is known that SARS-CoV-2 infection directly affects the central nervous system. It also produces indirect neurotoxicity with systemic immune hyperinflammation [13]. Infections damage the endothelium in cerebral vascular structures as well as systemic vascular endothelial structures and blood-brain barrier (BBB). As a result, neurological symptoms are associated with this neuroinflammatory process [14]. Previous studies have reported a relationship between chronic infection and hippocampal atrophy [15]. These results support the relationship between infections and cognitive dysfunction.

Patients with severe respiratory symptoms should be frequently evaluated for neurocognitive dysfunction during the COVID-19 disease process. Particularly, patients with cerebrovascular disease and other neurological complications should be evaluated more frequently. Detailed cognitive evaluation including long-term neurological and psychiatric symptoms should be performed on these patients. We aim to evaluate

"Cognitive COVID" and its neuropathological process in this chapter. In addition, we aim to discuss the clinical features and etiopathogenetic process of the disease with the current literature and to present the results associated with treatment.

2. Neurocognitive impairment in the previous coronavirus outbreaks

Two major coronavirus outbreaks were reported before the SARS-CoV-2 infection. These outbreaks were acute respiratory distress syndrome (ARDS) associated with SARS-CoV and Middle East respiratory Syndrome (MERS) associated with MERS-CoV virus [6, 16]. Neurocognitive disorders during the COVID-19 pandemic process have often been compared with these outbreaks. It has been reported that neurocognitive impairment is dominant in the COVID-19 process. These results were explained by the psychosocial effect of the disease and social isolation [12]. However, neurocognitive impairment is not only associated with psychosocial processes. Because the induced systemic inflammatory process contributes to neurocognitive dysfunction [14]. In a study of MERS-CoV patients, confusion was indicated to be associated with magnetic resonance imaging (MRI) results [17]. It was reported that approximately 25.7% of the patients had confusion [18].

Confusion, neurocognitive and neuropsychiatric symptoms are not only present in coronavirus infection. Inattention, memory and learning defects have been reported in human immunodeficiency virus (HIV) and Zika virus (ZIKV) diseases [19, 20]. Influenza virus may also cause cognitive dysfunction. The clinical presentation of the disease may progress from mild cognitive impairment to seizure and/or severe encephalopathy [21]. Influenza-associated neurological clinical manifestation is not common compared to coronavirus. In a national study conducted in Malaysia, the rate of neurological manifestation was detected as 8.3%. The hospitalization rate is higher in this patient group. However, long-term cognitive deficits are rare in patients with influenza [21, 22].

3. Neuropsychiatric and neurocognitive effects of the disease in the acute and chronic periods and its clinical manifestations

During the COVID-19 pandemic, social restrictions and the fear of contact with a COVID-19 patient have created a serious social panic. This is a cause for many psychological disorders [11, 23]. Anxiety and depression are the most common psychiatric disorders in this process [24]. In some studies, it has been demonstrated that the incidence of post-traumatic stress disorder (PTSD) is between 7 and 53.8% during the pandemic process [25]. Especially in elderly patients, cognitive dysfunction is associated with social isolation and psychological disorder [26]. In a recent population-based study, the effect of psychological stressors on the general cognitive functions of the population was evaluated. The results demonstrated that these factors cause cognitive dysfunction. In addition, it has been demonstrated that the psychological disorders associated with the pandemic are induced by anxiety and depression [27].

Cognitive disorders after viral infections have a complex presentation [12, 28]. There are some publications about neurocognitive effects of the COVID-19 pandemic. Acute impairment in neurocognitive functions during the COVID-19 disease is associated with metabolic disorder. Other neuropathological mechanisms are neurotropism of SARS-CoV-2, mechanical ventilation and adverse effect of neuro-sedative treatments [29].

In a study during the initial period of the pandemic, many neurological symptoms have been reported in patients with COVID-19. Dizziness, headache and neurocognitive deficits were detected in 24.8% of the patients [7]. In a study reported from the UK, behavioural and cognitive impairments were detected in 31% of the patients. Major neurocognitive disorders were determined in approximately 5% of total patients. Some cases of acute viral encephalitis have been reported during or after COVID-19. Transient or persistent neurocognitive disorders were determined in patients with encephalitis [3, 30]. These symptoms are called dysexecutive syndrome. Approximately 25% of COVID-19 patients presenting with ARDS had dysexecutive syndrome. Executive dysfunction predominates in these patients [8, 31]. It has been reported that neurocognitive disorder symptoms are more common in the elderly patients with severe respiratory/systemic symptoms [3]. Many mental disorders have been reported in the acute or chronic period of COVID-19 disease. In addition, post-infection cognitive disorders continue with long-term inattention and memory problems.

The long-term effects of COVID-19 disease were investigated in some studies. In a study by Woo et al., cognitive functions of COVID-19 patients were evaluated after being discharged from the intensive care unit. A lower cognitive function score was detected in the patients. More than one cognitive disorder, such as inattention (50%) and memory disorders (44.4%) was detected [32]. Lu et al. evaluated 60 patients during the early stage of SARS-CoV-2 infection and at a 3-month follow-up. Cognitive impairment increased during the process in this study [33].

4. Pathophysiology of neurocognitive disorders in COVID-19

The pathophysiological mechanisms of neurocognitive impairment after COVID-19 disease have not been determined definitively. SARS-CoV-2 infection causes deficits in the central nervous system by direct and/or indirect mechanisms. The induced psychosocial process contributes to neurocognitive dysfunction. This disease is a complex process with vascular and metabolic disorders. All factors associated with neurocognitive dysfunctions are summarized in **Figure 1**. There are 4 main pathophysiological mechanisms in this process. They are vascular, inflammatory, psychosocial factors and direct neurotropism.

4.1 Cerebrovascular diseases

The risk of acute cerebrovascular disease increased in COVID-19 disease after SARS-CoV-2 infection. In studies, cerebrovascular disease was detected with a frequency of 2–6% in hospitalized patients with the diagnosis of COVID-19 [12]. In a study reported from Spain, stroke was determined in 23 (1.4%) of 1683 patients. Approximately 75% of stroke patients were ischemic stroke [34]

It has been detected that cerebrovascular diseases are more common in COVID-19 patients with neurological complications. The incidence of stroke is higher in elderly patients with severe disease activity. This rate is higher, especially in patients with comorbid diseases, such as hypertension, diabetes mellitus and cerebrovascular disease [30]. However, stroke associated with large vessel disease after COVID-19 disease may be detected in young adults [35].

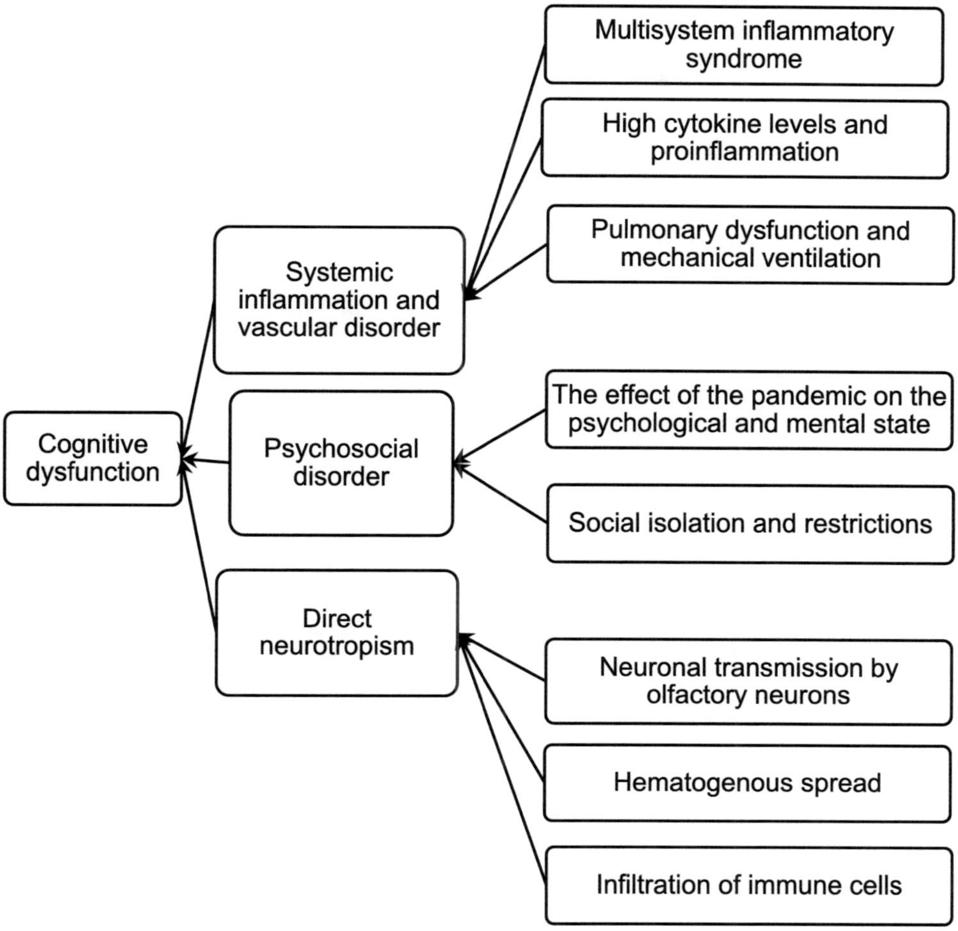

Figure 1.
Possible causal factors of cognitive symptoms associated with COVID-19 (coronavirus disease 2019).

Neurocognitive disorders associated with cerebrovascular diseases occur in COVID-19 patients. The pathophysiological mechanism of this process has not been definitively defined. This process is associated with systemic inflammation and disseminated intravascular coagulation (DIC) [36]. In patients with ARDS associated with COVID-19, a series of reactions including endothelial cell dysfunction, vascular leakage and dysregulated immune activation have been demonstrated for the mechanism of DIC. Activation of kallikrein-bradykinin system, leukocyte adhesion molecules, platelets and neutrophils increase inflammation. This process potentially causes vascular and neuronal damage in patients with COVID-19. SARS-CoV-2 infection damages vascular endothelial structures in cerebral vascular and many other tissues [37]. In many studies, major neurological complications after COVID-19 disease have been associated with cerebral vascular injury and ischemia.

Postmortem neuropathological autopsy studies in COVID-19 patients identified acute hypoxic-ischemic brain injury and perivascular inflammation in the cerebrum and cerebellum. However, SARS-CoV-2 virus could not be isolated in the central nervous system [38]. In the early postmortem period, hemorrhagic lesions and evidence of posterior reversible encephalopathy syndrome (PRES) were detected in patients with COVID-19 [39].

The results of the studies describe that COVID-19 process causes deficits in the central nervous system. The pathophysiological mechanisms of neurocognitive dysfunction in COVID-19 disease are systematically summarized in **Table 1**. It has been demonstrated that brain damage and cognitive impairment are associated with ischemic and inflammatory processes. Cognitive dysfunction associated with hypoxic-ischemic brain injury is explained by these mechanisms.

4.2 Systemic inflammation and acute respiratory distress syndrome

During the COVID-19 disease process, cytokine storm causes severe systemic inflammation [14]. Increased interleukin-1 (IL-1) and other mediators in the systemic circulation are major factors in systemic inflammation associated with COVID-19 [40, 41]. Increased proinflammation causes a vasculitic process, impaired capillary permeability and diffuse vascular thrombosis. This process causes damage to the blood-brain barrier. In addition, microglial inflammation is activated [42]. Neurological symptoms occur as a result of all these mechanisms. In the early period, delirium and seizures have been described [3]. Besides, increased inflammation may be associated with cerebrovascular diseases. As a result, a cerebral hypoxic-ischemic process is induced [5]. The possible causal elements of inflammatory factors on cognitive symptoms associated with COVID-19 disease are figured (**Figure 2**).

It is known that there is a relationship between cognitive disorders and increased inflammation. In a study evaluating Alzheimer's patients and the control group, a correlation was detected between cognitive impairment and increased systemic inflammation [43]. Long-term cognitive dysfunction is more common in patients with severe inflammatory disease. In addition, neurocognitive dysfunction associated with inflammation is higher in patients with neurodegenerative disease [44, 45].

The relationship between C-reactive protein (CRP) level and cognitive dysfunction was investigated in patients with COVID-19 disease. A positive correlation was determined between increased CRP level and cognitive impairment [46].

No.	Factor	Mechanisms
1.	Cardiorespiratory failure	Cerebral hypoperfusion Hypoxic-ischemic brain injury Diffuse white matter damage
2.	Coagulation disorder	Cerebral artery thrombosis Disseminated intravascular coagulation
3.	Cerebral microvascular dysfunction	Endothelial damage Pericytes damage Blood-brain barrier leakiness Neurovascular dysfunction Impaired autoregulation Impaired vascular/para-vascular drainage
4.	Renin-angiotensin system (RAS) dysregulation	RAS dysregulation RAS signal hyperactivity
5.	Encephalitis	Neuroinvasion via olfactory nerve Indirect inflammatory or vascular system

Table 1.
The pathophysiological mechanisms of neurocognitive dysfunction in COVID-19 disease.

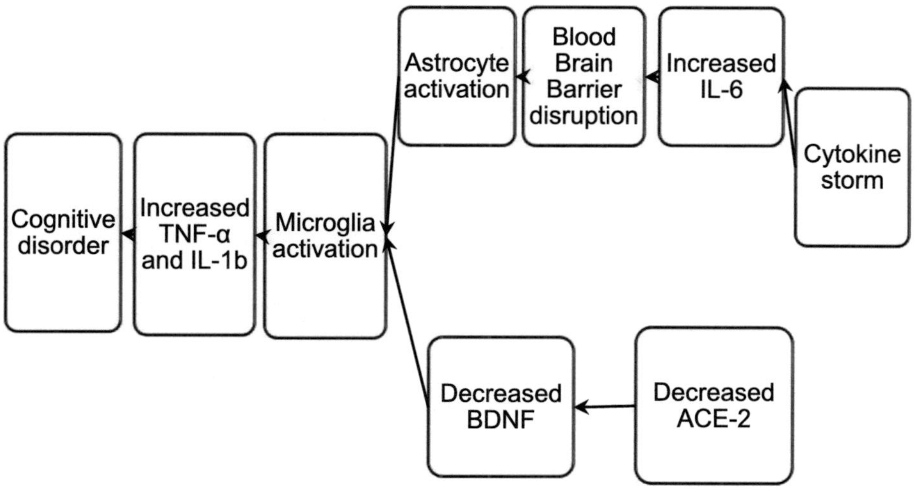

Figure 2.
The possible causal elements of inflammatory factors on cognitive symptoms associated with COVID-19.

These results were evaluated in another study. The relationship between CRP levels and cognitive impairment was confirmed. In the same study, the relationship between cognitive dysfunction and CRP level was also demonstrated over a long period. Disease-related respiratory failure and hypercapnia are the causes of increased IL-1 levels. These results are associated with cognitive impairment [47].

In a study from China with a large patient population, hospitalization was indicated in 19% of COVID-19 patients. In addition, ARDS was detected as a major indication for hospitalization associated with COVID-19 disease [48]. Post-ARDS cognitive impairment is not only associated with COVID-19 disease. Other diseases can also cause cognitive impairment after ARDS [49]. Neurocognitive impairment after ARDS is associated with hypoxia, induced hyperinflammation, and hemodynamic instability. Meta-analyses and studies have reported that neurocognitive dysfunction after ARDS has a high incidence. The incidence of neurocognitive dysfunction is 70–100% at the time of hospital discharge, 46–80% one year after discharge and 20% five years after discharge [49]. In addition, mechanical ventilation without ARDS is associated with long-term cognitive dysfunction and poor quality of life. Sedative treatments for mechanical ventilation are also associated with long-term cognitive impairment [50]. The evidence for the isolation of the virus directly from the cerebrospinal fluid (CSF) is insufficient [14]. There is a relationship between all these pathophysiological mechanisms. These mechanisms are complex and they create cognitive dysfunction.

4.3 Direct neurotropism

The investigations are limited about the direct invasion of the SARS-CoV-2 virus to central nervous system. However, it is thought that SARS-CoV-2 may invade neuronal tissue similar to other coronaviruses [51, 52]. Rare investigations have reported evidence of SARS-CoV-2 in the CSF examination [30, 53]. There are some mechanisms for the invasion of the virus (SARS-CoV-2) into the central nervous system However; these mechanisms are not definitive evidence. All mechanisms are explained in 3 main pathways.

The first pathway is direct retrograde neuronal transmission via olfactory neurons. It is known that the sense of smell and taste associated with SARS-CoV-2 is reduced. This is the first symptom of the disease in some COVID-19 patients. The smell impairment is explained by direct invasion of the mucosal epithelium and olfactory nerves [54]. Direct invasion is associated with angiotensin-converting enzyme 2 (ACE2) and transmembrane protease serine 2 (TMPRSS2) receptors. SARS-CoV-2 has a high affinity for ACE2 receptors [55]. Experimental studies about SARS-CoV confirmed neuronal transmission to the brain via the olfactory bulb. Structural and/or functional changes associated with COVID-19 have been reported in several areas of the brain (entorhinal cortex and hippocampus). Neuronal dysfunction associated with this process has been demonstrated [24].

The second pathway is hematogenous spreading. Some researchers report that the virus may cause cognitive disorders by direct hematogenous spread via the cerebrovascular pathway [5]. There is some data that SARS-CoV-2 has been detected in the blood samples of some COVID-19 patients. Functional (ACE2) receptors of SARS-CoV-2 are higher in endothelial cells and pericytes [56, 57]. The interaction of the virus with these receptors is the first step towards neuronal dysfunction. Delayed neurotropic features of SARS-CoV-2 induce major etiopathogenetic mechanisms for cognitive deficits and neurological symptoms [3]. Induced interleukins, tumour necrosis factor (TNF) and other inflammatory cytokines associated with SARS-CoV-2 may disrupt the endothelial structure of the blood-brain barrier [58]. This process contributes to a major neuroinvasion.

The third pathway is immune-mediated neuronal spreading. In a SARS-CoV-related study published in 2005, it was demonstrated that viral particles were detected in monocytes and lymphocytes [59]. Immune system cells may cause direct brain damage via ACE-2 receptors [60]. However, direct immune cell infiltration was not detected in the brain with pathological investigation after autopsy [60].

5. The relationship between COVID-19 vaccination and cognitive functions

Major neurocognitive disorders are higher in the elderly population. This disease is higher in patients over 60 years old, especially over 80 years of age. In addition, this age group is more sensitive to infections. Immune dysregulation causes a decreased vaccine-associated immune reaction in these patients. Increased age is associated with decreased immunity and increased risk of complications. International investigations have been initiated to accelerate the development of vaccines and medications for the COVID-19 pandemic. These results suggest a different vaccination protocol, especially with increased age. Because this group is highly sensitive to major neurocognitive disorders and other diseases [61].

More cases of adverse reactions after COVID-19 vaccination are being reported. One of the adverse reactions is neurocognitive disorders after vaccination. However, neurocognitive disorders are lower after COVID-19 vaccines. In a recent case report, two cases of encephalopathy were reported within one week after mRNA vaccination [62]. In addition, delirium was reported in an 89-year-old patient after the first dose of the mRNA vaccine [63]. The mechanism of the disease is systemic inflammation associated with anti-spike antibodies and macrophage activation after mRNA vaccines [62–64]. However, there is no case-control study on this subject.

Most of the immunogenic epitopes of SARS-CoV-2 are similar to human proteins. Vaccines with these epitopes have more risk for autoimmunity [65]. Increased inflammation and biochemical reactions associated with autoimmunity can cause neuroinflammation and cognitive impairment [66]. Experimental studies have demonstrated that there is a relationship between increased autoimmunity and cognitive impairment [67]. However, all these evaluations demonstrate that there is no definite relationship between vaccination and cognitive dysfunction.

6. Etiopathogenetic evaluation for understanding and treatment of the disease

It is important to know the causality and etiopathogenesis of COVID-19-related cognitive impairment before the treatment phase. All mechanisms are explained in 3 major pathways. The first is the direct neurotropism of SARS-CoV-2 and is explained by past SARS-CoV studies. The virus may invade the brain by direct neuronal or indirect immune cells-mediated hematogenous pathway. One of the main steps of treatment is to prevent the infiltration of virus-infected immune cells into the central nervous system. It is aimed to prevent cytokine storm with immunosuppression treatment. However, it is important that immunosuppression therapy does not induce infection. The second important step is to prevent the invasion of infiltrating cells with SARS-CoV-2 into the impaired blood-brain barrier structure. At this stage, it should be aimed to stabilize the blood-brain barrier structure [57, 58]. The main aim of treatment is to prevent immune reactivation. Viruses can cause retrograde brain invasion via olfactory neurons. However, there is not enough data about this subject. Invasion has been demonstrated to be associated with ACE2 and TMPRSS2 [12]. Therefore, these proteins and receptors should be targeted in therapy to prevent direct neuronal invasion [12]. Therefore, these proteins and receptors should be targeted during the treatment phase to prevent direct neuronal invasion.

Increased hyperinflammation is detected after cytokine storm in patients with COVID-19. Cytokine storm causes systemic inflammation and vascular damage. Thus, over-induced neuroinflammation is triggered. In addition, mechanical ventilation, cardiopulmonary failure and hypoxia also induce the neuropathological process. Prevention of hypoxia and increased proinflammation is important in the prevention of cognitive impairment. As a result of these mechanisms, cerebral microvascular dysfunction is tried to be prevented [57, 58].

Neuropsychiatric factors have been demonstrated to be important in the pathogenesis. Evaluation of neuropsychiatric disorders in the treatment phase is one of the main strategic steps. Therefore, all patients with and without neurological diseases should be evaluated for neuropsychiatric diseases. The major neuropsychiatric disorders in the COVID-19 disease process are anxiety and depression. These diseases should also be treated [6, 45, 68]. Evaluation of psychiatric and neurocognitive status is important in these patients.

The most important step of this process is the prevention of viral transmission. SARS-CoV-2 spread primarily via respiratory droplets during close face-to-face contact. Personal hygiene, social distance (at least 1 meter, optimum 2 meters) and personal protective equipment are important for protection from COVID-19 disease [57].

Neurocognitive disorders associated with coronavirus infection may have iatrogenic aetiology. Favipiravir and hydroxychloroquine are safe drugs for cognitive dysfunction. No cognitive impairment has been reported as an adverse reaction to tocilizumab. Azithromycin may cause somlonans, insomnia or agitation [57].

7. Approach to cognitive disorders in COVID-19 disease

The primary cause of cognitive impairment and the etiopathogenetic process should be investigated in patients with COVID-19. It is important to investigate systemic and metabolic causes. Activation of the renin-angiotensin system may also impair the metabolic process. Therefore, patients should also be evaluated for endocrinological status [69, 70]. Cardiopulmonary failure and hemodynamic disorders that cause cognitive impairment should be evaluated in patients with COVID-19. Hypoxic ischemic brain injury and diffuse white matter injury associated with hypoxemia are important for treatment and etiopathogenetic process [38, 39, 57].

Hypercoagulability-related cerebrovascular disease should be considered in COVID-19 patients with acute neurological clinical symptoms. Ischemic stroke in a COVID-19 patient is associated with indirect intravascular coagulation or direct cerebral arterial thrombosis after DIC [36, 71]. Brain neuroradiological imaging is indicated for these patients (Computed tomography (CT) and/or magnetic resonance imaging (MRI)).

Encephalitis may be detected as a result of direct or indirect neuronal invasion in patients with COVID-19. In these patients, diffusion restriction in the central nervous system, particularly in the corpus callosum splenium, has been reported. Patients usually have encephalopathy and neurocognitive symptoms. The neurological examination should be repeated periodically. CT and/or MRI neuroimaging is required. Electroencephalography (EEG) and CSF examination should be performed in some patients [3, 72, 73].

Hyperactive delirium is more common than hypoactive delirium in COVID-19 disease. Treatment and management of this clinical symptom are difficult. Scales associated with cognitive dysfunction and delirium should be applied periodically during the COVID-19 process. Control of risk factors associated with this process, optimum blood oxygenation, fluid and calorie support and cognitive behavioural therapy are important [2, 42].

It should be recommended not to change the living environment of patients during the COVID-19 disease process. Chronic diseases, alcohol and drugs may precipitate cognitive dysfunction. Therefore, it is important to evaluate these factors. Anticholinergic adverse effects of treatments for COVID-19 disease should be evaluated. In addition, anticholinergic adverse effects of treatments for chronic diseases should be evaluated [57, 74]. Agitation and cognitive changes are treated with haloperidol and benzodiazepines. However, these treatments have the potential for respiratory depression and extrapyramidal adverse reactions.

8. COVID-19 pandemic and major neurocognitive disorder

The COVID-19 pandemic has different effects on patients with Alzheimer's disease and other major neurocognitive disorders. These effects are not only associated with SARS-CoV-2 infection. On the other hand, the psychosocial process of the pandemic process also has negative effects. In some clinical studies, patients with major neurocognitive disorder and non-major neurocognitive disorder have been compared. Patients with major neurocognitive disorders have higher risk for COVID-19 disease. There are many etiological risk factors for the COVID-19 disease in patients with major neurocognitive disorder. First, cognitive impairment and neuropsychiatric symptoms are common in patients with major neurocognitive disorders. Therefore, protective factors and their management are difficult in patients with COVID-19 [75]. Moreover, it is not possible for these patients to fulfil the requirements of quarantine.

The potential for the APOE ε4 genetic allele is higher in patients with major neurocognitive disorders. This condition damages the blood-brain barrier and precipitates cognitive dysfunction. It is also known that APOE ε4 induces cognitive dysfunction associated with microglia. This process produces neuroinflammation and neurodegeneration [76]. In addition, APOE ε4 is associated with increased cytokine after inflammation. Cytokine storm is induced by these mechanisms. Cytokine storm is directly associated with serious COVID-19 disease complications, such as lung injury and multi-organ failure [77].

There are severe individual and social isolation precautions in many countries to control the pandemic. Pandemic precautions are higher in patients with major neurocognitive disorders. This situation causes neuropsychiatric effects. Especially social isolation causes serious psychiatric symptoms in this patient group. In addition, the incidence of stress, anxiety and depression has increased [75–78]. Social isolation is higher in patients with major neurocognitive disorders in the care centres. Therefore, these patients have more exposed to neuropsychiatric and neurocognitive effects. This is one of the reasons for increased neuropsychiatric symptoms in patients with major neurocognitive disorders [75, 76]. Social isolation in patients with major neurocognitive disorders has been associated with neuropsychiatric and neurocognitive disorders.

Social isolation causes more agitation and cognitive impairment in major neurocognitive disorder patients than in other patient groups. The neurocognitive dysfunction correlates with the duration of social isolation. Neurocognitive dysfunction, especially in the quarantine period, may be permanent. Older patients with major neurocognitive disorders have higher risk for COVID-19 disease. These patients have more severe disease outcomes than other patients without major neurocognitive disorders [79–81]. A large-scale cohort study in the UK has demonstrated that patients diagnosed with major neurocognitive disorders are at three times higher risk for severe COVID-19 disease than other patients [80]. Risk factors for major neurocognitive disorders – age, obesity, cardiovascular disease, hypertension and diabetes mellitus – are also risk factors for SARS-CoV-2 infection and severe COVID-19 disease [81]. Some genetic risk factors for COVID-19 have been determined. In particular, a study reported from the United Kingdom demonstrated that homozygous genetic mutations for APOE ε4 are a risk factor for hospitalization associated with COVID-19 [82].

In summary, the pieces of evidence demonstrate that: First, older patients with major neurocognitive disorders are at higher risk for COVID-19 disease. These patients are also at higher risk of disease-related morbidity and mortality after COVID-19 infection. Second, major neurocognitive disorder patients were isolated for a long period to control SARS-CoV-2 infection. These patients have a higher risk for neuropsychiatric and severe neurocognitive disorders. Consequently, social networks, occupational therapy, caregivers and staff education are important during and after the pandemic in patients with major neurocognitive disorders.

9. Conclusion

There are limited studies about cognitive dysfunction in COVID-19 disease in the literature. However, the negative effects of the pandemic have decreased. There is some evidence about the long-term cognitive effects of the COVID-19 disease in the literature. Therefore, it is necessary to plan more investigations about cognitive dysfunction and COVID-19 disease. Understanding the etiopathogenesis is important for diagnosis and treatment modality.

All results demonstrate that it is not possible to explain "cognitive COVID-19" with a single scenario. Etiopathogenesis has multifactorial effects. The disease has a complex nature. Understanding the disease and its treatment is not easy. This complex interaction makes it difficult to determine a single cause or effect. Understanding the etiopathogenesis of this process will decrease the risk of "cognitive COVID-19." It is known that most of this process is at the micromolecular part with inflammatory mechanisms. In addition, interactions at the receptor level are also important in this process. Therefore, determination of the etiopathogenetic process is essential for detection of treatment options.

Conflict of interest

The authors declare no conflict of interest.

Author details

Serefnur Ozturk* and Fettah Eren
Selcuk University Faculty of Medicine, Department of Neurology, Konya, Turkey

*Address all correspondence to: serefnur@yahoo.com

References

[1] Jaywant A, Vanderlind WM, Alexopoulos GS, Fridman CB, Perlis RH, Gunning FM. Frequency and profile of objective cognitive deficits in hospitalized patients recovering from COVID-19. Neuropsychopharmacology. 2021;**46**:2235-2240. DOI: 10.1038/s41386-021-00978-8

[2] Barbosa-Silva MC, Lima MN, Battaglini D, et al. Infectious disease-associated encephalopathies. Critical Care. 2021;**25**:236. DOI: 10.1186/s13054-021-03659-6

[3] Kumar S, Veldhuis A, Malhotra T. Neuropsychiatric and Cognitive Sequelae of COVID-19. Frontiers in Psychology. 2021;**12**:577529. DOI: 10.3389/fpsyg.2021.577529

[4] Rabinovitz B, Jaywant A, Fridman CB. Neuropsychological functioning in severe acute respiratory disorders caused by the coronavirus: Implications for the current COVID-19 pandemic. The Clinical Neuropsychologist. 2020;**34**:1453-1479. DOI: 10.1080/13854046.2020.1803408

[5] Miners S, Kehoe PG, Love S. Cognitive impact of COVID-19: Looking beyond the short term. Alzheimer's Research & Therapy. 2020;**12**:170. DOI: 10.1186/s13195-020-00744-w

[6] Ksiazek TG, Erdman D, Goldsmith CS, et al. A novel coronavirus associated with severe acute respiratory syndrome. The New England Journal of Medicine. 2003;**348**:1953-1966. DOI: 10.1056/NEJMoa030781

[7] Mao L, Jin H, Wang M, et al. Neurologic manifestations of hospitalized patients with coronavirus disease 2019 in Wuhan, China. JAMA Neurology. 2020;**77**:683-690. DOI: 10.1001/jamaneurol.2020.1127

[8] Helms J, Kremer S, Merdji H, et al. Neurologic features in severe SARS-CoV-2 infection. The New England Journal of Medicine. 2020;**382**:2268-2270. DOI: 10.1056/NEJMc2008597

[9] Varatharaj A, Thomas N, Ellul MA, et al. Neurological and neuropsychiatric complications of COVID-19 in 153 patients: A UK-wide surveillance study. Lancet Psychiatry. 2020;**7**:875-882. DOI: 10.1016/S2215-0366(20)30287-X

[10] Pereira A. Long-term neurological threats of COVID-19: A call to update the thinking about the outcomes of the coronavirus pandemic. Frontiers in Neurology. 2020;**11**:308. DOI: 10.3389/fneur.2020.00308

[11] Dubey S, Biswas P, Ghosh R, et al. Psychosocial impact of COVID-19. Diabetes and Metabolic Syndrome: Clinical Research and Reviews. 2020;**14**:779-788. DOI: 10.1016/j.dsx.2020.05.035

[12] Ellul MA, Benjamin L, Singh B, et al. Neurological associations of COVID-19. Lancet Neurology. 2020;**19**:767-783. DOI: 10.1016/S1474-4422(20)30221-0

[13] Desforges M, Le Coupanec A, Dubeau P, et al. Human coronaviruses and other respiratory viruses: Underestimated opportunistic pathogens of the central nervous system? Viruses. 2019;**12**:14. DOI: 10.3390/v12010014

[14] Heneka MT, Golenbock D, Latz E, Morgan D, Brown R. Immediate and long-term consequences of COVID-19 infections for the development of neurological disease. Alzheimer's Research & Therapy. 2020;**12**:69. DOI: 10.1186/s13195-020-00640-3

[15] Lindlau A, Widmann CN, Putensen C, Jessen F, Semmler A, Heneka MT. Predictors of hippocampal atrophy in critically ill patients. European Journal of Neurology. 2015;**22**:410-415. DOI: 10.1111/ene.12443

[16] Al-Osail AM, Al-Wazzah MJ. The history and epidemiology of Middle East respiratory syndrome corona virus. Multidisciplinary Respiratory Medicine. 2017;**12**:20. DOI: 10.1186/s40248-017-0101-8

[17] Arabi YM, Harthi A, Hussein J, et al. Severe neurologic syndrome associated with Middle East respiratory syndrome corona virus (MERS-CoV). Infection. 2015;**43**:495-501. DOI: 10.1007/s15010-015-0720-y

[18] Saad M, Omrani AS, Baig K, et al. Clinical aspects and outcomes of 70 patients with Middle East respiratory syndrome coronavirus infection: A single-center experience in Saudi Arabia. International Journal of Infectious Diseases. 2014;**29**:301-306. DOI: 10.1016/j.ijid.2014.09.003

[19] Kanmogne GD, Fonsah JY, Umlauf A, et al. Attention/working memory, learning and memory in adult Cameroonians: Normative data, effects of HIV infection and viral genotype. Journal of the International Neuropsychological Society. 2020;**26**:607-623. DOI: 10.1017/S1355617720000120

[20] Raper J, Kovacs-Balint Z, Mavigner M, et al. Long-term alterations in brain and behavior after postnatal Zika virus infection in infant macaques. Nature Communications. 2020;**11**:2534. DOI: 10.1038/s41467-020-16320-7

[21] Ekstrand JJ. Neurologic complications of influenza. Seminars in Pediatric Neurology. 2012;**19**:96-100. DOI: 10.1016/j.spen.2012.02.004

[22] Muhammad Ismail HI, Teh CM, Lee YL, National Paediatric H1N1 Study Group. Neurologic manifestations and complications of pandemic influenza A H1N1 in Malaysian children: What have we learnt from the ordeal? Brain & Development. 2015;**37**:120-129. DOI: 10.1016/j.braindev.2014.03.008

[23] Ammar A, Mueller P, Trabelsi K, et al. Psychological consequences of COVID-19 home confinement: The ECLB-COVID19 multicenter study. PLoS One. 2020;**15**:e0240204. DOI: 10.1371/journal.pone.0240204

[24] Ritchie K, Chan D, Watermeyer T. The cognitive consequences of the COVID-19 epidemic: Collateral damage? Brain Communication. 2020;**2**:fcaa069

[25] Xiong J, Lipsitz O, Nasri F, et al. Impact of COVID-19 pandemic on mental health in the general population: A systematic review. Journal of Affective Disorders. 2020;**277**:55-64. DOI: 10.1016/j.jad.2020.08.001

[26] Qureshi SU, Long ME, Bradshaw MR, et al. Does PTSD impair cognition beyond the effect of trauma? The Journal of Neuropsychiatry and Clinical Neurosciences. 2011;**23**:16-28. DOI: 10.1176/jnp.23.1.jnp16

[27] Fiorenzato E, Zabberoni S, Costa A, Cona G. Cognitive and mental health changes and their vulnerability factors related to COVID-19 lockdown in Italy. PLoS One. 2021;**16**:e0246204. DOI: 10.1371/journal.pone.0246204

[28] Rogers JP, Chesney E, Oliver D, et al. Psychiatric and neuropsychiatric presentations associated with severe coronavirus infections: A systematic review and meta-analysis with

comparison to the COVID-19 pandemic. Lancet Psychiatry. 2020;7:611-627. DOI: 10.1016/S2215-0366(20)30203-0

[29] Filatov A, Sharma P, Hindi F, Espinosa PS. Neurological complications of coronavirus disease (COVID-19): Encephalopathy. Cureus. 2020;**12**:7352. DOI: 10.7759/cureus.7352

[30] Moriguchi T, Harii N, Goto J, et al. A first case of meningitis/encephalitis associated with SARS-Coronavirus-2. International Journal of Infectious Diseases. 2020;**94**:55-58. DOI: 10.1016/j.ijid.2020.03.062

[31] Ardila A, Lahiri D. Executive dysfunction in COVID-19 patients. Diabetes and Metabolic Syndrome: Clinical Research and Reviews. 2020;**14**:1377-1378. DOI: 10.1016/j.dsx.2020.07.032

[32] Woo MS, Malsy J, Pöttgen J, et al. Frequent neurocognitive deficits after recovery from mild COVID-19. Brain Communication. 2020;**2**:fcaa205

[33] Lu Y, Li X, Geng D, et al. Cerebral micro-structural changes in COVID-19 patients – An MRI-based 3-month follow-up study. EClinicalMedicine. 2020;**25**:100484. DOI: 10.1016/j.eclinm.2020.100484

[34] Hernández-Fernández F, Sandoval Valencia H, Barbella-Aponte RA, et al. Cerebrovascular disease in patients with COVID-19: Neuroimaging, histological and clinical description. Brain. 2020;**143**:3089-3103. DOI: 10.1093/brain/awaa239

[35] Aggarwal G, Lippi G, Michael HB. Cerebrovascular disease is associated with an increased disease severity in patients with Coronavirus Disease 2019 (COVID-19): A pooled analysis of published literature. International Journal of Stroke. 2020;**15**:385-389. DOI: 10.1177/1747493020921664

[36] Reddy ST, Garg T, Shah C, et al. Cerebrovascular disease in patients with COVID-19: A review of the literature and case series. Case Reports in Neurology. 2020;**12**:199-209. DOI: 10.1159/000508958

[37] Varga Z, Flammer AJ, Steiger P, et al. Endothelial cell infection and endotheliitis in COVID-19. Lancet. 2020;**395**:1417-1418. DOI: 10.1016/S0140-6736(20)30937-5

[38] Solomon IH, Normandin E, Bhattacharyya S, et al. Neuropathological features of Covid-19. The New England Journal of Medicine. 2020;**383**:989-992. DOI: 10.1056/NEJMc2019373

[39] Coolen T, Lolli V, Sadeghi N, et al. Early postmortem brain MRI findings in COVID-19 non-survivors. Neurology. 2020;**95**:2016-2027. DOI: 10.1212/WNL.0000000000010116

[40] Wang J, Jiang M, Chen X, Montaner LJ. Cytokine storm and leukocyte changes in mild versus severe SARS-CoV-2 infection: Review of 3939 COVID-19 patients in China and emerging pathogenesis and therapy concepts. Journal of Leukocyte Biology. 2020;**108**:17-41. DOI: 10.1002/JLB.3COVR0520-272R

[41] Bülow Anderberg S, Luther T, Berglund M, et al. Increased levels of plasma cytokines and correlations to organ failure and 30-day mortality in critically ill Covid-19 patients. Cytokine. 2021;**138**:155389. DOI: 10.1016/j.cyto.2020.155389

[42] Boldrini M, Canoll PD, Klein RS. How COVID-19 Affects the Brain. JAMA Psychiatry. 2021;**78**:682-683. DOI: 10.1001/jamapsychiatry.2021.0500

[43] Shen XN, Niu LD, Wang YJ, et al. Inflammatory markers in Alzheimer's disease and mild cognitive impairment: A meta-analysis and systematic review of 170 studies. Journal of Neurology, Neurosurgery, and Psychiatry. 2019;**90**:590-598. DOI: 10.1136/jnnp-2018-319148

[44] Iwashyna TJ, Ely EW, Smith DM, Langa KM. Long-term cognitive impairment and functional disability among survivors of severe sepsis. Journal of the American Medical Association. 2010;**304**:1787-1794. DOI: 10.1001/jama.2010.1553

[45] Chakrabarty T, Torres IJ, Bond DJ, Yatham LN. Inflammatory cytokines and cognitive functioning in early-stage bipolar I disorder. Journal of Affective Disorders. 2019;**245**:679-685. DOI: 10.1016/j.jad.2018.11.018

[46] Zhou H, Lu S, Chen J, et al. The landscape of cognitive function in recovered COVID-19 patients. Journal of Psychiatric Research. 2020;**129**:98-102. DOI: 10.1016/j.jpsychires.2020.06.022

[47] Ding HG, Deng YY, Yang RQ, et al. Hypercapnia induces IL-1β overproduction via activation of NLRP3 inflammasome: Implication in cognitive impairment in hypoxemic adult rats. Journal of Neuroinflammation. 2018;**15**:4. DOI: 10.1186/s12974-017-1051-y

[48] Wu Z, McGoogan JM. Characteristics of and Important Lessons From the Coronavirus Disease 2019 (COVID-19) Outbreak in China: Summary of a Report of 72 314 Cases From the Chinese Center for Disease Control and Prevention. Journal of the American Medical Association. 2020;**323**:1239-1242. DOI: 10.1001/jama.2020.2648

[49] Sasannejad C, Ely EW, Lahiri S. Long-term cognitive impairment after acute respiratory distress syndrome: A review of clinical impact and pathophysiological mechanisms. Critical Care. 2019;**23**:352. DOI: 10.1186/s13054-019-2626-z

[50] Girard TD, Thompson JL, Pandharipande PP, et al. Clinical phenotypes of delirium during critical illness and severity of subsequent long-term cognitive impairment: A prospective cohort study. The Lancet Respiratory Medicine. 2018;**6**:213-222. DOI: 10.1016/S2213-2600(18)30062-6

[51] Ng Kee Kwong KC, Mehta PR, Shukla G, Mehta AR. COVID-19, SARS and MERS: A neurological perspective. Journal of Clinical Neuroscience. 2020;**77**:13-16. DOI: 10.1016/j.jocn.2020.04.124

[52] Valiuddin HM, Kalajdzic A, Rosati J, Boehm K, Hill D. Update on neurological manifestations of SARS-CoV-2. The Western Journal of Emergency Medicine. 2020;**21**:45-51. DOI: 10.5811/westjem.2020.8.48839

[53] Lewis A, Frontera J, Placantonakis DG, et al. Cerebrospinal fluid in COVID-19: A systematic review of the literature. Journal of the Neurological Sciences. 2021;**421**:117316. DOI: 10.1016/j.jns.2021.117316

[54] Mehraeen E, Behnezhad F, Salehi MA, Noori T, Harandi H, SeyedAlinaghi S. Olfactory and gustatory dysfunctions due to the coronavirus disease (COVID-19): A review of current evidence. European Archives of Oto-Rhino-Laryngology. 2021;**278**:307-312. DOI: 10.1007/s00405-020-06120-6

[55] Wrapp D, Wang N, Corbett KS, et al. Cryo-EM structure of the 2019-nCoV spike in the prefusion

conformation. Science. 2020;**367**:1260-1263. DOI: 10.1126/science.abb2507

[56] Baig AM, Khaleeq A, Ali U, Syeda H. Evidence of the COVID-19 virus targeting the CNS: Tissue distribution, host-virus interaction, and proposed neurotropic mechanisms. ACS Chemical Neuroscience. 2020;**11**:995-998. DOI: 10.1021/acschemneuro.0c00122

[57] Acar T, Acıman Demirel E, Afşar N, et al. The COVID-19 from neurological overview. Turkey Journal of Neurology. 2020;**26**:58-108. DOI: 10.4274/tnd.2020.73669

[58] Teuwen LA, Geldhof V, Pasut A, Carmeliet P. COVID-19: The vasculature unleashed. Nature Reviews. Immunology. 2020;**20**:389-391. DOI: 10.1038/s41577-020-0343-0

[59] Gu J, Gong E, Zhang B, et al. Multiple organ infection and the pathogenesis of SARS. The Journal of Experimental Medicine. 2005;**202**:415-424. DOI: 10.1084/jem.20050828

[60] Iadecola C, Anrather J, Kamel H. Effects of COVID-19 on the nervous system. Cell. 2020;**183**:16

[61] Palermo S. Covid-19 pandemic: Maximizing future vaccination treatments considering aging and frailty. Frontier in Medicine. 2020;**7**:558835

[62] Liu BD, Ugolini C, Jha P. Two cases of post-moderna COVID-19 vaccine encephalopathy associated with nonconvulsive status epilepticus. Cureus. 2021;**13**:e16172. DOI: 10.7759/cureus.16172

[63] Zavala-Jonguitud LF, Pérez-García CC. Delirium triggered by COVID-19 vaccine in an elderly patient. Geriatrics & Gerontology International. 2021;**21**:540. DOI: 10.1111/ggi.14163

[64] Jiang L, Tang K, Levin M, et al. COVID-19 and multisystem inflammatory syndrome in children and adolescents. The Lancet Infectious Diseases. 2020;**20**:276-288. DOI: 10.1016/S1473-3099(20)30651-4

[65] Lyons-Weiler J. Pathogenic priming likely contributes to serious and critical illness and mortality in COVID-19 via autoimmunity. J Transl Autoimmun. 2020;**3**:100051. DOI: 10.1016/j.jtauto.2020.100051

[66] Terrando N, Pavlov VA. Editorial: Neuro-immune interactions in inflammation and autoimmunity. Frontiers in Immunology. 2018;**9**:772. DOI: 10.3389/fimmu.2018.007727

[67] Lal H, Forster MJ. Autoimmunity and age-associated cognitive decline. Neurobiology of Aging. 1988;**9**:733-742. DOI: 10.1016/s0197-4580(88)80141-6

[68] Yalcın GY, Polat Dunya C, Tulek Z, Kurtuncu M, Eraksoy M. Evaluation of depression and anxiety of patients with multiple sclerosis during the COVID-19 pandemic: A comparison with the general population. Turkey Journal of Neurology. 2021;**27**:31-39. DOI: 10.4274/tnd.2021.63444

[69] Zoufaly A, Poglitsch M, Aberle JH, et al. Human recombinant soluble ACE2 in severe COVID-19 [published correction appears in Lancet Respir Med. 2020 Nov;8(11):e78]. The Lancet Respiratory Medicine. 2020;**8**:1154-1158. DOI: 10.1016/S2213-2600(20)30418-5

[70] Abd El-Aziz TM, Al-Sabi A, Stockand JD. Human recombinant soluble ACE2 (hrsACE2) shows promise for treating severe COVID-19. Signal Transduction and Targeted Therapy. 2020;**5**:258. DOI: 10.1038/s41392-020-00374-6

[71] Eren F, Demir A. Acute ischemic stroke in patient with coronavirus disease. Turkey Journal of Neurology. 2020;**26**:258-259. DOI: 10.4274/tnd.2020.42966

[72] Turkmen N, Bugrul A, Genc BO. Electroencephalographic findings in patients with COVID-19: A single-center experience. Turket Journal of Neurology. 2021;**27**:26-30. DOI: 10.4274/tnd.2021.76329

[73] Eren F, Ozdemir G, Ildız OF, Ergun D, Ozturk S. Mild encephalopathy with reversible splenial lesion associated with SARS-CoV-2 infection: A case report. Neurology Asia. 2021;**26**:825

[74] Reis J, Ozturk S, Tulek Z, Spencer P. The COVID-19 pandemic, a risk management approach. Turkey Journal of Neurology. 2021;**27**:1-5. DOI: 10.4274/tnd.2021.93296

[75] Mok VCT, Pendlebury S, Wong A, et al. Tackling challenges in care of Alzheimer's disease and other dementias amid the COVID-19 pandemic, now and in the future. Alzheimer's & Dementia. 2020;**16**:1571-1581. DOI: 10.1002/alz.12143

[76] Brown EE, Kumar S, Rajji TK, Pollock BG, Mulsant BH. Anticipating and Mitigating the Impact of the COVID-19 Pandemic on Alzheimer's Disease and Related Dementias. The American Journal of Geriatric Psychiatry. 2020;**28**:712-721. DOI: 10.1016/j.jagp.2020.04.010

[77] Ragab D, Salah Eldin H, Taeimah M, Khattab R, Salem R. The COVID-19 cytokine storm: What we know so far. Frontier in Immunology. 2020;**11**:1446. DOI: 10.3389/fimmu.2020.01446

[78] Manca R, De Marco M, Venneri A. The impact of COVID-19 infection and enforced prolonged social isolation on neuropsychiatric symptoms in older adults with and without dementia: A review. Frontiers in Psychiatry. 2020;**11**:585540. DOI: 10.3389/fpsyt.2020.585540

[79] Atkins JL, Masoli JAH, Delgado J, et al. Preexisting comorbidities predicting COVID-19 and mortality in the UK Biobank Community Cohort. The Journals of Gerontology. Series A, Biological Sciences and Medical Sciences. 2020;**75**:2224-2230. DOI: 10.1093/gerona/glaa183

[80] Onder G, Rezza G, Brusaferro S. Case-fatality rate and characteristics of patients dying in relation to COVID-19 in Italy. Journal of the American Medical Association. 2020;**323**:1775-1776. DOI: 10.1001/jama.2020.4683

[81] Williamson EJ, Walker AJ, Bhaskaran K, et al. Factors associated with COVID-19-related death using OpenSAFELY. Nature. 2020;**584**:430-436. DOI: 10.1038/s41586-020-2521-4

[82] Kuo CL, Pilling LC, Atkins JL, et al. APOE e4 genotype predicts severe COVID-19 in the UK Biobank Community Cohort. The Journals of Gerontology. Series A, Biological Sciences and Medical Sciences. 2020;**75**:2231-2232. DOI: 10.1093/gerona/glaa131

Chapter 5

Perspective Chapter: New Use of the SSRI Fluvoxamine in the Treatment of COVID-19 Symptoms

Jawza F. Alsabhan and Tahani K. Alshammari

Abstract

From the perspective of repurposing medication, recent evidence suggests that the use of selective serotonin reuptake inhibitor antidepressants (SSRIs) can help reduce the severity of symptoms and death associated with SARS-CoV-2 infection. To focus more, COVID-19 is a viral disease with potentially high risk of symptoms. There is presently no cure. However, there are specific treatments that may help manage the condition. Since the SSRI fluvoxamine has a unique mechanism of action in reducing cytokine production, researchers have started to relate the antiviral effects via modulation of sigma-1 receptors with the vision of treatment options for COVID-19 patients. The scope of this chapter is to examine different mechanisms of fluvoxamine in relation to immune response, including both the serotonin and the sigma-1 receptor-related mechanisms. Addressing the impact of fluvoxamine in minimizing possible complications during COVID-19 infection.

Keywords: fluvoxamine, anti-inflammatory, coronavirus disease 2019, sigma-1 receptor, clinical studies, preclinical studies

1. Introduction – COVID-19 options for treatment

The coronavirus disease 2019 (COVID-19) is an acute respiratory infection related to the new RNA virus coronavirus 2, that produces severe acute respiratory syndrome (SARS-CoV-2) [1]. Since the first SARS-CoV-2-infected patients were reported in Wuhan, China, in December 2019, the number of individuals infected with COVID-19 has risen significantly around the world [2]. In January 2020, the World Health Organization (WHO) announced that COVID-19 had been labeled as a public health pandemic disease worldwide [3]. Likewise, during the last three years, individuals worldwide face a large wave of COVID-19 produced by SARS-CoV-2 variants (i.e., delta, lambda, mu, and omicron) on a widespread globe. In January 2022, the World Health Organization (WHO) published an updated report about enhancing the response to the new mutation called Omicron SARS-CoV-2 variant [4]. To focus more on COVID-19 symptoms, after the incubation period (2–14 days), three phases of COVID-19 symptoms appeared [1]. The first stage, known as the acute COVID-19 stage (stage I) characterized by mild to moderate symptoms including fever or chills, cough, shortness of breath fatigue, muscle or body aches, headache, new loss of taste or smell, sore throat, congestion or running nose, nausea, and diarrhea [2]. The prevalence of mild to moderate symptoms is significant in SARS-CoV-2-infected individuals [5]. Post-acute viral syndromes are acknowledged as prolonged and multi-organ effects [6]. The second stage (stage II) is less common and characterized by severe clinical stages such as dyspnea accompanied by hypoxemia [7, 8]. As a consequence of severe clinical symptoms, stage III can occur, including serious difficulties such as arrhythmias, septic shock, and multi-organ failures, ultimately resulting in intubation or death [2]. A high proportion of COVID-19 non survivors had pre-existing cardiovascular illness and multi organ dysfunction [9].

SARS-CoV-2 infection appears to have harmful effects on the central nervous system (CNS), leading to psychiatric and neurological symptoms [10]. Brain-related manifestations were reported in individuals with and without neuropsychiatric diseases [11]. Existing in vitro and in vivo studies support the notion of SARS-CoV-2-related neuroinvasive risks. These risks were transported mainly through olfaction and the trigeminal pathways [12]. According to national longitudinal research in China, depression, anxiety, and insomnia were the most common psychiatric disorders associated with the COVID-19 pandemic [13]. Another study indicated that the prevalence of neurological manifestations was reasonably noted, including encephalopathy, delirium, seizures, Guillain-Barré-syndrome, and motor dysfunctions [14]. Another review reported that the emergence of psychiatric disorders occurs within three months in COVID-19 survivors [6].

COVID-19 outbreaks present challenges for therapeutic and drug management in clinical conditions and complications. Recently, several researchers emphasized medication repurposing as an approaching method to establish a fast-track line for discovering therapeutic treatments for COVID-19 patients worldwide [15–18]. Drug repurposing, also known as drug reuse, is defined as exploring new indications for existing drugs. This approach limits the cost of both research and development significantly [19]. Serendipitously revealed a substantial number of current identified repurposed drugs [20]. The repurposing strategy provided promising treatment candidates in other viral pandemics outbreaks, including ZIKA, Ebola, and dengue [21].

Zhang et al summarized the current potential therapeutic approaches for diseases related to COVID-19 infection and explain their mechanisms of action, safety, and effectiveness such as antiviral drugs, convalescent plasma, spike Protein-Angiotensin-Converting enzyme 2 blockers, chloroquine, hydroxychloroquine, human monoclonal antibody, mesenchymal stem cells, inhaled nitric oxide (iNO), and corticosteroids [22]. Another review highlighted alternative treatment approaches such as mesenchymal stem cells, human monoclonal antibodies, and complementary Chinese medicine [20].

A comprehensive and systematic research about the repurposing of drugs in COVID-19 was conducted by Srivastava and Singh (2021), the results revealed that no drugs passed clinical trials or were approved by the FDA for COVID-19 [23]. In fact, various reports that clinical trials regarding the potential therapeutic possibilities, such as hydroxychloroquine, lopinavir-ritonavir, and ivermectin, showed that choices were unsuccessful in the treatment of COVID-19 patients [24–27]. Although COVID-19 vaccines were successfully developed and massively distributed, there is a lack of effective treatment [28].

Most significantly, there are cumulative clinical data linked with the use of antidepressants, including the selective serotonin reuptake inhibitor (SSRI) and the serotonin-norepinephrine reuptake inhibitor (SNRI) with a reduced risk of clinical complications in SARS-CoV-2-infected patients [18]. In line with this, a randomized controlled trial showed that patients who received fluvoxamine had a decreased risk of clinical deterioration compared to those who received placebo during the early period of infection [29]. Following that, an observational study done by Hoertel et al. discovered that the antidepressants, such as SSRIs and SNRIs, may be associated with a lower risk of intubation or death in SARS-CoV-2-infected hospitalized patients [30]. This advantage was not reported with other antipsychotics. For example, a multicenter observational study indicated that administration of haloperidol was not associated with a reduced risk of intubation or death in hospitalized COVID-19 patients [31].

Fluvoxamine has advantages over other repurposing drugs such as positive safety profiles, widespread availability, inexpensive, accessible mode of administration as immediate-release tablets and controlled-release capsules, and use for children and adolescents [32, 33]. The available dosage form of fluvoxamine is both immediate-release tablets and controlled-release capsules. The main therapeutic indication of fluvoxamine is to treat patients with obsessive-compulsive disorder (OCD). The pharmacokinetic properties of fluvoxamine include long half-life of about 9–28 hours according to its dosage form. The clinical guideline recommended the therapeutic dose of fluvoxamine between 100–300 mg/day [34]. Fluvoxamine indication is related to COVID-19 was clarified on the US National Institutes of Health (NIH) COVID-19 Guidelines Panel on April 23, 2021, despite the fact that evidence for fluvoxamine effectiveness was lacking. Recently, a retrospective cohort study of COVID-19 patients treated with SSRIs using electronic health records of 87 health care centers across the US was done in November 2021 by Oskotsky et al. [35]. The study participants were COVID-19 patients receiving fluoxetine only (n = 470), COVID-19 patients receiving fluoxetine or fluvoxamine (n = 481), and COVID-19 patients receiving other SSRIs (n = 2898) compared with matched untreated control COVID-19 patients. The results showed that the patients who received any SSRI had a lower risk of death. In contrast, there was no significant relationship between SSRIs other than fluoxetine or fluvoxamine and the risk of mortality [35]. Finally, fluvoxamine might be used as a preventive medication for patients infected with SARS-CoV-2 in the early stages [16, 36]. In this chapter, we review the fluvoxamine mechanisms of action in COVID-19 and discuss the studies that focus on the impact of the use of fluvoxamine in minimizing the possible complication during COVID-19 infection. Here, we review two main mechanisms mediated by fluvoxamine, the serotonin and the sigma-1 receptor-related mechanisms.

2. Mechanism of fluvoxamine

2.1 Inhibition of serotonin transporter

The main mechanism of action for fluvoxamine, as a selective serotonin-reuptake inhibitor (SSRIs), in the brain is to inhibit the serotonin transporter (SERT) on the 5-HT neuron in the synaptic cleft leading to an increase in the level of the neurotransmitter serotonin [33, 37].

The serotonin transporter is also located on the platelet membranes [38] and in the gut. The serotonin plasma-platelet regulation is a complex biphasic mechanism. Specifically, an elevation in plasma serotonin is associated with reducing platelet SERT surface expression [39]. As a consequence of serotonin transporter inhibition in the platelets by fluvoxamine, this could reduce platelet aggregation [40]. In support of this, elevated circulating serotonin was reported in hypertensive patients [41]. In fact, previously proven that fluvoxamine should be used with caution in patients receiving NSAIDs, aspirin, or other drugs that may impair coagulation and peptic ulcer patients due to the antiplatelet activity mechanism SSRIs that can increase the risk of bleeding [42, 43]. Interestingly, a previous report indicated that transgenic mice harboring SERT construct mutation exhibited altered platelet aggregation [44]. Overall, the physiological role of SERT in Platelets includes maintaining system homeostasis, regulation of drugs' concentration, and function [39, 45].

Besides, the antiplatelet activity mechanism of fluvoxamine has a protective effect against myocardial infarction (MI) and a promising role for patients with thrombotic risk [46]. Clearly, fluvoxamine has anti-inflammatory properties in several animal and clinical studies through the mechanism of serotonin transporter inhibition [47, 48]. For instance, in a Parkinson's disease model, fluvoxamine has been shown to reduce inflammation in injured striatal neurons by elevating anti-inflammatory cytokines and lowering inflammatory cytokines and lipid peroxidation in a 6-hydroxydopamine (6-OHDA) lesion-induced rat model [49]. In line with this, chronic administration of fluvoxamine to the 6-OHDA Parkinsonism model improves the Parkinson's-like symptoms, including a reduction in the dopaminergic neuronal degeneration, improvement in motor dysfunction, and normalization of corticosterone levels in the circuitry [50]. Another preclinical setting utilized the same model, the 6-OHDA Parkinsonism model, which indicated that chronic fluvoxamine treatment alters inflammatory hallmarks of Parkinsonism centrally using both the mRNA and the protein level analysis. The level of IL-1β, IL-6, and TNF-α was reduced following one month of Fluvoxamine treatment [49]. Highlighting the fluvoxamine-mediated pharmacological link between serotonin – anti-inflammatory mechanisms at central and peripheral levels.

Likewise, another study revealed that fluvoxamine inhibits inflammation genes in *in vitro* settings [32]. In multiple sclerosis, fluvoxamine reduced the lymphocyte infiltration and the circulating IFN-γ in experimental autoimmune encephalomyelitis. It further affects the pathological demyelination of lumbar spinal cord in multiple sclerosis animal models [51]. In the context of dementia, a previous review highlighted the anti-inflammatory effects of SSRIs, and the evidence provided indicated that introducing SSRIs in neurodegenerative dementias has beneficial effects [52]. Previous studies have proven that fluvoxamine has potent anti-inflammatory properties in vitro and in vivo models. Besides being an effective anti-inflammatory agent, fluvoxamine was found to have antioxidant effects. In a rat model of ulcers, the stress-induced peptic ulcer model, compared to the control group, the fluvoxamine-treated group exhibited reduced biochemical measurements representing oxidative stress [53]. Most significantly, the serotonin transporter in rodents and humans is highly expressed by the lung, demonstrating that the serotonin transporter in lung endothelium controls the bioavailability of the potent vasoconstrictor serotonin [54, 55]. It was reported that inhibiting gut- and lung-serotonin modulates pulmonary hypertension [56]. Additionally, fluvoxamine can positively improve the lung function of chronic obstructive pulmonary disease (COPD) [57]. For depressed COPD patients, SSRIs are the first-line treatment [58]. However, there is a need for a further clinical study to clarify more about the role of fluvoxamine in the treatment of COVID-19 patients. Although other antidepressants can act on serotonin transporter as an inhibitor, they did not have the same favorable impact on COVID-19 patients [57]. As a result, it is unclear whether fluvoxamine's blockage of serotonin transporters plays a substantial role in its positive benefits for COVID-19 patients. The anti-inflammatory effects of serotonin transporter inhibition, on the other hand, may play a role in its positive benefits [55]. To support the potential use of SSRIs in the treatment of post-COVID-19 depression, a recent observational study showed that treatment with different SSRIs antidepressants has positive effects in patients with post-COVID-19 depression [59]. In support of this, another report highlighted that SSRIs might decrease the rate of mortality in COVID-19 patients [35]. However, different mechanism of action needs to be clarified more about the role of fluvoxamine in the treatment of COVID-19 patients. These mechanisms might be acid sphingomyelinase mediated [60], or melatonin receptor-mediated [61].

2.2 The Sigma-1 receptor-mediated mechanism

Several studies established the role of the sigma-1 receptor in the replication of SARS-CoV-2. Initially, it was recognized by its action as a cellular factor known as endoplasmic reticulum (ER) protein sigma-1 receptor that mediates the early steps of viral RNA replication but not the persistent hepatitis C virus (HCV) RNA replication [62]. The ER chaperones are required to control the production of glycosylated proteins in the cell, including those required for viral infection phases and those involved in immune escape [63]. Therefore, they play various important roles at various stages of the infectious cycle. A recent study recognized protein-protein interactions between SARS-CoV-2 and human proteins including the sigma-1 and sigma-2 receptors [64]. In line with this, a recent report linked this molecular pathway and SARS-CoV-2 replication [65]. Moreover, sigma-1 receptor agonists may protect against mitochondrial damage and ER stress in response to SARS-CoV-2 infection [66]. For that reason, the use of drugs with sigma-1 receptor ligand properties may enhance additive value in early intervention for COVID-19 patients [67].

Previous reports have linked sigma-1 receptor and psychiatric disorders, including anxiety [68], depression [69], and schizophrenia [70].

Cognitive deficit is a core feature of psychiatric disorders, including depression. Reports highlighted the role of the sigma-1 receptor in the fluvoxamine antidepressant mediated mechanism [71]. First, Sigma-1 receptors are expressed abundantly in cortical and motor brain regions [72], indicating functional involvement in the pathology of depression. Additionally, electrophysiological studies indicated that sigma-1 receptor modulated glutamatergic transmission in primary hippocampal neurons. Besides, they were found to be highly expressed in the olfactory bulb [72], a brain region involved in adult neurogenesis. Adult neurogenesis is involved in modulating synaptic plasticity [73] and disrupted in preclinical models of depression [74]. A previous study reported sigma-1 receptor's functional involvement in modulating adult neurogenesis [75]. In a model of Alzheimer's with cognitive impairment, sigma-1 receptors were found to promote spines' maintenance and maturation [76]. Recent studies highlight the role of spine modulation in promoting fast-acting antidepressant effects [77], signifying the role of Sigma-1 receptors in tacking pathological mechanisms of depression.

Besides, sigma-1 receptors were reported to modulate protein kinase signaling (pERK) molecularly in a neuropathic pain animal model [78], and this kinase pathway was found to be involved in depression [79].

In addition, a recent review found that the significant potentiation of the nerve growth factor (NGF) by SSRIs including fluvoxamine leading to induced neurite outgrowth in cell culture and brain plasticity via selective sigma-1 receptor agonistic activity [80]. In clinical settings, NGF was reported to be reduced in depressed patients [81], this reduction was correlated with suicidal tendencies [82]. Moreover, preclinical studies in animal models of depression reported reduced NGF levels [83–85].

Additionally, modulation of the sigma-1 receptor pathway positively impacted inflammatory pathways such as IL-6 tumor necrosis factor-α (TNFα) [86]. In line with this, sigma-1 receptor agonist (the pRE-084) presented neuroprotective effects measured by a decreased infarct volume in an embolic stroke model. This was mostly regraded y a reduction in inflammatory cytokines, including TNF-alpha and multiple isoforms of IL in cortical tissues [87]. In another study utilizing a stroke model in rats, the sigma-1 receptor was reported to exert neuroprotective effects, and these modulations were mediated via targeting glutamate-induced excitotoxicity [88]. Also, in a rat model of renal ischemia, the fluvoxamine mediated sigma-1 receptor mechanism was reported to enhance the survival rate, renal function, and histological characteristics [89]. All these evidence suggest that molecular modulation of the sigma-1 receptor has beneficial effects. It further confirms that the neuroprotective effects of fluvoxamine render it to be considered a prophylactic therapeutic candidate to prevent COVID-19 risks. However, further studies are required to answer whether the anti-inflammatory and other fluvoxamine neuroprotective effects of fluvoxamine are clinically relevant for COVID-19 patients.

Antidepressants	Affinity to sigma 1 receptor	Action at sigma receptor	Anti-inflammatory effect	Reference
Fluvoxamine (SSRI)	Potent	Agonist	Beneficial effect in both preclinical and clinical models of inflammation.	[40, 62, 86, 90]
Sertraline (SSRI)	High to moderate	Antagonist	Strong anti-inflammatory effects by lowering and controlling pro-inflammatory cytokines.	[18, 71]
Fluoxetine (SSRI)	High to moderate	Agonist	Anti-inflammatory effects of fluoxetine in lipopolysaccharide (LPS)-stimulated microglial cells.	[91, 92]
Escitalopram (SSRI)	High to moderate	Agonist	Beneficial effect as an anti-inflammatory in the preclinical module.	[66, 93]
Citalopram(SSRI)	High to moderate	Agonist	Beneficial effect in both preclinical and clinical models of inflammation.	[48, 92]
Paroxetine (SSRI)	Very weak		Partial anti-inflammatory effect.	[48]
Imipramine (TCA)	Very weak	Agonist	Weak inflammatory effect.	[48, 94]
Venlafaxine (SNRI)	Very weak		Weak inflammatory effect.	[94]
Mirtazapine (NaSSA)	Very weak		No sufficient evidence in clinical studies.	[95]

TCA: Tricyclic antidepressants; SSRI: Selective serotonin reuptake inhibitor; SNRI: Serotonin norepinephrine reuptake inhibitor; NaSSA: Noradrenaline specific serotonergic antidepressant. The measure for sigma affinity indicates that potent = 17 nM, high to moderate = 30–400 nM, very week > 10,000 nM.

Table 1.
Affinity of the antidepressants for sigma-1 receptor.

For the most important part, which is the relation between the use of antidepressants and sigma-1 receptor, a study examined in an animal model the SSRIs binding affinity to the sigma-1 receptor [71]. As a result, the study revealed that different SSRIs, including sertraline, fluoxetine, citalopram, and fluvoxamine, have a significant functional impact ranging from high to moderate affinity for sigma-1 receptors in the rat brain (**Table 1**).

3. Conclusion

In this chapter, we reviewed the mechanisms of action of fluvoxamine, including the serotonergic and the sigma-1 mediated mechanisms with regard to COVID-19 infection. Fluvoxamine is not FDA-approved for the treatment of any infection-related disorder. However, accumulated evidence highlighted potential beneficial effects.

To sum up, fluvoxamine could help to improve the clinical deterioration associated with COVID-19 symptoms. However, it is for future studies to mechanistically examine the potential mechanisms and profile consequences related to preventive measures of fluvoxamine in treating COVID-19 patients.

Funding

Not funded

Conflicts of interest

The authors declare that there is no conflict of interest.

Author details

Jawza F. Alsabhan[1*] and Tahani K. Alshammari[2]

1 Department of Clinical Pharmacy, King Saud University, Riyadh, Saudi Arabia

2 Department of Pharmacology and Toxicology, College of Pharmacy, King Saud University, Saudi Arabia

*Address all correspondence to: jawza@ksu.edu.sa

References

[1] Wiersinga WJ, Rhodes A, Cheng AC, Peacock SJ, Prescott HC. Pathophysiology, transmission, diagnosis, and treatment of coronavirus disease 2019 (COVID-19): A review. JAMA – Journal of American Medical Association. 2020;**324**(8):782-793

[2] Guan W, Ni Z, Hu Y, Liang W, Ou C, He J, et al. Clinical characteristics of coronavirus. The New England Journal of Medicine. 2020;**382**(18):1708-1720

[3] Novel Coronavirus (2019-nCoV). In: WHO. 2020. pp. 1-5

[4] WHO. Enhancing response to Omicron SARS-CoV-2 Variant: Technical brief and priority actions for Member States. WHO; 2022. pp. 1-28

[5] Chen N, Zhou M, Dong X, Qu J, Gong F, Han Y, et al. Epidemiological and clinical characteristics of 99 cases of 2019 novel coronavirus pneumonia in Wuhan, China: A descriptive study. Lancet. 2020;**395**(10223):507-513

[6] Nalbandian A, Sehgal K, Gupta A, Madhavan MV, McGroder C, Stevens JS, et al. Post-acute COVID-19 syndrome. Nature Medicine. 2021;**27**(4):601-615

[7] Zhou F, Yu T, Du R, Fan G, Liu Y, Liu Z, et al. Clinical course and risk factors for mortality of adult inpatients with COVID-19 in Wuhan , China: A retrospective cohort study. Lancet. 2020;**395**(10229):1054-1062

[8] Chaudhary S, Benzaquen S, Woo JG, Rubinstein J, Matta A, Albano J, et al. Clinical characteristics, respiratory mechanics, and outcomes in critically ill individuals with COVID-19 infection in an underserved urban population. Respiratory Care. 2021;**66**(6):897-907

[9] Zaim S, Chong JH, Sankaranarayanan V, Harky A. COVID-19 and multiorgan response. Current Problems in Cardiology. 2020;**45**(8):100618

[10] Guerrero JI, Barragán LA, Martínez JD, Montoya JP, Peña A, Sobrino FE, et al. Central and peripheral nervous system involvement by COVID-19: A systematic review of the pathophysiology, clinical manifestations, neuropathology, neuroimaging, electrophysiology, and cerebrospinal fluid findings. BMC Infectious Diseases. 2021;**21**(1):1-16

[11] Panariello F, Cellini L, Speciani M, De Ronchi D, Atti AR. How does SARS-CoV-2 affect the central nervous system? A working hypothesis. Frontiers in Psychiatry. 2020;**19**(11):582345

[12] Liu JM, Tan BH, Wu S, Gui Y, Le SJ, Li YC. Evidence of central nervous system infection and neuroinvasive routes, as well as neurological involvement, in the lethality of SARS-CoV-2 infection. Journal of Medical Virology. 2021;**93**(3):1304-1313

[13] Shi L, Lu ZA, Que JY, Huang XL, Lu QD, Liu L, et al. Long-term impact of covid-19 on mental health among the general public: A nationwide longitudinal study in China. International Journal of Environmental Research and Public Health. 2021;**18**(16):8790

[14] Najjar S, Najjar A, Chong DJ, Pramanik BK, Kirsch C, Kuzniecky RI, et al. Central nervous system complications associated with SARS-CoV-2 infection: Integrative concepts of pathophysiology and case reports. Journal of Neuroinflammation. 2020;**17**(1):1-14

[15] Hsieh K, Wang Y, Chen L, Zhao Z, Savitz S. Drug repurposing for COVID - 19 using graph neural network and harmonizing multiple evidence. 2021;1-14

[16] Hashimoto K. Repurposing of CNS drugs to treat COVID-19 infection: Targeting the sigma-1 receptor. European Archives of Psychiatry and Clinical Neuroscience. 2021;**271**(2):249-258

[17] Barghash RF, Fawzy IM, Chandrasekar V, Singh AV, Katha U, Mandour AA. In silico modeling as a perspective in developing potential vaccine candidates and therapeutics for COVID-19. Coatings. 2021;**11**(1273):1-26

[18] Gaber M, Hamed M, Samir R. The possible immunoregulatory and anti-inflammatory effects of selective serotonin reuptake inhibitors in coronavirus disease patients. Medical Hypotheses. 2020;**144**(110140):1-5

[19] Pushpakom S, Iorio F, Eyers PA, Escott KJ, Hopper S, Wells A, et al. Drug repurposing: Progress, challenges and recommendations. Nature Reviews. Drug Discovery. 2018;**18**(1):41-58

[20] Parvathaneni V, Gupta V. Utilizing drug repurposing against COVID-19 – Efficacy, limitations, and challenges. Life Sciences. 2020;**15**(259):118275

[21] Mani D, Wadhwani A, Krishnamurthy PT. Drug repurposing in antiviral research: A current scenario. Journal of Young Pharmacists. 2019;**11**(2):117-121

[22] Zhang J, Xie B, Hashimoto K. Brain, behavior , and immunity current status of potential therapeutic candidates for the COVID-19 crisis. Brain, Behavior, and Immunity. 2020;**87**(April):59-73

[23] Srivastava K, Singh MK. Drug repurposing in COVID-19: A review with past , present and future. Metab Open. 2021;**12**(August):100121

[24] Self WH, Semler MW, Leither LM, Casey JD, Angus DC, Brower RG, et al. Effect of hydroxychloroquine on clinical status at 14 days in hospitalized patients with COVID-19: A Randomized Clinical Trial. JAMA – Journal of American Medical Association. 2020;**324**(21):2165-2176

[25] López-Medina E, López P, Hurtado IC, et al. Effect of ivermectin on time to resolution of symptoms among adults with mild COVID-19: A Randomized Clinical Trial. 2021;**325**(14):1426-1435

[26] Abayomi A, Osibogun A, Ezechi O, Wright K, Ola B, Ojo O, et al. A multi-centre, randomized, double-blind, placebo-controlled clinical trial of the efficacy and safety of chloroquine phosphate, hydroxychloroquine sulphate and lopinavir/ritonavir for the treatment of COVID-19 in Lagos State: Study protocol for a randomi. Trials. 2021;**22**(869):1-19

[27] Asili P, Mirahmad M, Tabatabaei-Malazy O, Manayi A, Haghighat E, Mahdavi M, et al. Characteristics of published/ registered clinical trials on COVID-19 treatment: A systematic review. Journal of Pharmaceutical Sciences. 2021;**29**:449-467

[28] Khataniar A, Pathak U, Rajkhowa S, Jha AN. A comprehensive review of drug repurposing strategies against known drug targets of COVID-19. Covid. 2022;**2**(2):148-167

[29] Lenze EJ, Mattar C, Zorumski CF, Stevens A, Schweiger J, Nicol GE, et al. Fluvoxamine vs Placebo and clinical deterioration in outpatients with symptomatic COVID-19: A Randomized Clinical Trial. JAMA – Journal of American Medical Association. 2020;**324**(22):2292-2300

[30] Hoertel N, Sánchez-Rico M, Vernet R, Beeker N, Jannot AS, Neuraz A,

et al. Association between antidepressant use and reduced risk of intubation or death in hospitalized patients with COVID-19: Results from an observational study. Molecular Psychiatry. 2021;**26**(9):5199-5212

[31] Hoertel N, Sa M, Neuraz A, Blanco C, Jannot S, Paris N, et al. Observational study of haloperidol in hospitalized patients with COVID-19. PLoS One. 2021;**16**(2):e0247122

[32] Hashimoto Y, Suzuki T, Hashimoto K. Old drug fluvoxamine, new hope for COVID-19. European Archives of Psychiatry and Clinical Neuroscience. 2022;**272**(1):161-163

[33] Cheer SM, Figgitt DP. A review of its therapeutic potential in the management of anxiety disorders in children and adolescents. Paediatric Drugs. 2001;**3**(10):763-781

[34] FDA. Fluvoxamine Maleate Tablets Label. 2012. pp. 1-35

[35] Oskotsky T, Marić I, Tang A, Oskotsky B, Wong RJ, Aghaeepour N, et al. Mortality risk among patients with COVID-19 prescribed selective serotonin reuptake inhibitor antidepressants. JAMA Neurology. 2021;**4**(11):1-11

[36] Gordon DE, Jang GM, Bouhaddou M, Xu J, Obernier K, White KM, et al. A SARS-CoV-2 protein interaction map reveals targets for drug repurposing. Nature. 2020;**583**(7816):459-468

[37] Al-timimi SJ, Jamil NF. Current pharmacological treatment of obsessive-compulsive disorder. Arabian Journal of Psychiatry. 2020;**31**(2):98-104

[38] De Abajo FJ. Effects of selective serotonin reuptake inhibitors on platelet function: Mechanisms, clinical outcomes and implications for use in elderly patients. Drugs & Aging. 2011;**28**(5):345-367

[39] Mercado CP, Kilic F. Molecular mechanisms of sert in platelets: Regulation of plasma serotonin levels. Molecular Interventions. 2010;**10**(4):231-241

[40] Sukhatme VP, Reiersen AM, Vayttaden SJ, Sukhatme VV. Fluvoxamine: A review of its mechanism of action and its role in COVID-19. Frontiers in Pharmacology. 2021;**12**(April):1-9

[41] Brenner B, Harney JT, Ahmed BA, Jeffus BC, Unal R, Mehta JL, et al. Plasma serotonin levels and the platelet serotonin transporter. Journal of Neurochemistry. 2007;**102**(1):206-215

[42] Howland RH. Exploring psychotherapeutic issues and agents in clinical practice. Journal of Psychosocial Nursing. 2004;**45**(4):15-22

[43] Laursen SB, Leontiadis GI, Stanley AJ, Hallas J, Schaffalitzky de Muckadell OB. The use of selective serotonin receptor inhibitors (SSRIs) is not associated with increased risk of endoscopy-refractory bleeding, rebleeding or mortality in peptic ulcer bleeding. Alimentary Pharmacology & Therapeutics. 2017;**46**(3):355-363

[44] Carneiro AMD, Cook EH, Murphy DL, Blakely RD. Interactions between integrin αIIbβ3 and the serotonin transporter regulate serotonin transport and platelet aggregation in mice and humans. The Journal of Clinical Investigation. 2008;**118**(4):1544-1552

[45] Jedlitschky G, Greinacher A, Kroemer HK. Transporters in human platelets: Physiologic function and impact for pharmacotherapy. Blood. 2012;**119**(15):3394-3402

[46] Yang Y, Li X, Chen S, Xiao M, Liu Z, Li J, et al. Mechanism and therapeutic strategies of depression after myocardial infarction. Psychopharmacology. 2021;**238**(6):1401-1415

[47] Rafiee L, Hajhashemi V, Javanmard SH. Fluvoxamine inhibits some inflammatory genes expression in LPS / stimulated human endothelial cells, U937 macrophages , and carrageenan-induced paw edema in rat. Iranian Journal of Basic Medical Sciences. 2016;**19**:977-984

[48] Arteaga-henríquez G, Simon MS, Burger B, Weidinger E, Wijkhuijs A, Arolt V, et al. Low-grade inflammation as a predictor of antidepressant and anti- inflammatory therapy response in MDD Patients: A systematic review of the literature in combination with an analysis of experimental data collected in the EU-MOODINFLAME consortium. Frontiers in Psychiatry. 2019;**10**(458):1-15

[49] Dallé E, Daniels WMU, Mabandla MV. Fluvoxamine maleate normalizes striatal neuronal inflammatory cytokine activity in a Parkinsonian rat model associated with depression. Behavioural Brain Research. 2017;**316**:189-196

[50] Dallé E, Daniels WMU, Mabandla MV. Long-term treatment with fluvoxamine decreases nonmotor symptoms and dopamine depletion in a postnatal stress rat model of Parkinson's disease. Oxidative Medicine and Cellular Longevity. 2020;**20**:1-15

[51] Gharghani M. Fluvoxamine-An antidepressant drug with anti-inflammatory and oligodendrogenesis effects in rat model of monophasic multiple sclerosis: Studies in vivo and in vitro. Journal of Neurology and Neurophysiology. 2016;**2016**:9562

[52] Abanmy N, Alsabhan J, Gard P, Scutt G. Association between the Val66Met polymorphism (rs6265 / G196A) of the BDNF gene and cognitive performance with SSRI use in Arab Alzheimer's disease patients. Saudi Pharmaceutical Journal. 2021;**29**(12): 1392-1398

[53] Elsaed WM, Alahmadi AM, Al-Ahmadi BT, Taha JA, Tarabishi RM. Gastroprotective and antioxidant effects of fluvoxamine on stress-induced peptic ulcer in rats. Journal of Taibah University Medical Science. 2018;**13**(5):422-431

[54] Castro ECC, Sen P, Parks WT, Langston C, Galambos C. The role of serotonin transporter in human lung development and in neonatal lung disorders. Canadian Respiratory Journal. 2017;**2017**:1-10

[55] Meikle C, Creeden J, McCullumsmith C, Worth R. SSRIs : Applications in inflammatory lung disease and implications for COVID-19. Neuropsychopharmacol Reports. 2021;**41**(3):325-335

[56] Abid S, Houssaini A, Chevarin C, Marcos E, Tissot CM, Gary-Bobo G, et al. Inhibition of gut- and lung-derived serotonin attenuates pulmonary hypertension in mice. American Journal of Physiology. Lung Cellular and Molecular Physiology. 2012;**303**(6):500-508

[57] Pollok J, JEM VA, Carson-Chahhoud KV. Pharmacological interventions for the treatment of depression in chronic obstructive pulmonary disease. Cochrane Database of Systematic Reviews. 2018;**2018**:1-53

[58] Cafarella PA, Effing TW, Usmani ZA, Frith PA. Treatments for anxiety and depression in patients with chronic obstructive pulmonary disease: A literature review. Respirology. 2012;**17**(4):627-638

[59] Mazza MG, Zanardi R, Palladini M, Rovere-Querini P, Benedetti F. Rapid response to selective serotonin reuptake inhibitors in post-COVID depression. European Neuropsychopharmacology. 2022;**54**:1-6

[60] Schloer S, Brunotte L, Goretzko J, Mecate-Zambrano A, Korthals N, Gerke V, et al. Targeting the endolysosomal host-SARS-CoV-2 interface by clinically licensed functional inhibitors of acid sphingomyelinase (FIASMA) including the antidepressant fluoxetine. Emerging Microbes and Infections. 2020;**9**(1):2245-2255

[61] Kuykendall J. Fluvoxamine strongly inhibits melatonin metabolism in a patient with low-amplitude melatonin profile. Day Care & Early Education. 2000;**20**

[62] Friesland M, Mingorance L, Chung J, Chisari FV, Gastaminza P. Sigma-1 receptor regulates early steps of viral RNA replication at the onset of hepatitis C virus infection. Journal of Virology. 2013;**87**(11):6377-6390

[63] Bagchi P. Endoplasmic reticulum in viral infection. International Review of Cell and Molecular Biology. 2020;**350**:265-284

[64] Spack NP, Shumer DE, NJN. A SARS-CoV-2 protein interaction map reveals targets for drug repurposing. Physiology & Behavior. 2017;**176**(12):139-148

[65] Gordon DE, Hiatt J, Bouhaddou M, Rezelj VV, Ulferts S, Braberg H, et al. Comparative host-coronavirus protein interaction networks reveal pan-viral disease mechanisms. Science (80-). 2020;**370**:6521

[66] Hashimoto K. Activation of sigma-1 receptor chaperone in the treatment of neuropsychiatric diseases and its clinical implication. Journal of Pharmacological Sciences. 2015;**127**(1):6-9

[67] Vela JM. Repurposing sigma-1 receptor ligands for COVID-19 therapy? Frontiers in Pharmacology. 2020;**11**:1-23

[68] Irons J. Fluvoxamine in the treatment of anxiety disorders. Neuropsychiatric Disease and Treatment. 2005;**1**(4):289-299

[69] Hindmarch I, Hashimoto K. Cognition and depression: The effects of fluvoxamine, a sigma-1 receptor agonist, reconsidered. Human Psychopharmacology: Clinical and Experimental. 2010;**25**(2):193-200

[70] Iyo M, Shirayama Y, Watanabe H, Fujisaki M, Miyatake R, Fukami G, et al. Fluvoxamine as a sigma-1 receptor agonist improved cognitive impairments in a patient with schizophrenia. Progress in Neuro-Psychopharmacology & Biological Psychiatry. 2008;**32**(4):1072-1073

[71] Ishima T, Fujita Y, Hashimoto K. Interaction of new antidepressants with sigma-1 receptor chaperones and their potentiation of neurite outgrowth in PC12 cells. European Journal of Pharmacology. 2014;**15**(727):167-173

[72] Alonso G, Phan VL, Guillemain I, Saunier M, Legrand A, Anoal M, et al. Immunocytochemical localization of the sigma1 receptor in the adult rat central nervous system. Neuroscience. 2000;**97**(1):155-170

[73] Alshammari MA, Alshammari TK, Nenov MN, Scala F, Laezza F. Fibroblast growth factor 14 modulates the neurogenesis of granule neurons in the adult dentate gyrus. PMol Neurobiology. 2016;**53**(10):7254-7270

[74] Sahay A, Hen R. Adult hippocampal neurogenesis in depression. Nature Neuroscience. 2007;**10**(9):1110-1115

[75] Moriguchi S, Shinoda Y, Yamamoto Y, Sasaki Y, Miyajima K, Tagashira H, et al. Stimulation of the sigma-1 receptor by DHEA enhances synaptic efficacy and neurogenesis in the hippocampal dentate gyrus of olfactory bulbectomized mice. PLoS One. 2013;**8**(4):e60863

[76] Ahn H, Weaver M, Lyon D, Choi E, Roger B, Fillingim P. Pridopidine stabilizes mushroom spines in mouse models of Alzheimer's disease by acting on the sigma-1 receptor. Physiology & Behavior. 2017;**176**(1):139-148

[77] Duman CH, Duman RS. Spine synapse remodeling in the pathophysiology and treatment of depression. Neuroscience Letters. 2015;**5**(601):20-29

[78] Castany S, Gris G, Vela JM, Verdú E, Boadas-Vaello P. Critical role of sigma-1 receptors in central neuropathic pain-related behaviours after mild spinal cord injury in mice. Scientific Reports. 2018;**8**(1):1-13

[79] Mao J, Hu Y, Ruan L, Ji Y, Lou Z. Role of endoplasmic reticulum stress in depression (Review). Molecular Medicine Reports. 2019;**20**(6):4774-4780

[80] Voronin MV, Vakhitova YV, Seredenin SB. Chaperone Sigma1R and antidepressant effect. International Journal of Molecular Sciences. 2020;**21**(7088):1-33

[81] Chen YW, Lin PY, Tu KY, Cheng YS, Wu CK, Tseng PT. Significantly lower nerve growth factor levels in patients with major depressive disorder than in healthy subjects: A meta-analysis and systematic review. Neuropsychiatric Disease and Treatment. 2015;**11**:925-933

[82] De Azevedo CT, Mondin TC, Wiener CD, Marques MB, Fucolo BDÁ, Pinheiro RT, et al. Neurotrophic factors, clinical features and gender differences in depression. Neurochemical Research. 2014;**39**(8):1571-1578

[83] Angelucci F, Aloe L, Jiménez-Vasquez P, Mathé AA. Lithium treatment alters brain concentrations of nerve growth factor, brain-derived neurotrophic factor and glial cell line-derived neurotrophic factor in a rat model of depression. The International Journal of Neuropsychopharmacology. 2003;**6**(3):225-231

[84] Song C, Xiang YZ, Manku M. Increased phospholipase A2 activity and inflammatory response but decreased nerve growth factor expression in the olfactory bulbectomized rat model of depression: Effects of chronic ethyl-eicosapentaenoate treatment. The Journal of Neuroscience. 2009;**29**(1):14-22

[85] Angelucci F, Aloe L, Jiménez-Vasquez P, Mathé AA. Electroconvulsive stimuli alter nerve growth factor but not brain-derived neurotrophic factor concentrations in brains of a rat model of depression. Neuropeptides. 2003;**37**(1):51-56

[86] Valdes R, Millner LM. Modulation of the Sigma-1 Receptor-IRE1 pathway is beneficial in preclinical models of inflammation and sepsis. Physiology & Behavior. 2019;**176**(3):139-148

[87] Allahtavakoli M, Jarrott B. Sigma-1 receptor ligand PRE-084 reduced infarct volume, neurological deficits, pro-inflammatory cytokines and enhanced anti-inflammatory cytokines after embolic stroke in rats. Brain Research Bulletin. 2011;**85**(3-4):219-224

[88] Shen YC, Wang YH, Chou YC, Liou KT, Yen JC, Wang WY, et al. Dimemorfan protects rats against ischemic stroke through activation of sigma-1 receptor-mediated mechanisms

by decreasing glutamate accumulation. Journal of Neurochemistry. 2008;**104**(2):558-572

[89] Hosszu A, Antal Z, Lenart L, Hodrea J, Koszegi S, Balogh DB, et al. Σ1-receptor agonism protects against renal ischemia-reperfusion injury. Journal of American Society of Nephrology. 2017;**28**(1):152-165

[90] Furuse T, Hashimoto K. Sigma-1 receptor agonist fluvoxamine for delirium in intensive care units: Report of five cases. Annals of General Psychiatry. 2010;**9**:2-5

[91] Tynan RJ, Weidenhofer J, Hinwood M, Cairns MJ, Day TA, Walker FR. A comparative examination of the anti-inflammatory effects of SSRI and SNRI antidepressants on LPS stimulated microglia. Brain, Behavior, and Immunity. 2012;**26**(3):469-479

[92] Sacre S, Medghalchi M, Gregory B, Brennan F, Williams R. Fluoxetine and citalopram exhibit potent antiinflammatory activity in human and murine models of rheumatoid arthritis and inhibit toll-like receptors. Arthritis and Rheumatism. 2010;**62**(3):683-693

[93] Abdo SA, Wadie W, Abdelsalam RM, Khattab MM. Potential anti-inflammatory effect of escitalopram in iodoacetamide-induced colitis in depressed ovariectomized rats: Role of α7-nAChR. Inflammation. 2019;**42**(6):2056-2064

[94] Obuchowicz E, Bielecka-Wajdman A, Zieliński M, MacHnik G, Gołyszny M, Ludyga T. Imipramine and venlafaxine differentially affect primary glial cultures of prenatally stressed rats. Frontiers in Pharmacology. 2020;**10**(January):1-17

[95] El Awdan SA. Anti-inflammatory, anti-nociceptive and anti-arthritic effects of antidepressants in rats. Journal of Pharma Care Health System. 2015;**4**(2):86

Chapter 6

Olfaction and Depression: Does the Olfactory Bulbectomized Rat Reflect a Translational Model for Depression?

Berend Olivier, Megan E. Breuer, Christiaan H. Vinkers and Jocelien D.A. Olivier

Abstract

The olfactory bulbectomized (OBX) rat is extensively used as an animal model to detect putative antidepressant drugs. The model has some unusual characteristics, as it detects antidepressant activity of drugs only after medium to long-term administration, thereby reflecting the human situation, as antidepressants do not work acutely but only after long-term administration. The slow onset of action of antidepressants is a major drawback of current antidepressants and the availability of an animal depression model that potentially reveals rapid onset of antidepressant activity might be a great asset. Although an animal model of depression ideally should reflect correlates of human depression, several 'surrogate' parameters, like 'hyperactivity', reflect astonishingly well the 'antidepressant' profile of antidepressants in human depression. Using a new environment (open field) and a home cage to measure activity, imipramine, a classic tricyclic antidepressant, reduced hyperactivity in OBX rats, both in home cage and open field. Telemetrically measured, OBX-induced hyperactivity was already found after a couple of days and indicated that the OBX model is able to detect early (days) effects of (classic) antidepressants. Although imipramine treatment for 3, 7 and 14 days reduced OBX-induced hyperactivity, daily treatment with imipramine for 14 days, but not for 3 or 7 days, reduced hyperactivity (both in home cage and open field) of OBX rats up to 6 weeks after cessation of treatment, indicating neuroplastic changes in the brain. The attractiveness of the OBX model for detection of antidepressants lies in the resemblance to the human situation (onset of action). Moreover, the model suggests that long-term antidepressant treatment (in rats at least 14 days) leads to long-term behavioral changes that far outlast the presence of the antidepressant in the body. Whether this aspect contributes to efficient antidepressant effects needs further investigation.

Keywords: depression, olfaction, olfactory bulbectomy, animal model, hyperactivity, pharmacology, antidepressants, onset of action, long-lasting effects

1. Introduction

Depression is a prevalent and severe brain disorder that hits many people; it is estimated that it occurs at a 12 months prevalence rate of 7% in Europe [1]. Major depression is mainly characterized by depressed mood, anhedonia, loss of general interest and fatigue. Depression is associated with brain changes in various areas of the prefrontal limbic network [2]. This network involves the orbitofrontal cortex, anterior and posterior cingulate cortex, insula, amygdala, hippocampus and thalamus [3]. Regions associated with olfactory processes have a large overlap with those areas in the prefrontal limbic network and it has been suggested that (reduced) olfaction might be a (cognitive) marker for depression [4]. Croy et al. [5] showed that reduction of olfactory associated functions in the brain of depressed women improved with antidepressant (psycho) therapy to normal control levels, indicating that olfaction may represent a marker for depression. A connection between olfaction and depressive behavior has come strongly forward with the introduction of the olfactory bulbectomized (OBX) rat (see reviews by refs. [6, 7]).

The OBX rat has been strongly advocated as an animal model of depression for various reasons. Rajkumar and Dawe [8] gave an extensive overview and critical discussion on the commonalities between the OBX model and perturbations in the frontal cortex of the human depressed brain. Although it is clear that the brain and behavioral changes in the OBX-brain (of rats) are not directly comparable to the changes in the brain (in particular the frontal cortical areas) of depressed humans, there are considerable similarities that support at least a (partial) role of the OBX rat as modeling (part of) human depressive behaviors [7, 9]. In this paper, the OBX model as used for almost two decades in our laboratory is used. Activity as parameter for detecting 'depression' aspects in rats is widely used and accepted as a sensitive measure of antidepressant effects of various manipulations (antidepressants). Standard use is the measurement of the activity of rats in an Open Field (open arena) during a short test (lasting between 10 and 30 minutes in general). In our research, we also applied telemetric measurements (heart rate, body temperature and activity) in the home cage to measure more refined parameters like day-night rhythms. The present paper is in particular a reflection of our scientific work on the OBX rat model as one of the best (if not the best animal model) model of human depression that can be used to study aspects of the process of depression that cannot be directly studied in humans.

2. Olfactory bulbectomy (OBX) in rats as a depression model

The OBX rat has been extensively used for testing potential antidepressant effects of new and existent drugs [6, 7]. After olfactory bulbectomy in rats, a variety of behavioral changes emerge, including, for example, increased activity, disturbed sexual behavior [10, 11], reduced taste aversion, passive avoidance deficits, impaired spatial learning and impaired food-motivated behavior [12–18]. Following chronic (weeks), but not acute treatment with clinically established antidepressants with various mechanisms of action, normalization of these disturbed behaviors occurs [13–15, 19]. The OBX model therefore is one of the very few (if not only) animal models that share the typical slow onset of action of antidepressants as seen in human depressed patients [20, 21].

One of the most used and validated parameters to study pharmacological effects of putative antidepressants is the hyperactivity induced by olfactory bulbectomy

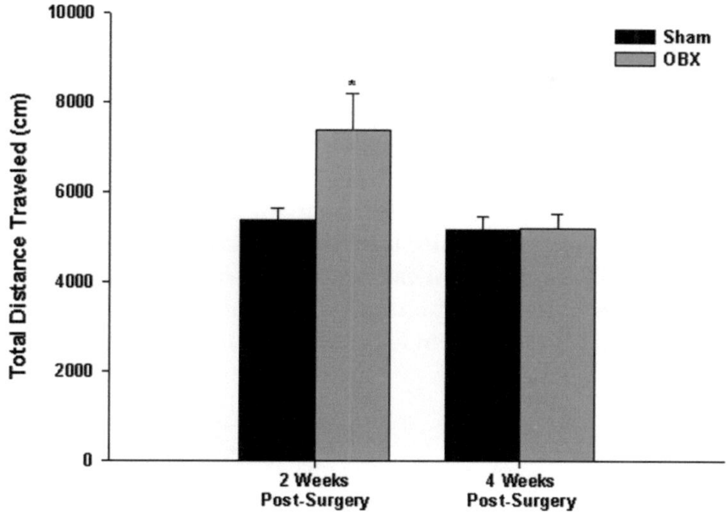

Figure 1.
*Post-surgical hyperactivity in Wistar rats. Total distance traveled (cm ± SEM) in the open field 2 and 4 weeks post-surgery. Bulbectomized Wistar animals are significantly more active than shams 2 weeks after surgery, but this effect is no longer present 4 weeks after surgery. * = $p < 0.05$ compared to shams. For methods used we refer to refs. [25–29].*

in rats [6, 7], both in an open field test (new environment) and in the home cage [22]. Most OBX studies in rats have been performed in Spague-Dawley (SD) and Wistar (Wi) strains. Because SD rats are considerably more active after olfactory bulbectomy than Wi rats [23] and this hyperactivity after OBX is present for at least 5 months, but possibly lifelong in SD rats [24]. This is not the case in Wi rats, which show hyperactivity 2 weeks after OBX, but not anymore after 4 weeks post-surgery (**Figure 1**), which in our hands makes the SD strain more attractive for OBX studies.

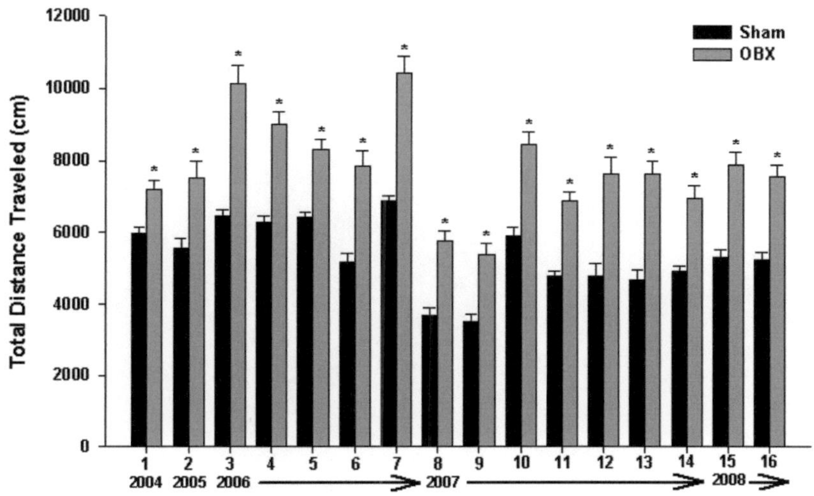

Figure 2.
*Post-surgical open field comparisons over 5 years. Total distance traveled (cm, ± SEM) in the open field 2 weeks post-surgery for 16 different groups of animals. Animals were placed in the open field and allowed to explore for 15 minutes. In total, the N was approximately 750 for both OBX and sham groups. * = $p < 0.05$ compared to shams. For methods used we refer to refs. [25–29].*

Hyperactivity after OBX is always found in our experiments performed over several years as shown in **Figure 2**, portraying the activity of male Sprague-Dawley rats 2 weeks after sham or OBX surgery over a period of 5 years. Animals were tested in an open field for 15 minutes and the total distance traveled (cm) was measured. Although the level of activity varied over time, OBX always induced hyperactivity.

Although almost all OBX experiments are performed in male rats, whereas depression is more prevalent in the female than in the male human population [30], it is of note that OBX in female rats also leads to enhanced activity [31]. Although the hyperactivity after OBX is generally measured in a new environment (often an Open Field test), this hyperactivity is also present in the home cage and emerges approx. 2–3 days after surgery [22] as shown in **Figure 3**. Although circadian rhythmicity is

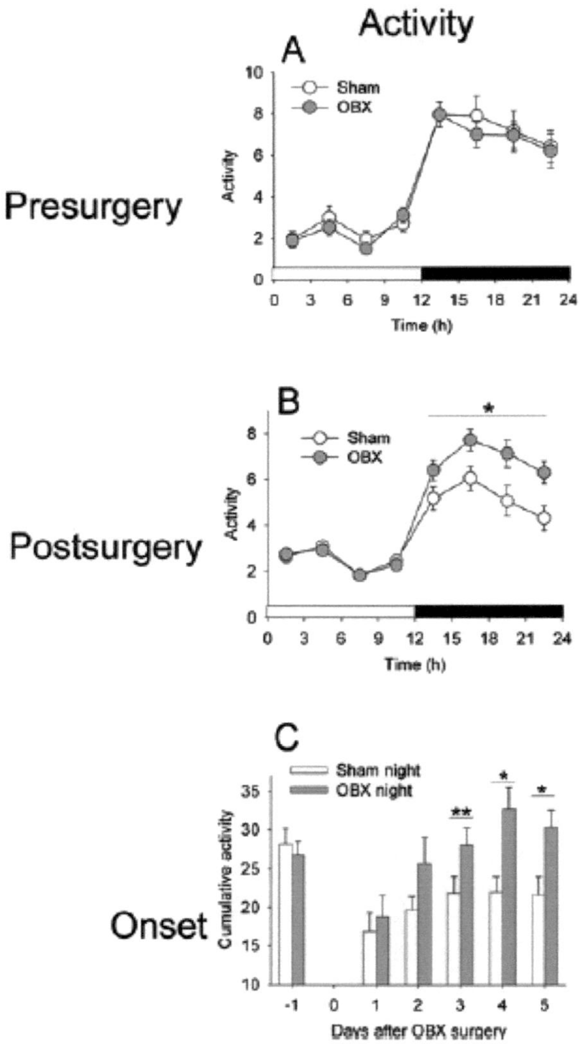

Figure 3.
Circadian rhythmicity of locomotor activity (A, B) before (A) and after olfactory bulbectomy (B). Postsurgical data reflect the average over 14 days starting immediately after surgery. (C) represents the onset of the changes in locomotor activity induced by OBX (day 0) over the first 5 days during the nocturnal phase. For methods used we refer to ref. [22].

not affected, OBX rats display several changes in basal circadian amplitudes in the home cage, besides increased nocturnal activity, enhanced nocturnal body temperature and decreased heart rate, confirming earlier findings [19, 32].

Although olfaction is clearly abolished after complete OBX, several aspects of OBX-induced changes cannot be simply explained by loss of olfaction persé. Anosmia in rats, induced by rinsing the olfactory epithelium with zinc sulphate ($ZnSO_4$), does not lead to hyperactivity in an open field [33, 34]. This lends support to the notion that dysfunctional systems in the brain and particularly the limbic system that involves a variety of neurochemical and pharmacological changes in various neurotransmitter systems are involved, including, for example, the serotonergic and noradrenergic systems [7].

Remarkably, many of the behavioral and biochemical changes induced by OBX can be reversed by chronic administration of almost all antidepressants [6, 35]. Moreover, several more recently developed or applied techniques or models to treat depression in humans, also appear to work in the OBX model in rats, like deep brain stimulation of the infralimbic prefrontal cortex [36], a multi-targeted food intervention [16] and environmental enrichment [37].

The OBX model in male rats has received its 'fame' as depression model, because of the activity of antidepressants in it [35]. Antidepressants with various mechanisms of action (SSRIs, SNRIs, NRIs, TCAs and others) exert inhibition of OBX-induced hyperactivity [38]. Characteristically, this inhibition does not occur after acute, but after (sub) chronic administration of antidepressants. This pattern of activity follows the human situation, where antidepressants only work after chronic administration (weeks-months [39]). The OBX model in rats accordingly is very efficient and reliable in predicting putative antidepressant activity of new psychoactive drugs or substances, although the model is also generating false positive and false negative results [35].

3. Does the OBX model in rats detect fast-onset antidepressants?

The question is whether the OBX model in rats can be used for detection of fast-onset antidepressants, that is, compounds that exert antidepressant activity acutely or after a short interval (hours or days; not weeks). Clinical studies have indicated that low doses of intravenous ketamine and one of its enantiomers (esketamine) exert antidepressant effects, especially in treatment-resistant depression [40, 41]. However, studies on (es)ketamine in the OBX model are scarce. In one study [42] a single intraperitoneal injection of ketamine 24 h before testing did not affect hyperactivity in an Open Field in mice, although some other anhedonic-like behaviors were reversed. Similarly, ketamine did not inhibit hyperactivity in OBX rats 24 h after 10-mg/kg IP injections [43].

Although several other potential strategies for fast-onset antidepressants are in development [44] no emerging data are available yet in the olfactory bulbectomized rat model. Still, theoretically, the OBX model in rats should be able to detect fast(er) onset of antidepressant activity, but more fundamental research should be performed into the early changes in the brain after such a drastic phenomenon as ablation of the complete olfactory machinery.

4. Imipramine: onset of action and long-term effects in the OBX rat model

Although the OBX model seems to generate an 'ideal' model to accurately predict the antidepressant onset, this is in particular based on the effects of classical antidepressants (see [35]). However, in using the tricyclic antidepressant imipramine as standard antidepressant in our OBX rat research [25–29], we did interesting observations. Most OBX/antidepressant studies measure effects 14 days after starting treatment in behaviourally stable (hyperactive in an Open Field) animals. However, imipramine (20 mg/kg, IP) already reduced activity to sham-control levels after 7 days of IMI treatment [25]. Although not tested after 7 days, the SSRI escitalopram (5 and 10 mg/kg, PO) like imipramine (20 mg/kg, PO) reduced hyperactivity to sham-operated rat levels, showing the 'classical' effects of SSRI- and TCA-antidepressants [25].

The finding that imipramine has already inhibitory effects on OBX-induced hyperactivity after 7 days of treatment, indicates that the OBX hyperactivity model is very sensitive to antidepressant effects. Probably, disturbed systems in the brain after olfactory bulbectomy, which lead to almost immediate behavioral and physiological effects [22] are influenced in such a way by certain drugs (e.g. antidepressants) that hyperactivity is quite rapidly depressed to normal levels. It is completely unknown what underlies these processes and future research is needed to unravel possible mechanisms.

The classical OBX model uses a 14 days treatment period to find putative antidepressiant drug effects. The question arose whether drug treatment for a long period (e.g. 14 days) led to sustained effects on activity if drug treatment is stopped. In other words, is hyperactivity returning rapidly or delayed after discontinuation of the antidepressant [25]. In the latter study, the activity of sham and OBX rats was measured 1, 2, 6 and 10 weeks after cessation of the tricyclic antidepressant imipramine (20 mg/kg, PO) or escitalopram (5 and 10 mg/kg, PO) treatment. After these periods of drug cessation, no drug levels are present anymore in the experimental rats. One, 2 and 3 weeks after stopping 14 days of treatment with vehicle, escitalopram (5 and 10 mg/kg) and imipramine (20 mg/kg), the three antidepressant-treated groups still showed comparable activity levels as the sham-operated groups; 6 weeks after stopping treatment the escitalopram-treated animals returned to their initial hyperactivity-level as observed 14 days after OBX. In contrast, the imipramine group still did not differ from the sham group. Only 10 weeks after cessation of treatment the imipramine group (and both escitalopram groups also) showed hyperactivity like before.

In a separate study, we examined the onset of action of imipramine (10 mg/kg, IP) and vehicle measuring activity in an Open Field test. First, 120 Wistar male rats were run in an open field and were assigned, based on their basal activity into equal activity groups. Half of the animals were olfactory bulbectomized, and half obtained sham surgery. After surgery, animals recovered for 2 weeks. Animals were then assigned to four groups with regard to their post-surgical open field activity so that there were equal numbers of more or less active animals in each treatment group (N = 15–20 animals per group).

All animals received one intraperitoneal injection per day for 3, 7 or 14 days. On days 1, 3, 7 and 14, animals were tested in the open field, 30 minutes after injection, to observe the onset of action of imipramine. All animals were also tested 1, 2 and 6 weeks after cessation of treatment to observe any long-lasting effects of imipramine treatment. No acute effects of imipramine were found on day 1 after the very first injection in all three groups (**Table 1**). Bulbectomized rats in all groups remained significantly more active compared to sham-operated groups.

After 3 days of treatment, imipramine significantly reduced the hyperactivity of the OBX group, towards the sham level (**Figure 4** top). This effect of imipramine was short-lived: 1, 2 and 6 weeks after cessation of treatment olfactory bulbectomized animals returned to their enhanced OBX level. Bulbectomy-induced hyperactivity

	Group 1 (3 days treatment)	Group 2 (7 days treatment)	Group 3 (14 days treatment)
Sham vehicle	4411 ± 317.3	4999 ± 430.2	3992 ± 355.7
OBX vehicle	6703 ± 523.4*	6915 ± 387.8*	6202 ± 596.9*
Sham imipramine	3530 ± 213.3	3531 ± 219.9	3633 ± 352.5
OBX imipramine	4818 ± 262.9*	5535 ± 855.4*	5194 ± 592.5*

*Data are expressed as mean distance traveled (cm) ± SEM. Group 1 = animals receiving imipramine or vehicle for 3 days; group 2 = animals receiving imipramine or vehicle for 7 days; and group 3 = animals receiving imipramine or vehicle for 14 days. Methods as described in refs. [25–29]. * = $p < 0.05$ compared to the corresponding sham group.*

Table 1.
Acute effects (on day 1 of all three groups) of imipramine on vehicle treatment or sham-bulbectomized activity and olfactory bulbectomy-induced hyperactivity in an open field (15 minutes in a 70 × 70 × 45 cm chamber under fluorescent lighting using Noldus Etho Vision[R] during the light period (9–13 h)).

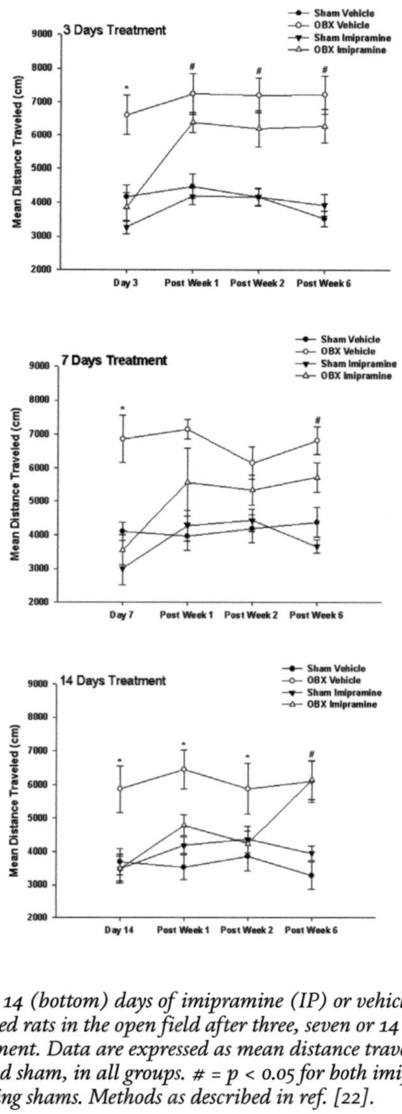

Figure 4.
*Effects of 3 (top), 7 (middle) and 14 (bottom) days of imipramine (IP) or vehicle treatment (IP) on sham-operated or olfactory bulbectomized rats in the open field after three, seven or 14 days of treatment as well as 1, 2, 6 weeks after cessation of treatment. Data are expressed as mean distance traveled (cm) ± SEM. * = $p < 0.05$ compared to all animals, OBX and sham, in all groups. # = $p < 0.05$ for both imipramine and vehicle OBX animals, compared to corresponding shams. Methods as described in ref. [22].*

was clearly present up to 6 weeks after cessation of 3 days of imipramine treatment. No effect of habituation to the open field was seen. After 7 days of treatment, imipramine significantly reduced the hyperactivity of the OBX group, towards the sham level (**Figure 4** middle). Like after 3 days of treatment, no effects of imipramine were found 1, 2 or 6 weeks after cessation of the 7-day treatment.

After 14 days of treatment, imipramine significantly reduced the hyperactivity of the OBX group, towards the sham level (**Figure 4** bottom). However, this effect was still present 1–2 weeks after cessation of the treatment. Six weeks after cessation the level of (hyper) activity of the imipramine pretreated group had returned to the OBX sham level.

The results of this experiment show that the olfactory bulbectomy model is suitable to detect the onset of action of antidepressants, and also for examining the lasting behavioral effects after cessation of sub-chronic treatment, an effect that has hardly been examined. Interestingly, our results indicate that while treatment for 3 or 7 days may be behaviourally effective, these effects are less stable and treatment should continue for 14 days or more to allow for long-term antidepressant effects (which may be dependent on changes in brain plasticity) to take place. This makes the bulbectomy model attractive for observing not only the onset of action of antidepressants but also the optimal dose duration for long-term therapeutic effects after cessation of treatment.

For quite some time, it was suggested that the addition of $5\text{-}HT_{1A}$ receptor antagonists to settled antidepressants might facilitate a shorter onset of action than the antidepressants alone [20]. Cryan et al. [45] found that the addition of pindolol, a β-adrenoceptor antagonist and partial $5\text{-}HT_{1A}$ receptor (ant) agonist, did not affect the onset time when given for 3, 7 and 14 days in combination with the SSRI paroxetine, indicating that the olfactory bulbectomy model may not be suitable for the detection of onset of action. However, since paroxetine was given at a dose of 2.5 mg/kg, this dose may have been too low to elicit any behavioral effects before day 14 of treatment. Moreover, the quality of pindolol as $5\text{-}HT_{1A}$ receptor antagonist is also questionable. In a subsequent study examining the highly selective $5\text{-}HT_{1A}$ receptor antagonist WAY100635, Cryan et al. [46] found that the addition of WAY100635 to paroxetine treatment did not alter onset of action (after 3 and 7 days of treatment), nor did the drug, when given alone, affect the onset time. Like earlier found in human depression, the addition of a $5\text{-}HT_{1A}$ receptor antagonist, at least in the bulbectomy model, does not facilitate a shorter onset of action compared to animals treated with an antidepressant alone.

Several studies have examined the effects of antidepressants with combined mechanisms of action (like SNRIs or NDRIs) or combination of different antidepressants on olfactory bulbectomy-induced behaviors. For example, it has been proposed that triple reuptake inhibitors (TUIs), inhibiting serotonin, noradrenaline and dopamine transporters would have a faster onset [47]. Quite to the contrary however, Breuer et al. [27] found that TUIs have a slower onset of action compared to imipramine, which was already active after 3 days of administration (see **Figure 4**). Similarly, in a study examining the effects of dual treatment with sertraline (an SSRI) and reboxetine (a selective noradrenaline reuptake inhibitor), Harkin et al. [9] found that treatment had no added effect on bulbectomy-induced hyperactivity in the open field; the drugs, either alone or in combination, did not have any behavioral effect until day 14 of treatment. The current experiment has shown that bulbectomized animals do respond to 10 mg/kg imipramine treatment after 3, 7 and 14 days and that these effects, after cessation of treatment, are dependent upon treatment duration. Interestingly, we have shown previously that treatment with imipramine at 20 mg/kg significantly altered bulbectomy-induced hyperactivity for up to 10 weeks after cessation of treatment [25]. Also, when observing the lasting effects of pramipexole, a dopamine D_2/D_3 receptor agonist, on bulbectomy-induced hyperactivity, we found that while treatment with 1.0 mg/kg did not elicit any behavioral changes during the treatment period of 14 days (perhaps because this dose may have increased activity in the bulbectomy animals), this dose did have a behavioral effect after cessation of treatment [29]. Thus, normalization of hyperactivity may not only be dependent upon the duration of treatment but also upon the dosage used.

It has been previously shown that chronic treatment, whether with SSRIs or TCAs, leads to a sustainable effect in the open-field paradigm [25]. This suggests that antidepressant treatment may perhaps result in semi-permanent changes in brain plasticity. There is evidence that chronic antidepressant treatment may have a significant effect on NMDA receptors, an effect that has been shown to be sustainable for several days after cessation of treatment [47]. Bulbectomy leads to significant elevations in NMDA receptor levels in the rat prefrontal cortex, an effect that was sustainable until at least 5 weeks following bulbectomy [48]. In addition, Keilhoff et al. [49] also found that chronic imipramine treatment increased neurogenesis in the hippocampal subventricular zone and amygdala of bulbectomized animals, indicating that chronic antidepressant treatment may also have significant effects on neurogenesis in the adult brain and that therapeutic effects of antidepressants may be neurogenesis-dependent [50].

The fact that imipramine was active in the OBX model after only 3 days of once-daily administration is comparable to effects found with the 5-HT_4 receptor agonist RS 67333, in which the bulbectomized animals showed normalized activity in the open field after 3 days of treatment [51]. However, while bulbectomized animals in the current experiment showed normalized activity in the open field on day 3 or day 7 of treatment, the effect disappeared 1 week after cessation of treatment, suggesting that a longer treatment duration is needed for sustainable behavioral effects. That imipramine was behaviourally active after 3 days of treatment further supports the findings of Cryan et al. [45] which show that bulbectomized animals show attenuation of 8-OH-DPAT-induced hypothermia after only 3 days of combined treatment with pindolol and paroxetine, suggesting that these animals do show changes in 5-HT_{1A} receptor sensitivity. In an experiment examining the effects of WAY-163909 (3 mg/kg), a 5-HT_{2C} receptor agonist, Rosenzweig-Lipson et al. [52] found that this drug had a faster onset of action in the olfactory bulbectomy model, compared to traditional SSRIs, in that bulbectomy-induced hyperactivity was reduced after 5 days of treatment. Similarly, in a study examining the effects of pramipexole (a dopamine D_2/D_3 agonist) on bulbectomy-induced hyperactivity, pramipexole, at doses of 0.3 and 0.1 mg/kg, was also active in the olfactory bulbectomy model after 7 days of treatment, comparable to imipramine and 7 OH-DPAT [29]. The results of these studies therefore indicate that the onset of action may not be strictly and only regulated by 5-HT_{1A} receptors.

While we cannot completely rule out that treatment with 5-HT_{1A} receptor antagonists may help to facilitate a faster onset of action, more studies must be done to pinpoint the mechanism behind the onset phenomenon before better and perhaps faster, treatments can be found. It has previously been shown that antidepressant treatment may work relatively quickly for some patients, who report improvements in mood after only 1 week of treatment [53, 54], though there is much debate as to whether or not this early onset of action in patients is due to a placebo effect. However, what if the therapeutic effects of antidepressant treatment are entirely reliant upon neurogenesis? Alterations in neurogenesis in the human adult brain may only occur after chronic, but not acute, antidepressant treatment [55]. If the therapeutic action of antidepressants is indeed entirely dependent upon neurogenesis, it may be difficult to find new treatments with faster onset. However, this remains a subject for scrutiny, as the working mechanisms behind antidepressant efficacy are not yet fully understood and therefore must be further examined.

5. Effects of OBX and imipramine on activity in the home cage

Although olfactory bulbectomy leads to hyperactivity in a new environment (mostly an Open Field situation is used to measure activity), we have previously shown, using telemetric methods, that OBX-ed rats also display hyperactivity in their home cage that emerges already significantly 2–3 days after surgery (see **Figure 4** and [22]). A cohort

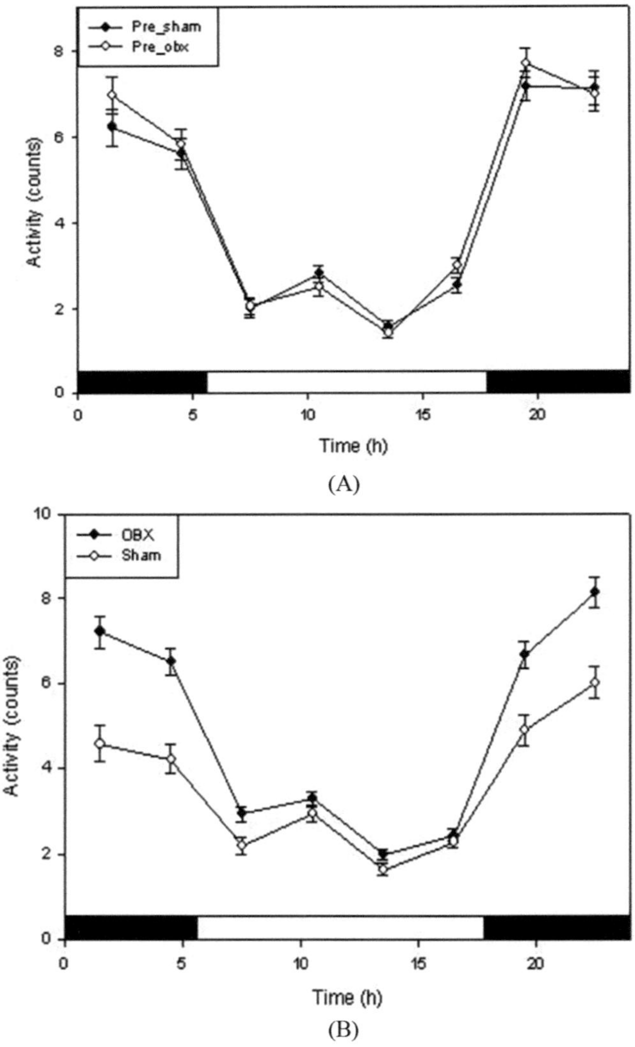

Figure 5.
(A) Presurgery 24 h baseline: Circadian rhythm of locomotor activity before OBX/sham surgery (3 h blocks). No differences exist between the group that will undergo OBX surgery (n = 21) and the group that will undergo sham surgery (n = 21). Black/white bar represents night/day cycle respectively. (B) 24 h curves of 19 days of post OBX/sham surgery, 3 h blocks. Methods as described in ref. [22].

of 48 male SD rats were implanted with radio-telemetric transmitters and after 2 weeks of recovery randomized into two groups that either were olfactory bulbectomized or sham-operated. During recovery from transmitter implantation for 4 days baseline telemetric measures were continuously measured (activity, heart rate and temperature) but only activity is shown here. After OBX- and sham-surgery telemetric measures were continuously measured for 19 days. Six months after OBX/sham surgery, a 14-day treatment period with either imipramine (10 mg/kg, IP) or vehicle (saline, IP) was given to either half of the OBX- and half of the sham-operated rats (**Figure 5**).

Figure 6 shows the circadian rhythms of locomotor activity in the home cage before OBX/sham surgery (5A) portrayed in 3 h blocks. No differences exist between the groups that will undergo OBX surgery (N = 21) and the sham surgery group (N = 21). **Figure 6B** shows the average circadian activity over 19 days of post-OBX (N = 19)/sham surgery (N = 17); OBX rats showed an overall increased activity (surgery main effect ($F(1,37) = 20.5$; $p < 0.001$), but mainly during the night (day: surgery main effect $F(1,37) = 4.412$, $p < 0.05$; night: surgery main effect $F(1,37) = 24.748$, $p < 0.001$).

After 14 days of vehicle, OBX rats receiving vehicle were still overall more active than shams receiving vehicle (main surgery effect, $F(1,19) = 5.391$, $p < 0.05$), which appeared a stronger nocturnal hyperactivity (vehicle night blocks: main operation effect $F(1,19) = 5.329$, $p < 0.05$; vehicle day blocks: effect $F(1,19) = 4.038$, $p = 0.059$,

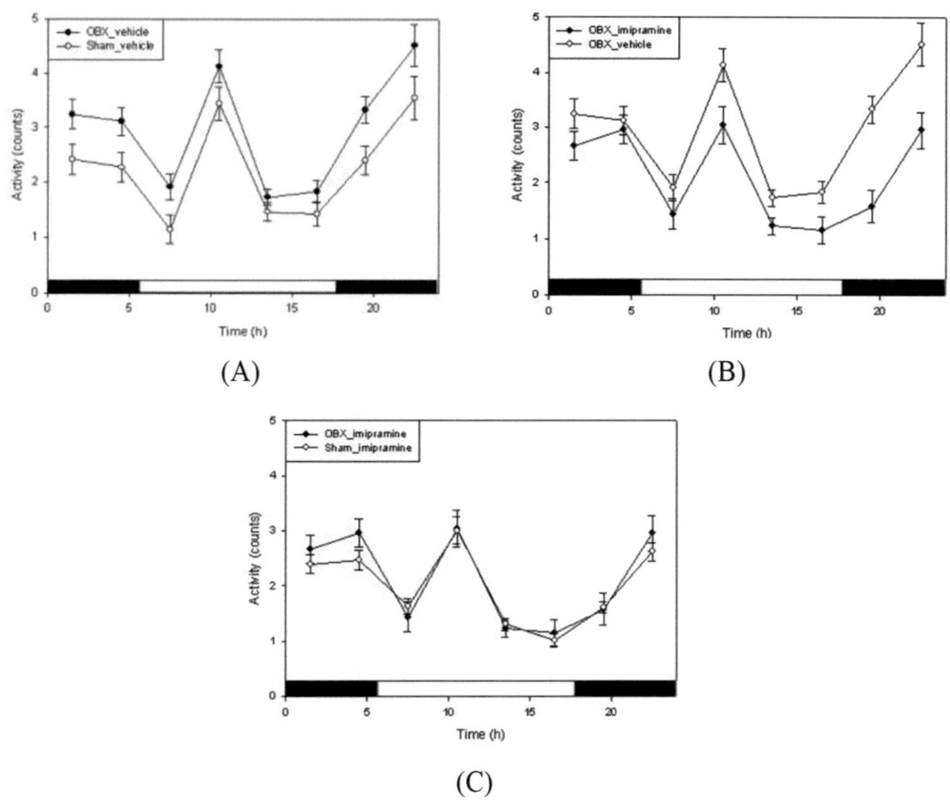

Figure 6.
*24 h activity pattern of 14 days imipramine administration, 3 h blocks (A) OBX vehicle vs. sham vehicle; (B) OBX imipramine vs. sham imipramine; (C) OBX vehicle vs. OBX imipramine. Black/white bar represents night/day cycle respectively. The peak in activity seen around 10 h is due to the daily injection stress (compare the peak in **Figure** 5 vs. **Figure** 6). Methods as described in ref. [22].*

NS) (see **Figure 6A**). OBX animals that were treated with imipramine were however no longer different from sham animals treated with imipramine (surgery effect $F(1,17) = 0.588$, $p = 0.454$, NS) (see **Figure 6C**). As a result, OBX animals receiving imipramine were no longer identical to OBX animals getting vehicle (main treatment effect $F(1,18) = 8.832$, $p < 0.01$), the diminished activity in imipramine OBX rats being present during day as well as night (see **Figure 6B**).

Over the 2 weeks after imipramine treatment stopped, OBX rats that had received imipramine increased their nocturnal activity, almost being different again from sham animals that had received imipramine (imipramine group: surgery effect $F(1,17) = 3.482$, $p = 0.079$, NS, see **Figure 7**). OBX animals that were in the vehicle group still displayed overall (but mainly nocturnal) hyperactivity (sham group: surgery effect $F(1,19) = 5.687$, $p < 0.05$). Whereas during treatment, imipramine OBX rats were less active than vehicle OBX rats, 2 weeks after cessation they were no longer different (OBX group: treatment effect $F(1,18) = 1.182$, $p = 0.291$, NS, see **Figure 7C**).

Unfortunately, we have not tested all these parameters in the various groups at later stages (weeks 6 and 10). We assume that the home cage activities in the various treatment groups show a comparable pattern as observed in the Open Field (as described earlier). The telemetric data (we also gathered body temperature and heart rate-not used here) on activity in the home cage strongly reflect similar findings when OBX- and sham-operated animals are tested in the Open Field, although the effects

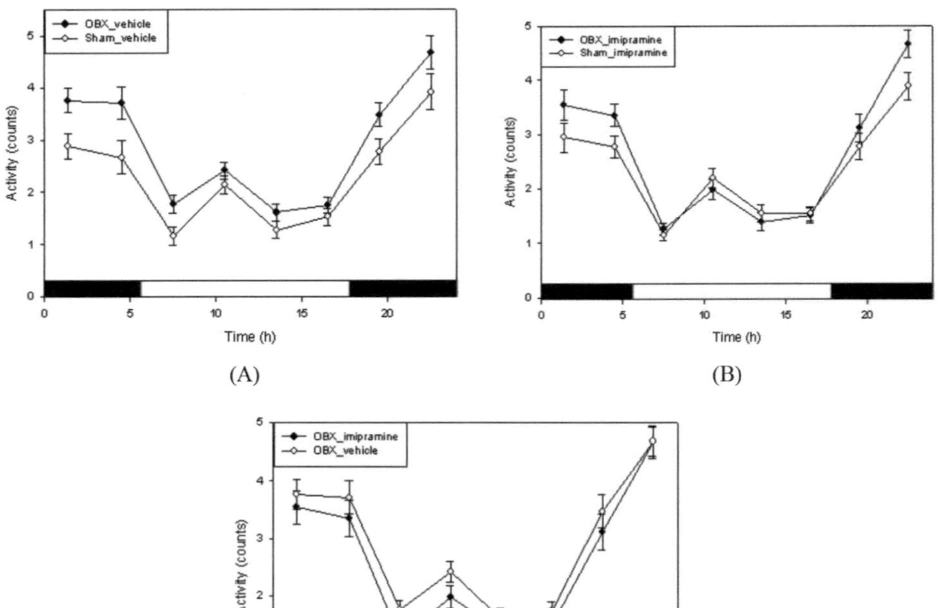

Figure 7.
Average 24 h activity circadian rhythm of the 2-week period after stopping imipramine treatment, 3 h blocks (A) OBX vehicle vs. sham vehicle; (B) Sham-imipramine vs. OBX imipramine. (C) OBX imipramine vs. OBX vehicle. Black/white bar represents night/day cycle respectively. Methods as described in ref. [22].

are more pronounced. This possibly reflects that a new environment induces additional stress that enhances activity, both in sham and OBX rats, which was already found earlier [22].

6. The olfactory bulbectomy model in rats: a model of what?

Although the OBX model in rats (and to a lesser extent mice) is primarily known for its detection of antidepressant activity in a molecule, the model has several other interesting features, in particular, to study degenerative processes in the brain after removing the olfactory bulbs. OBX leads to widespread trans-neuronal degeneration, cognitive decline, reduced volumes of several brain structures (hippocampus, nucleus caudatus and amygdala), disruption of the blood-brain barrier and several other serious changes [7, 15]. All these aspects make the OBX model in rats attractive, as has also been illustrated in the present chapter with regard to onset of behavioral changes after OBX, but also neuroplastic changes after long-term administration of antidepressants. Whether these changes reflect effects on neurodegenerative processes is not clear yet. Much research using the model is needed to show its further contribution to neuroscience.

Author details

Berend Olivier[1,2]*, Megan E. Breuer[1], Christiaan H. Vinkers[1,3] and Jocelien D.A. Olivier[4]

1 Department of Psychopharmacology, Utrecht Institute for Pharmaceutical Sciences (UIPS), Utrecht University, Utrecht, Netherlands

2 Department of Psychiatry, Yale University School of Medicine, New Haven, USA

3 Department of Psychiatry, Amsterdam UMC, Location VUmc, Amsterdam, Netherlands

4 Neurobiology, Groningen Institute of Evolutionary Life Sciences (GELIFES), Rijksuniversiteit Groningen, Groningen, Netherlands

*Address all correspondence to: b.olivier@uu.nl

References

[1] Wittchen HU, Jacobi F, Rehm J, Gustavsson A, Svensson M, Jönsson B, et al. The size and burden of mental disorders and other disorders of the brain in Europe 2010. European Neuropsychopharmacology. 2011;**21**(9):655-679. DOI: 10.1016/j.euroneuro.2011.07.018

[2] Liu CH, Ma X, Wu X, Li F, Zhang Y, Zhou FC, et al. Resting-state abnormal baseline brain activity in unipolar and bipolar depression. Neuroscience Letters. 2012;**516**(2):202-206. DOI: 10.1016/j.neulet.2012.03.083

[3] Höflich A, Baldinger P, Savli M, Lanzenberger R, Kasper S. Imaging treatment effects in depression. Reviews in the Neurosciences. 2012;**23**(3):227-252. DOI: 10.1515/revneuro-2012-0038

[4] Atanasova B, Graux J, El Hage W, Hommet C, Camus V, Belzung C. Olfaction: A potential cognitive marker of psychiatric disorders. Neuroscience and Biobehavioral Reviews. 2008;**32**(7):1315-1325. DOI: 10.1016/j.neubiorev.2008.05.003

[5] Croy I, Symmank A, Schellong J, Hummel C, Gerber J, Joraschky P, et al. Olfaction as a marker for depression in humans. Journal of Affective Disorders. 2014;**160**:80-86. DOI: 10.1016/j.jad.2013.12.026

[6] Kelly JP, Wrynn AS, Leonard BE. The olfactory bulbectomized rat as a model of depression: An update. Pharmacology & Therapeutics. 1997;**74**(3):299-316. DOI: 10.1016/s0163-7258(97)00004-1

[7] Song C, Leonard BE. The olfactory bulbectomised rat as a model of depression. Neuroscience and Biobehavioral Reviews. 2005;**29**(4-5):627-647. DOI: 10.1016/j.neubiorev.2005.03.010

[8] Rajkumar R, Dawe GS. OBscure but not OBsolete: Perturbations of the frontal cortex in common between rodent olfactory bulbectomy model and major depression. Journal of Chemical Neuroanatomy. 2018;**91**:63-100. DOI: 10.1016/j.jchemneu.2018.04.001

[9] Harkin A, Kelly JP, McNamara M, Connor TJ, Dredge K, Redmond A, et al. Activity and onset of action of reboxetine and effect of combination with sertraline in an animal model of depression. European Journal of Pharmacology. 1999;**364**(2-3):123-132. DOI: 10.1016/s0014-2999(98)00838-3

[10] Chambliss HO, Van Hoomissen JD, Holmes PV, Bunnell BN, Dishman RK. Effects of chronic activity wheel running and imipramine on masculine copulatory behavior after olfactory bulbectomy. Physiology & Behavior. 2004;**82**(4):593-600. DOI: 10.1016/j.physbeh.2004.04.064

[11] Oral E, Aydin MD, Aydin N, Ozcan H, Hacimuftuoglu A, Sipal S, et al. How olfaction disorders can cause depression? The role of habenular degeneration. Neuroscience. 2013;**240**:63-69. DOI: 10.1016/j.neuroscience.2013.02.026

[12] Bijlsma EY, Oosting RS, Olivier B, Groenink L. Disrupted startle modulation in animal models for affective disorders. Behavioural Brain Research. 2010;**208**(2):383-390. DOI: 10.1016/j.bbr.2009.12.007

[13] Borre Y, Sir V, de Kivit S, Westphal KG, Olivier B, Oosting RS. Minocycline restores spatial but not fear

memory in olfactory bulbectomized rats. European Journal of Pharmacology. 2012;**697**(1-3):59-64. DOI: 10.1016/j.ejphar.2012.09.005

[14] Borre Y, Bosman E, Lemstra S, Westphal KG, Olivier B, Oosting RS. Memantine partly rescues behavioral and cognitive deficits in an animal model of neurodegeneration. Neuropharmacology. 2012;**62**(5-6):2010-2017. DOI: 10.1016/j.neuropharm.2011.12.034

[15] Borre Y, Lemstra S, Westphal KG, Morgan ME, Olivier B, Oosting RS. Celecoxib delays cognitive decline in an animal model of neurodegeneration. Behavioural Brain Research. 2012;**234**(2):285-291. DOI: 10.1016/j.bbr.2012.07.007

[16] Borre YE, Panagaki T, Koelink PJ, Morgan ME, Hendriksen H, Garssen J, et al. Neuroprotective and cognitive enhancing effects of a multi-targeted food intervention in an animal model of neurodegeneration and depression. Neuropharmacology. 2014;**79**:738-749. DOI: 10.1016/j.neuropharm.2013.11.009

[17] Prins J, Westphal KG, Korte-Bouws GA, Quinton MS, Schreiber R, Olivier B, et al. The potential and limitations of DOV 216,303 as a triple reuptake inhibitor for the treatment of major depression: A microdialysis study in olfactory bulbectomized rats. Pharmacology, Biochemistry, and Behavior. 2011;**97**(3):444-452. DOI: 10.1016/j.pbb.2010.10.001

[18] Prins J, Denys DA, Westphal KG, Korte-Bouws GA, Quinton MS, Schreiber R, et al. The putative antidepressant DOV 216,303, a triple reuptake inhibitor, increases monoamine release in the prefrontal cortex of olfactory bulbectomized rats. European Journal of Pharmacology. 2010;**633**(1-3):55-61. DOI: 10.1016/j.ejphar.2010.02.009

[19] van Riezen H, Leonard BE. Effects of psychotropic drugs on the behavior and neurochemistry of olfactory bulbectomized rats. Pharmacology & Therapeutics. 1990;**47**(1):21-34. DOI: 10.1016/0163-7258(90)90043-2

[20] Blier P. Possible neurobiological mechanisms underlying faster onset of antidepressant action. The Journal of Clinical Psychiatry. 2001;**62**(Suppl 4):7-11; discussion 37-40

[21] Coppola DM, Parrish WR. The olfactory bulbectomy disease model: A Re- evaluation. Physiology & Behavior. 2021;**240**:113548. DOI: 10.1016/j.physbeh.2021.113548

[22] Vinkers CH, Breuer ME, Westphal KG, Korte SM, Oosting RS, Olivier B, et al. Olfactory bulbectomy induces rapid and stable changes in basal and stress-induced locomotor activity, heart rate and body temperature responses in the home cage. Neuroscience. 2009;**159**(1):39-46. DOI: 10.1016/j.neuroscience.2008.12.009

[23] Roche M, Harkin A, Kelly JP. Chronic fluoxetine treatment attenuates stressor-induced changes in temperature, heart rate, and neuronal activation in the olfactory bulbectomized rat. Neuropsychopharmacology. 2007;**32**(6):1312-1320. DOI: 10.1038/sj.npp.1301253

[24] van der Stelt HM, Breuer ME, Olivier B, Westenberg HG. Permanent deficits in serotonergic functioning in olfactory bulbectomized rats: An in vivo microdialysis study. Biological Psychiatry. 2005;**57**(9):1061-1067. DOI: 10.1016/j.biopsych.2004.12.040

[25] Breuer ME, Groenink L, Oosting RS, Westenberg HG, Olivier B. Long-term behavioral changes after cessation of chronic antidepressant treatment in

olfactory bulbectomized rats. Biological Psychiatry. 2007;**61**(8):990-995. DOI: 10.1016/j.biopsych.2006.08.032

[26] Breuer ME. Depression's Next Top Model: Pharmacology of Olfactory Bulbectomy-Induced Behaviors. PhD-thesis. Utrecht University. Wageningen: Ponsen & Loyen B.V.; 2008. pp. 1-183

[27] Breuer ME, Chan JS, Oosting RS, Groenink L, Korte SM, Campbell U, et al. The triple monoaminergic reuptake inhibitor DOV 216,303 has antidepressant effects in the rat olfactory bulbectomy model and lacks sexual side effects. European Neuropsychopharmacology. 2008;**18**(12):908-916. DOI: 10.1016.j.euroneuro.2008.07.011

[28] Breuer ME, van Gaalen MM, Wernet W, Claessens SE, Oosting RS, Behl B, et al. SSR149415, a non-peptide vasopressin V_{1b} receptor antagonist, has long-lasting antidepressant effects in the olfactory bulbectomy-induced hyperactivity depression model. Naunyn-Schmiedeberg's Archives of Pharmacology. 2009;**379**(1):101-106. DOI: 10.1007/s00210-008-0336-1

[29] Breuer ME, Groenink L, Oosting RS, Buerger E, Korte M, Ferger B, et al. Antidepressant effects of pramipexole, a dopamine D_3/D_2 receptor agonist, and 7-OH-DPAT, a dopamine D_3 receptor agonist, in olfactory bulbectomized rats. European Journal of Pharmacology. 2009;**616**(1-3):134-140. DOI: 10.1016/j.ejphar.2009.06.029

[30] Malhi GS, Mann JJ. Depression. Lancet. 2018;**392**(10161):2299-2312. DOI: 10.1016/S0140-6736(18)31948-2

[31] Stock HS, Hand GA, Ford K, Wilson MA. Changes in defensive behaviors following olfactory bulbectomy in male and female rats. Brain Research. 2001;**903**(1-2):242-246. DOI: 10.1016/s0006-8993(01)02421-0

[32] Giardina WJ, Radek RJ. Effects of imipramine on the nocturnal behavior of bilateral olfactory bulbectomized rats. Biological Psychiatry. 1991;**29**(12):1200-1208. DOI: 10.1016/0006-3223(91)90327-i

[33] Mar A, Spreekmeester E, Rochford J. Antidepressants preferentially enhance habituation to novelty in the olfactory bulbectomized rat. Psychopharmacology. 2000;**150**(1):52-60. DOI: 10.1007/s002130000400

[34] Cryan JF, Mombereau C. In search of a depressed mouse: Utility of models for studying depression-related behavior in genetically modified mice. Molecular Psychiatry. 2004;**9**(4):3

[35] Ramaker MJ, Dulawa SC. Identifying fast-onset antidepressants using rodent models. Molecular Psychiatry. 2017;**22**(5):656-665. DOI: 10.1038/mp.2017.36

[36] Jiménez-Sánchez L, Linge R, Campa L, Valdizán EM, Pazos Á, Díaz Á, et al. Behavioral, neurochemical and molecular changes after acute deep brain stimulation of the infralimbic prefrontal cortex. Neuropharmacology. 2016;**108**:91-102. DOI: 10.1016/j.neuropharm.2016.04.02026-57

[37] Hendriksen H, Meulendijks D, Douma TN, Bink DI, Breuer ME, Westphal KG, et al. Environmental enrichment has antidepressant-like action without improving learning and memory deficits in olfactory bulbectomized rats. Neuropharmacology. 2012;**62**(1):270-277. DOI: 10.1016/j.neuropharm.2011.07.018

[38] Besson A, Haddjeri N, Blier P, de Montigny C. Effects of the co-administration of mirtazapine and paroxetine on serotonergic neurotransmission in the rat brain.

European Neuropsychopharmacology. 2000;**10**(3):177-188. DOI: 10.1016/s0924-977x(00)00069-9

[39] Harmer CJ, Duman RS, Cowen PJ. How do antidepressants work? New perspectives for refining future treatment approaches. Lancet Psychiatry. 2017;**4**(5):409-418. DOI: 10.1016/S2215-0366(17)30015-9

[40] Bahji A, Vazquez GH, Zarate CA Jr. Comparative efficacy of racemic ketamine and esketamine for depression: A systematic review and meta-analysis. Journal of Affective Disorders. 2021;**278**: 542-555. DOI: 10.1016/j.jad.2020.09.071

[41] Swainson J, Thomas RK, Archer S, Chrenek C, MacKay MA, Baker G, et al. Esketamine for treatment resistant depression. Expert Review of Neurotherapeutics. 2019;**19**(10):899-911. DOI: 10.1080/14737175.2019.1640604

[42] de Almeida RF, Pocharski CB, Rodrigues ALS, Elisabetsky E, Souza DO. Guanosine fast onset antidepressant-like effects in the olfactory bulbectomy mice model. Scientific Reports. 2020;**10**(1):8429. DOI: 10.1038/s41598-020-65300-w

[43] Holubova K, Kleteckova L, Skurlova M, Ricny J, Stuchlik A, Vales K. Rapamycin blocks the antidepressant effect of ketamine in task-dependent manner. Psychopharmacology. 2016;**233**(11):2077-2097. DOI: 10.1007/s00213-016-4256-3

[44] Li YF. A hypothesis of monoamine (5-HT)—Glutamate/GABA long neural circuit: Aiming for fast-onset antidepressant discovery. Pharmacology & Therapeutics. 2020;**208**:107494. DOI: 10.1016/j.pharmthera.2020.107494

[45] Cryan JF, McGrath C, Leonard BE, Norman TR. Combining pindolol and paroxetine in an animal model of chronic antidepressant action—Can early onset of action be detected? European Journal of Pharmacology. 1998;**352**(1):23-28. DOI: 10.1016/s0014-2999(98)00402-6

[46] Cryan JF, McGrath C, Leonard BE, Norman TR. Onset of the effects of the 5-HT_{1A} antagonist, WAY-100635, alone, and in combination with paroxetine, on olfactory bulbectomy and 8-OH-DPAT-induced changes in the rat. Pharmacology, Biochemistry, and Behavior. 1999;**63**(2):333-338. DOI: 10.1016/s0091-3057(98)00245-7

[47] Stahl SM, Pradko JF, Haight BR, Modell JG, Rockett CB, Learned-Coughlin S. A review of the neuropharmacology of bupropion, a dual norepinephrine and dopamine reuptake inhibitor. Primary Care Companion to the Journal of Clinical Psychiatry. 2004;**6**(4):159-166. DOI: 10.4088/pcc.v06n0403

[48] Webster HH, Flores G, Marcotte ER, Cecyre D, Quirion R, Srivastava LK. Olfactory bulbectomy alters NMDA receptor levels in the rat prefrontal cortex. Synapse. 2000;**37**(2):159-162. DOI: 10.1002/1098-2396(200008)37:2<159::AID-SYN9>3.0.CO;2-N

[49] Keilhoff G, Becker A, Grecksch G, Bernstein HG, Wolf G. Cell proliferation is influenced by bulbectomy and normalized by imipramine treatment in a region-specific manner. Neuropsychopharmacology. 2006;**31**(6):1165-1176. DOI: 10.1038/sj.npp.1300924

[50] Santarelli L, Saxe M, Gross C, Surget A, Battaglia F, Dulawa S, et al. Requirement of hippocampal neurogenesis for the behavioral effects of antidepressants. Science. 2003;**301**(5634):805-809. DOI: 10.1126/science.1083328

[51] Lucas G, Rymar VV, Du J, Mnie-Filali O, Bisgaard C, Manta S, et al. Serotonin(4) (5-HT(4)) receptor agonists are putative antidepressants with a rapid onset of action. Neuron. 2007;**55**(5):712-725. DOI: 10.1016/j.neuron.2007.07.041

[52] Rosenzweig-Lipson S, Sabb A, Stack G, Mitchell P, Lucki I, Malberg JE, et al. Antidepressant-like effects of the novel, selective, 5-HT_{2C} receptor agonist WAY-163909 in rodents. Psychopharmacology. 2007;**192**(2):159-170. DOI: 10.1007/s00213-007-0710-6

[53] Taylor MJ, Freemantle N, Geddes J, Bhagwagar Z. Early onset of selective serotonin reuptake inhibitor antidepressant action: Systematic review and meta-analysis. Archives of General Psychiatry. 2006;**63**:1217-1223. DOI: 10.1001/archpsyc.63.11.1217

[54] Tollefson GD. Holman SL (1994): How long to onset of antidepressant action. International Clinical Psychopharmacology. 1994;**9**(4):245-250. DOI: 10.1097/00004850-199400940-00003

[55] Malberg JE. Implications of adult hippocampal neurogenesis in antidepressant action. Journal of Psychiatry & Neuroscience. 2004;**29**(3):196-205

Chapter 7

Role of Zinc and Zinc Ionophores in Brain Health and Depression Especially during the COVID-19 Pandemic

Amr Ahmed, Amr Ghit, Asmaa Houjak and Mahmoud Elkazzaz

Abstract

Zinc is a trace metal ion that has a role in both physiological and pathological processes, making it one of the most common and necessary components involved in brain function. Besides, zinc is required for cell proliferation control in a variety of mechanisms, including hormonal regulation of cell division. Also, zinc serves as a biochemical signal to immune cells and transcription factors involved in the synthesis of inflammatory cytokines. On the other hand, zinc has a variety of crucial roles in neurogenesis and also acts as a neuromodulator on a wide range of membrane receptors, ion channels, and transporters. Zinc is produced by neurons under several conditions to activate microglia. The link between zinc dysregulation and psychiatric disorder was that zinc acts as an inhibitory modulator at the N-methyl-D aspartic acid (NMDA) glutamate receptor. Ionophores are ion carrier molecules that reversibly bind and transport ions through biological membranes. Ionophores can be natural or synthetic products. Zinc ionophores such as quercetin, epigallocatechin gallate (EGCG), hinokitol, and proanthocyanidins have been shown to protect brain health, particularly in depression clinically significant depression and depressive symptoms in post-COVID-19 syndrome may have severe implications as it relates to life outcomes quality, herein according to previous research studies, we showed zinc deficiency as a possible risk factor for depression symptoms, which were commonly observed following severe infection of COVID-19.

Keywords: ionophore, zinc, cytokines, quercetin, EGCG, hinokitol, proanthocyanidins

1. Introduction

Zinc is a trace metal ion that has a role in both physiological and pathological processes, making it one of the most common and necessary components involved in brain function. The cortex, amygdala, olfactory bulb, and hippocampus neurons all carry “free ionic zinc” (Zn^{2+}), which appears to have the largest concentration of zinc in the brain. Zinc is involved in the physiochemical function of enzymes, proteins, and signal transcription factors, as well as the maintenance of numerous homeostatic systems, functioning as structural, regulatory, and catalytic cofactors for enzymes including DNA and RNA polymerases, histone deacetylases, and DNA ligases. Zinc is also required for cell proliferation and genomic integrity [1–5].

As a neuromodulator, zinc is produced during synaptic transmission and attaches to presynaptic or postsynaptic membrane receptors, allowing it to translocate from presynaptic terminals to postsynaptic neurons [6, 7]. Zinc can be found in glutamatergic neurons' synaptic vesicles. Zinc is therefore liberated from glutamatergic synaptic vesicles and then interacts with excitatory and inhibitory amino acid receptors (N-methyl-D aspartic acid (NMDA), α-amino-3-hydroxy-5-methyl-4-isoxazolepropionic acid (AMPA), and γ-aminobutyric acid (GABA) [8–10]. Because of its actions on numerous voltage-gated ion channels, extracellular Zn^{2+} can modify the excitability of nerve cells [11–13].

Besides, zinc is required for cell proliferation control in a variety of mechanisms, including hormonal regulation of cell division. Also, zinc serves as a biochemical signal to immune cells and transcription factors involved in the synthesis of inflammatory cytokines. Zinc supplementation has been proven in trials to reduce rates of infection and proinflammatory cytokine secretion. Zinc also possesses metal-binding characteristics and is widely recognized for its antioxidant qualities [14, 15]. Zinc deficiency causes apoptosis in neurons via the mitochondrial pathway [16, 17]. Zinc has just lately been discovered to have a role in intracellular signaling as a second messenger. It is also used by immune cells as a molecular signal. Zinc controls a variety of transcription factors that control gene expression and are engaged in the signal transduction of inflammatory cytokines and adhesion molecules. Zinc helps to preserve genomic stability by regulating redox homeostasis, DNA repair, synthesis, and methylation [18, 19].

2. Role of zinc in the brain

2.1 Role of zinc in neurogenesis and synaptic transmission

Zinc has a variety of crucial roles in neurogenesis [4]. Zinc deficiency decreases the neurogenesis process and impairs the expression of genes involved in hippocampus proliferation and neuronal development in the postnatal rat cerebellum [20]. Further, zinc deficiency reduces the proliferation of the human neuroblastoma cell line, promotes apoptosis, and inhibits retinoic-acid-induced neuronal development in cultured cells [1, 21].

Of note, zinc is found in the presynaptic glutamatergic vesicles across the brain, including the cerebral cortex, limbic system, hippocampus, and olfactory bulb [22].

It acts as a neuromodulator on a wide range of membrane receptors, ion channels, and transporters [23]. Synaptic zinc, in particular, is enhanced via a specialized zinc transporter, ZnT3, and is coreleased with glutamate during action potential-induced exocytosis [24]. These also have an impact on synaptic transmission, which interacts with receptors and channels that regulate auditory processing [25, 26]. Synaptic zinc has been discovered to inhibit NMDA receptors, GABA-A receptors, and calcium channels while activating AMPA and glycine receptors [27–30]. Zinc also has vital effects on other kinds of receptors, including serotonin, dopamine, and acetylcholine receptors, as well as voltage-gated ion channels for sodium, potassium, calcium, and chlorine [29, 31].

Synaptic zinc regulates sensory processing and improves acuity in the discrimination of different sensory stimuli. Synaptic zinc plasticity leads to prolonged adaptations and sense memories. Recently, the mechanism of this long-term synaptic zinc plasticity has been described as being due to group 1 metabotropic glutamate receptors (G1 mGluRs)-dependent mechanism that triggers a bidirectional long-term change in synaptic zinc signaling [32].

2.2 Role of zinc at depression

No one denies that depression treatment is a gateway to overcoming many social and psychological problems that affect millions of people all over the world. Many factors play a role in depressive-like behaviors, such as impairment of functions of the hippocampus and the prefrontal cortex. These brain parts play an important role in decision-making processes, so any dysfunction at this area can induce a predisposition to negative feelings, and many glucocorticoid receptors are involved in these areas [33].

In terms of both pharmacological and clinical/epidemiological data, recent years have provided additional evidence confirming the role of zinc in depression. Zinc demonstrated antidepressant-like efficacy in preclinical studies and depressive models. Clinical evidence suggested that zinc supplementation might be beneficial in people suffering from depression. Zinc supplementation has been demonstrated to be beneficial as adjuvant therapy or as a stand-alone intervention for depression. Furthermore, zinc consumption has been linked to an increased risk of depression. Dietary zinc restriction was found to be a causal factor in the development of depressive-like symptoms or anhedonia in mouse studies [34]. Some epidemiological studies have reported that reduced nutritional zinc consumption is related to depression in females but not in males [35]. Even though the first prospective study examining the relationship between zinc intake and depression risk found a small but significant inverse correlation between them, a 20-year follow-up study found that a reduced dietary zinc intake protects from depression in men who were not previously depressed. However, because the research participants were all men with a hospital discharge diagnosis of unipolar depression, the findings cannot be applied to women or patients who did not require hospitalization. On the contrary, a reduced nutritional zinc intake was found to be a risk factor for depression in a prospective analysis of both men and women [36]. Mice missing the G-protein-coupled receptor 39 (GPR39), a zinc-activated receptor, show depressive-like behavior [37]. TC-G-1008, a GPR39 agonist, was recently discovered to have antidepressant-like effects [38]. These findings add to the growing body of evidence that zinc is useful in the treatment of depression.

Meta-analyses support the use of zinc as a supplement in the treatment of severe depression, and single research currently supports the use of zinc for psychotic symptoms [39]. Zinc deficiency has also been linked to neuropsychiatric symptoms such as altered behavior and cognition, learning difficulties, and depression [40–42].

The link between zinc dysregulation and psychiatric disorder was that zinc acts as an inhibitory modulator at the NMDA glutamate receptor [43–45]. In addition, the inhibitory effects on the nicotinic acetylcholine receptor (nAChR), GSK3 (glycogen synthase kinase 3beta), and NOS (nitric oxide synthase) are also relevant to depressive processes [46, 47].

Numerous studies show lower zinc blood levels in depressed people compared with healthy people, with a meta-analysis showing depressive symptomatology at zinc serum levels of 1.8 M or below [48]. In several investigations, zinc supplementation enhanced mood in those who were suffering from treatment-resistant depression [41, 49].

Zinc's effect on the brain-derived neurotrophic factor (BDNF), a growth factor that promotes neurogenesis and differentiation, may be connected to depression. The hippocampus is a center of lifelong neurogenesis, and periods of significant depression are associated with reduced BDNF expression and neuro/synaptogenesis. Rodents on a zinc-deficient diet had lower zinc levels in the hippocampus vesicles, a part of the brain where zinc levels are generally greater, as well as lower amounts of progenitor cells and immature neurons. Zinc-rich diets, on the other hand, increased amounts of progenitor cells [3, 41]. The GPR39 receptor is most likely a critical connection in the interaction between zinc and the serotonergic system, which is required for antidepressants that affect the serotonin pathway to work [34].

2.3 Zinc and neuroimmunity

Of note, laboratory animal models showed that zinc insufficiency induces thymus and lymphoid tissue atrophy. It lowers the number of spleen cells and the sensitivity to antigens that are both T-cell-dependent and -independent [50]. Microglia is a kind of immune cell found in the central nervous system (CNS) [51]. The link between zinc and microglial activation reflects an undiscovered process that may play a role in neuropathy. However, zinc is produced by neurons under several conditions to activate microglial [52].

3. Zinc ionophores

Ionophores are ion carrier molecules that reversibly bind and transport ions through biological membranes. Many ionophores are lipid-soluble ion transporters that traverse the cell membrane. Ionophores accelerate ion transport through hydrophobic membranes such as liquid polymeric membranes (carrier-based ion-selective electrodes), lipid bilayers in live cells, or synthetic vesicles (liposomes). A hydrophilic core and a hydrophobic section interact with the membrane in the structure of an ionophore [53]. Many microorganisms, fungi, and plants naturally manufacture ionophores, which import ions into their cells and function as a defense against competing or harmful species. Ionophores made from synthetic materials have also been developed. Ionophores that select for cations and anions have a wide range of uses in the analysis [54]. When paired with the ion they bind, these chemicals have been proven to have a variety of biological effects as well as a synergistic impact [55]. Ionophores change the permeability of biological membranes in the direction of certain ions for which they have affinity and selectivity (**Figure 1**). An ionophore has a hydrophilic core and a hydrophobic section that interacts with the membrane in terms of structure. An ionophore-ion complex is formed when ions are bound to the hydrophilic center. X-ray crystallography has confirmed the structure of the ionophore-ion complex [58].

Zinc ionophores (**Table 1**; **Figure 2**) have been shown to inhibit replication of various viruses in vitro, including coxsackievirus [63, 65], equine arteritis virus [68], coronavirus [68], HCV [69], HSV [70], HCoV-229E [71], HIV [72, 73], mengovirus [63, 65], MERS-CoV [71], rhinovirus [65], SARS-CoV-1 [68], and Zika virus [74].

3.1 Examples of zinc ionophores and their role in brain health, depression as an example

3.1.1 Quercetin

Quercetin has attracted the attention of many researchers because of its capacity to pass the blood–brain barrier. It appears in the brain after hours of administration and plays a key function in the central nervous system [75]. Discoveries from animal

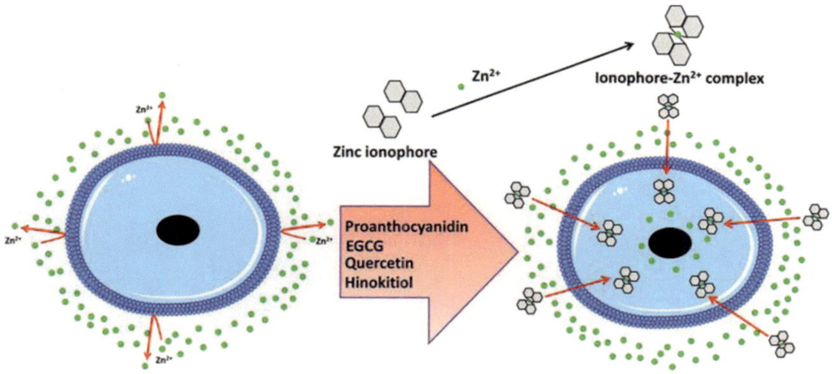

Figure 1.
Zinc ionophores mechanism in penetrating cell membranes. Two ionophore molecules can mediate intracellular zinc accumulation by exchanging extracellular Zn^{2+} with $2H^{+}$ [56]. Then, ionophore-zinc complex is taken up by endocytosis, followed by lysosomal disruption to release zinc into the cytoplasm [57].

Zinc Ionophore	Sources	References
Calcimycin	*Streptomyces chartreusensis*	[59, 60]
Chloroquine	*Cinchona officinalis*	[61]
Clioquinol	Synthetic ionophore	[55]
Diiodohydroxyquinoline	Synthetic ionophore	[62]
Dithiocarbamates	Synthetic ionophore	[63]
EGCG	*Camellia sinensis* (tea plant), apples, plums, onions	[64]
Hinokitiol	*Cupressaceae* species	[65]
Proanthocyanidins	Grape seed	[66]
PBT2	Synthetic analog of 8-hydroxyquinoline	[67]
Pyrithione	*Allium stipitatum*	[65]
Quercetin	Vegetables, fruits, berries, herbs, trees, and other plants	[64]
Zincophorin	*Streptomyces griseus*	[55]

Table 1.
Nature and synthetic zinc ionophores.

model research reported that antioxidant, anti-inflammatory, and neuroprotective effects of quercetin keep neurons in healthy condition by inhibiting the formation of hydroperoxide, reducing free radicals, and restoring antioxidant enzymes. Further, the study of quercetin at rat models proves its antidepressant action [76, 77]. Also, quercetin can reduce stress and depressive-like symptoms [75].

3.1.2 Epigallocatechin gallate (EGCG)

EGCG may act as a new antidepressant by inhibiting neuroinflammation, which may help to alleviate depression. Models of chronic unexpected mild stress (CUMS) in rats have been created in experimental investigations of depression [78]. Although the etiology of depression is not well understood, one popular theory is that depressed

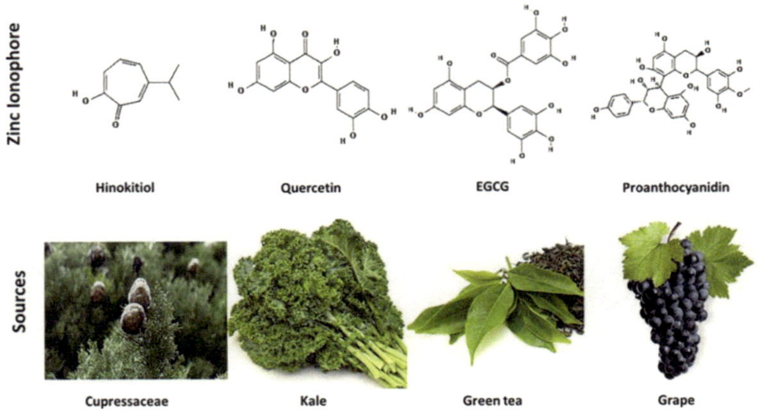

Figure 2.
Natural zinc ionophores and their sources. Chemical structures of ionophores obtained from Pubchem database (Hinokitiol, CID: 3611; quercetin, CID: 5280343; EGCG, CID: 65064; Proanthocyanidin, CID: 108065).

people have greater amounts of cytokines such as IL-6 due to lower levels of amines such as serotonin, noradrenaline, and dopamine [79]. EGCG injection improved depressed behavior in rats by reducing Il-6 levels in the hippocampus. As a result, EGCG was suggested to be used as a new antidepressant to reduce neuroinflammation, which could help to alleviate depression [80].

3.1.3 Hinokitol

Hinokitiol (β-thujaplicin) is a monoterpenoid that occurs naturally in the wood of Cupressaceae plants. It is a natural zinc ionophore that is safe to use. Because of its powerful, broad-spectrum antiviral, antibacterial, antifungal, anti-inflammatory, and anticancer effects, it is frequently employed in oral care and medicinal products. It is also a food additive that does not build up in the body. Throughout years of use, there have been no reports of allergic, poisonous, or adverse consequences in the literature. Hinokitiol is a safe zinc ionophore that increases the intracellular pool of labile zinc by facilitating zinc influx into cells [81].

3.1.4 Proanthocyanidins

Proanthocyanidins (GSPs), which comprise dimers, trimers, oligomers, and oligomers of catechin and epicatechin, are known to have antidepressant properties. Recent research has demonstrated the mechanism of GSPs' antidepressant effects in female juvenile prenatally stressed offspring rats. The main pathway was that GSPs work synergistically to inhibit oxidative stress and inflammatory response activator proteins [66].

4. Cross talk between zinc deficiency and depression caused by COVID-19

High rates of neuropsychiatric symptoms (e.g., depression) have been observed among patients affected by COVID-19, suggesting an effect of COVID-19 on the human central nervous system (CNS) [82–85]. It was showed globally that depression is a leading cause of disability [86]. Accordingly, clinically significant depression and depressive symptoms in post-COVID-19 syndrome may have severe implications as it relates to life outcomes quality [86]. Herein according to previous research studies, we showed zinc deficiency as a possible risk factor for depression symptoms, which were commonly observed following severe infection of COVID-19. A meta-analysis of 17 observational studies found that blood Zn^{2+} concentrations were lower in depressed subjects than in control subjects [48]. Interestingly, a recent study showed that a significant number of patients with COVID-19 were zinc-deficient [87], and a higher number of zinc-deficient COVID-19 patients had prolonged hospital stay when compared with those with normal zinc levels and required intensive care unit (ICU) [87]. A significant positive correlation was observed between the prevalence of zinc deficiency and COVID-19 cases [88]. A pooled analysis of 1532 COVID-19 patients suggested that zinc deficiency was associated with a sixfold increased risk of severe disease and 16-fold increased risk of death via elevating LDH [89]. The elevated LDH in the present study was probably indicative of severe disease [87]. Because zinc has a critical role in regulating functions of the human brain, many disorders have been linked with Zn^{2+} deficiency, including neurological diseases, such as psychiatric disorders, (depression) [48, 89] and schizophrenia [90]. Consequently, the clinical picture, which is common in severe COVID-19 patients and is referred to as "Depression" [82–85], is nothing more than depression seen in zinc deficiency [48, 87–89]. Most likely, depression and other mental problems in these patients also develop due to zinc deficiency in nerve cells in the brain.

The first study revealing a relationship between depression and dietary zinc deficiency was conducted by Amani et al. [90]. This study included 23 young females diagnosed with moderate and severe depression and 23 healthy volunteers who were age-matched. The findings revealed that the depressive group's daily zinc consumption and serum zinc concentration were both lower than the healthy women's. Moreover, an inverse correlation between serum zinc concentration and the depression scores was obtained [90]. According to the World Health Organization (WHO), zinc deficiency affects at least one-third of the world's population [91]. The fact that zinc deficiency is linked to the risk of infection and severe advancement of COVID-19 [91] gives a first significant clue on a link between zinc deficiency and the risk of infection as well as its symptoms with unknown etiology such as depression and suggests possible benefits of zinc supplementation. Owing to Zn^{2+} neuroprotective properties, it is not surprising that Zn^{2+} supplementation could be effective not only on COVID-19-related symptoms but also on virus replication, as well as on COVID-19-related inflammation and neurological damage [92]. In vitro, Zn^{2+} inhibits Coronavirus and Arter virus RNA polymerase activity, and zinc ionophores prevent these viruses from replicating in cell culture [93]. Zinc ionophore may play a role in therapeutic management for COVID-19 [94].

5. Conclusions

Zinc deficiency has been linked to different nervous system disorders. Because zinc is not fat-soluble, it requires transporters called zinc ionophores, which facilitate the entrance of zinc in cytoplasm increasing its level of concentration in the body after consumption. The role of zinc in protecting brain cells has been extensively studied recently particularly in depression treatment. Therefore, natural zinc ionophores plus zinc supplements, which are commercially available, could be a new way to treatment of many neuropsychiatric disorders. Zinc ionophore may play a role in therapeutic management for COVID-19 and postcovid-19 depression.

Abbreviations

AMPA	α-amino-3-hydroxy-5-methyl-4-isoxazolepropionic acid
BDNF	brain-derived neurotrophic factor
CUMS	chronic unexpected mild stress
EGCG	Epigallocatechin gallate
G1 mGluRs	group 1 metabotropic glutamate receptors
GABA	γ-aminobutyric acid, gamma-Aminobutyric acid
GPR39	G-protein coupled receptor 39
GSK3	glycogen synthase kinase 3beta
GSPs	Proanthocyanidins
nAChR	nicotinic acetylcholine receptor
NMDA	N-methyl-D aspartic acid
NOS	nitric oxide synthase
LDH	Lactate dehydrogenase

Author details

Amr Ahmed[1*], Amr Ghit[2,3*], Asmaa Houjak[4*] and Mahmoud Elkazzaz[5]

1 Public Health Department, First Health Cluster, Ministry of Health, Riyadh, Saudi Arabia

2 Department of Medicine and Aging Sciences, "G. d'Annunzio" University of Chieti-Pescara, Chieti, Italy

3 Center for Advanced Studies and Technology (CAST), "G. d'Annunzio" University of Chieti-Pescara, Chieti, Italy

4 Faculty of Science, Department of Chemistry, Princess Noura University (PNU), Riyadh, Saudi Arabia

5 Faculty of Science, Department of Chemistry and Biochemistry, Damietta University, Kafr Elsheikh, Egypt

*Address all correspondence to: drmedahmed@gmail.com; amr.ghit@unich.it and mahmoudelkazzaz2051@gmail.com

References

[1] Adamo AM, Zago MP, Mackenzie GG, et al. The role of zinc in the modulation of neuronal proliferation and apoptosis. Neurotoxicity Research. 2010;**17**:1-14. DOI: 10.1007/s12640-009-9067-4

[2] Gao H-L, Zheng W, Xin N, et al. Zinc deficiency reduces neurogenesis accompanied by neuronal apoptosis through caspase-dependent and -independent signaling pathways. Neurotoxicity Research. 2009;**16**:416-425. DOI: 10.1007/s12640-009-9072-7

[3] Suh SW, Won SJ, Hamby AM, et al. Decreased brain zinc availability reduces hippocampal neurogenesis in mice and rats. Journal of Cerebral Blood Flow and Metabolism. 2009;**29**:1579-1588. DOI: 10.1038/jcbfm.2009.80

[4] Corniola RS, Tassabehji NM, Hare J, et al. Zinc deficiency impairs neuronal precursor cell proliferation and induces apoptosis via p53-mediated mechanisms. Brain Research. 2008;**1237**:52-61. DOI: 10.1016/j.brainres.2008.08.040

[5] Moon M-Y, Kim HJ, Choi BY, et al. Zinc promotes adipose-derived mesenchymal stem cell proliferation and differentiation towards a neuronal fate. Stem Cells International. 2018;**2018**:5736535. DOI: 10.1155/2018/5736535

[6] Jan H-H, Chen I-T, Tsai Y-Y, Chang Y-C. Structural role of zinc ions bound to postsynaptic densities. Journal of Neurochemistry. 2002;**83**:525-534. DOI: 10.1046/j.1471-4159.2002.01093.x

[7] Grabrucker AM, Knight MJ, Proepper C, et al. Concerted action of zinc and ProSAP/shank in synaptogenesis and synapse maturation. The EMBO Journal. 2011;**30**:569-581. DOI: 10.1038/emboj.2010.336

[8] Draguhn A, Verdorn TA, Ewert M, et al. Functional and molecular distinction between recombinant rat GABAA receptor subtypes by Zn^{2+}. Neuron. 1990;**5**:781-788. DOI: 10.1016/0896-6273(90)90337-f

[9] Westbrook GL, Mayer ML. Micromolar concentrations of Zn^{2+} antagonize NMDA and GABA responses of hippocampal neurons. Nature. 1987; **328**:640-643. DOI: 10.1038/328640a0

[10] Tabata T, Ishida AT. A zinc-dependent Cl^- current in neuronal somata. The Journal of Neuroscience. 1999;**19**:5195-5204. DOI: 10.1523/JNEUROSCI.19-13-05195.1999

[11] Koh JY, Suh SW, Gwag BJ, et al. The role of zinc in selective neuronal death after transient global cerebral ischemia. Science. 1996;**272**:1013-1016. DOI: 10.1126/science.272.5264.1013

[12] Weiss JH, Hartley DM, Koh JY, Choi DW. AMPA receptor activation potentiates zinc neurotoxicity. Neuron. 1993;**10**:43-49. DOI: 10.1016/0896-6273(93)90240-r

[13] Sensi SL, Yin HZ, Carriedo SG, et al. Preferential Zn^{2+} influx through Ca^{2+}–permeable AMPA/kainate channels triggers prolonged mitochondrial superoxide production. Proceedings of the National Academy of Sciences of the United States of America. 1999;**96**:2414-2419. DOI: 10.1073/pnas.96.5.2414

[14] MacDonald RS. The role of zinc in growth and cell proliferation. The Journal of Nutrition. 2000;**130**:1500S-1508S. DOI: 10.1093/jn/130.5.1500S

[15] Jarosz M, Olbert M, Wyszogrodzka G, et al. Antioxidant

and anti-inflammatory effects of zinc. Zinc-dependent NF-κB signaling. Inflammopharmacology. 2017;**25**:11-24. DOI: 10.1007/s10787-017-0309-4

[16] Choi DW, Koh JY. Zinc and brain injury. Annual Review of Neuroscience. 1998;**21**:347-375. DOI: 10.1146/annurev.neuro.21.1.347

[17] Sensi SL, Paoletti P, Bush AI, Sekler I. Zinc in the physiology and pathology of the CNS. Nature Reviews. Neuroscience. 2009;**10**:780-791. DOI: 10.1038/nrn2734

[18] Prasad AS. Zinc in human health: Effect of zinc on immune cells. Molecular Medicine. 2008;**14**:353-357. DOI: 10.2119/2008-00033.Prasad

[19] Wessels I, Maywald M, Rink L. Zinc as a gatekeeper of immune function. Nutrients. 2017;**9**:1286, 2. DOI: 10.3390/nu9121286

[20] Dvergsten CL, Fosmire GJ, Ollerich DA, Sandstead HH. Alterations in the postnatal development of the cerebellar cortex due to zinc deficiency. II. Impaired maturation of Purkinje cells. Brain Research. 1984;**318**:11-20. DOI: 10.1016/0165-3806(84)90057-9

[21] Gower-Winter SD, Corniola RS, Morgan TJJ, Levenson CW. Zinc deficiency regulates hippocampal gene expression and impairs neuronal differentiation. Nutritional Neuroscience. 2013;**16**:174-182. DOI: 10.1179/1476830512Y.0000000043

[22] Frederickson CJ. Neurobiology of zinc and zinc-containing neurons. International Review of Neurobiology. 1989;**31**:145-238. DOI: 10.1016/s0074-7742(08)60279-2

[23] Blakemore LJ, Trombley PQ. Zinc as a neuromodulator in the central nervous system with a focus on the olfactory bulb. Frontiers in Cellular Neuroscience. 2017;**11**:297. DOI: 10.3389/fncel.2017.00297

[24] Qian J, Noebels JL. Exocytosis of vesicular zinc reveals persistent depression of neurotransmitter release during metabotropic glutamate receptor long-term depression at the hippocampal CA3-CA1 synapse. The Journal of Neuroscience. 2006;**26**:6089-6095. DOI: 10.1523/JNEUROSCI.0475-06.2006

[25] Li Y, Hough CJ, Suh SW, et al. Rapid translocation of Zn(2+) from presynaptic terminals into postsynaptic hippocampal neurons after physiological stimulation. Journal of Neurophysiology. 2001;**86**:2597-2604. DOI: 10.1152/jn.2001.86.5.2597

[26] Ketterman JK, Li YV. Presynaptic evidence for zinc release at the mossy fiber synapse of rat hippocampus. Journal of Neuroscience Research. 2008;**86**:422-434. DOI: 10.1002/jnr.21488

[27] Bitanihirwe BKY, Cunningham MG. Zinc: The brain's dark horse. Synapse. 2009;**63**:1029-1049. DOI: 10.1002/syn.20683

[28] Nakashima AS, Dyck RH. Zinc and cortical plasticity. Brain Research Reviews. 2009;**59**:347-373. DOI: 10.1016/j.brainresrev.2008.10.003

[29] Smart TG, Xie X, Krishek BJ. Modulation of inhibitory and excitatory amino acid receptor ion channels by zinc. Progress in Neurobiology. 1994;**42**:393-441. DOI: 10.1016/0301-0082(94)90082-5

[30] Mayer ML, Vyklicky LJ. The action of zinc on synaptic transmission and neuronal excitability in cultures of mouse hippocampus. The Journal of Physiology. 1989;**415**:351-365. DOI: 10.1113/jphysiol.1989.sp017725

[31] Frederickson CJ, Koh J-Y, Bush AI. The neurobiology of zinc in health and disease. Nature Reviews. Neuroscience. 2005;**6**:449-462. DOI: 10.1038/nrn1671

[32] Vogler NW, Betti VM, Goldberg JM, Tzounopoulos T. Mechanisms underlying long-term synaptic zinc plasticity at mouse dorsal Cochlear nucleus glutamatergic synapses. The Journal of Neuroscience. 2020;**40**:4981-4996. DOI: 10.1523/JNEUROSCI.0175-20.2020

[33] Silvestro S, Bramanti P, Mazzon E. Role of quercetin in depressive-like behaviors: Findings from animal models. Applied Science. 2021;**11**:7116

[34] Doboszewska U, Wlaź P, Nowak G, et al. Zinc in the monoaminergic theory of depression: Its relationship to neural plasticity. Neural Plasticity. 2017; **2017**:3682752. DOI: 10.1155/2017/3682752

[35] Maserejian NN, Hall SA, McKinlay JB. Low dietary or supplemental zinc is associated with depression symptoms among women, but not men, in a population-based epidemiological survey. Journal of Affective Disorders. 2012;**136**:781-788. DOI: 10.1016/j.jad.2011.09.039

[36] Milton AH, Vashum KP, McEvoy M, et al. Prospective study of dietary zinc intake and risk of cardiovascular disease in women. Nutrients. 2018;**10**:38. DOI: 10.3390/nu10010038

[37] Młyniec K, Budziszewska B, Holst B, et al. GPR39 (zinc receptor) knockout mice exhibit depression-like behavior and CREB/BDNF down-regulation in the hippocampus. The International Journal of Neuropsychopharmacology. 2014;**18**:3. DOI: 10.1093/ijnp/pyu002

[38] Starowicz G, Jarosz M, Frąckiewicz E, et al. Long-lasting antidepressant-like activity of the GPR39 zinc receptor agonist TC-G 1008. Journal of Affective Disorders. 2019;**245**:325-334. DOI: 10.1016/j.jad.2018.11.003

[39] Petrilli MA, Kranz TM, Kleinhaus K, et al. The emerging role for zinc in depression and psychosis. Frontiers in Pharmacology. 2017;**8**:414. DOI: 10.3389/fphar.2017.00414

[40] Nowak G. Does interaction between zinc and glutamate system play a significant role in the mechanism of antidepressant action? Acta Poloniae Pharmaceutica. 2001;**58**:73-75

[41] Nowak G, Siwek M, Dudek D, et al. Effect of zinc supplementation on antidepressant therapy in unipolar depression: A preliminary placebo-controlled study. Polish Journal of Pharmacology. 2003;**55**:1143-1147

[42] Howland JG, Wang YT. Synaptic plasticity in learning and memory: Stress effects in the hippocampus. Progress in Brain Research. 2008;**169**:145-158. DOI: 10.1016/S0079-6123(07)00008-8

[43] Frederickson CJ, Suh SW, Silva D, et al. Importance of zinc in the central nervous system: The zinc-containing neuron. The Journal of Nutrition. 2000;**130**:1471S-1483S. DOI: 10.1093/jn/130.5.1471S

[44] Paz RD, Tardito S, Atzori M, Tseng KY. Glutamatergic dysfunction in schizophrenia: From basic neuroscience to clinical psychopharmacology. European Neuropsychopharmacology. 2008;**18**:773-786. DOI: 10.1016/j.euroneuro.2008.06.005

[45] Szewczyk B, Poleszak E, Sowa-Kućma M, et al. The involvement of NMDA and AMPA receptors in the mechanism of antidepressant-like action of zinc in the forced swim test. Amino Acids. 2010;**39**:205-217. DOI: 10.1007/s00726-009-0412-y

[46] Nowak G. Zinc, future mono/adjunctive therapy for depression: Mechanisms of antidepressant action. Pharmacological Reports. 2015;**67**:659-662. DOI: 10.1016/j.pharep.2015.01.015

[47] Szewczyk B, Pochwat B, Rafało A, et al. Activation of mTOR dependent signaling pathway is a necessary mechanism of antidepressant-like activity of zinc. Neuropharmacology. 2015;**99**:517-526. DOI: 10.1016/j.neuropharm.2015.08.026

[48] Swardfager W, Herrmann N, Mazereeuw G, et al. Zinc in depression: A meta-analysis. Biological Psychiatry. 2013;**74**:872-878. DOI: 10.1016/j.biopsych.2013.05.008

[49] Siwek M, Dudek D, Paul IA, et al. Zinc supplementation augments efficacy of imipramine in treatment resistant patients: A double blind, placebo-controlled study. Journal of Affective Disorders. 2009;**118**:187-195. DOI: 10.1016/j.jad.2009.02.014

[50] Prasad AS. Zinc: Role in immunity, oxidative stress and chronic inflammation. Current Opinion in Clinical Nutrition and Metabolic Care. 2009;**12**:646-652. DOI: 10.1097/MCO.0b013e3283312956

[51] Lenz KM, Nelson LH. Microglia and beyond: Innate immune cells As regulators of brain development and behavioral function. Frontiers in Immunology. 2018;**9**:698. DOI: 10.3389/fimmu.2018.00698

[52] Kauppinen TM, Higashi Y, Suh SW, et al. Zinc triggers microglial activation. The Journal of Neuroscience. 2008;**28**:5827-5835. DOI: 10.1523/JNEUROSCI.1236-08.2008

[53] Bakker E, Bühlmann P, Pretsch E. Carrier-based ion-selective electrodes and bulk Optodes. 1. General Characteristics. Chemical Reviews. 1997;**97**:3083-3132. DOI: 10.1021/cr940394a

[54] Bühlmann P, Pretsch E, Bakker E. Carrier-based ion-selective electrodes and bulk Optodes. 2. Ionophores for potentiometric and optical sensors. Chemical Reviews. 1998;**98**:1593-1688. DOI: 10.1021/cr970113+

[55] Ding W-Q, Lind SE. Metal ionophores—An emerging class of anticancer drugs. IUBMB Life. 2009;**61**:1013-1018. DOI: 10.1002/iub.253

[56] Harbison-Price N, Ferguson SA, Heikal A, Taiaroa G, Hards K, Nakatani Y, et al. Multiple bactericidal mechanisms of the zinc ionophore PBT2. mSphere. 2022;**5**:e00157-e00120. DOI: 10.1128/mSphere.00157-20

[57] Samutprasert P, Chiablaem K, Teeraseranee C, et al. Epigallocatechin gallate-zinc oxide co-crystalline nanoparticles as an anticancer drug that is non-toxic to normal cells. RSC Advances. 2018;**8**:7369-7376. DOI: 10.1039/C7RA10997K

[58] Steinrauf LK, Hamilton JA, Sabesan MN. Crystal structure of valinomycin-sodium picrate. Anion effects on valinomycin-cation complexes. Journal of the American Chemical Society. 1982;**104**:4085-4091. DOI: 10.1021/ja00379a008

[59] Abbott BJ, Fukuda DS, Dorman DE, et al. Microbial transformation of A23187, a divalent cation ionophore antibiotic. Antimicrobial Agents and Chemotherapy. 1979;**16**:808-812. DOI: 10.1128/AAC.16.6.808

[60] Raatschen N, Wenzel M, Ole Leichert LI, et al. Extracting iron and manganese from bacteria with

ionophores—A mechanism against competitors characterized by increased potency in environments low in micronutrients. Proteomics. 2013;**13**:1358-1370. DOI: 10.1002/pmic.201200556

[61] Xue J, Moyer A, Peng B, et al. Chloroquine is a zinc ionophore. PLoS One. 2014;**9**:e109180. DOI: 10.1371/journal.pone.0109180

[62] Aggett PJ, Delves HT, Harries JT, Bangham AD. The possible role of diodoquin as a zinc ionophore in the treatment of acrodermatitis enteropathica. Biochemical and Biophysical Research Communications. 1979;**87**:513-517. DOI: 10.1016/0006-291x(79)91825-4

[63] Lanke K, Krenn BM, Melchers WJG, et al. PDTC inhibits picornavirus polyprotein processing and RNA replication by transporting zinc ions into cells. The Journal of General Virology. 2007;**88**:1206-1217. DOI: 10.1099/vir.0.82634-0

[64] Dabbagh-Bazarbachi H, Clergeaud G, Quesada IM, et al. Zinc ionophore activity of quercetin and epigallocatechin-gallate: From Hepa 1-6 cells to a liposome model. Journal of Agricultural and Food Chemistry. 2014;**62**:8085-8093. DOI: 10.1021/jf5014633

[65] Krenn BM, Gaudernak E, Holzer B, et al. Antiviral activity of the zinc ionophores pyrithione and hinokitiol against picornavirus infections. Journal of Virology. 2009;**83**:58-64. DOI: 10.1128/JVI.01543-08

[66] Sun Q, Jia N, Ren F, Li X. Grape seed proanthocyanidins improves depression-like behavior by alleviating oxidative stress and NLRP3 activation in the hippocampus of prenatally-stressed female offspring rats. Journal of Histotechnology. 2021;**44**:90-98. DOI: 10.1080/01478885.2020.1861907

[67] Bohlmann L, De Oliveira DMP, El-Deeb IM, et al. Chemical synergy between Ionophore PBT2 and zinc reverses antibiotic resistance. MBio. 2018;**9**:e02391-e02318. DOI: 10.1128/mBio.02391-18

[68] te Velthuis AJW, van den Worm SHE, Sims AC, et al. Zn(2+) inhibits coronavirus and arterivirus RNA polymerase activity in vitro and zinc ionophores block the replication of these viruses in cell culture. PLoS Pathogens. 2010;**6**:e1001176. DOI: 10.1371/journal.ppat.1001176

[69] Mizui T, Yamashina S, Tanida I, et al. Inhibition of hepatitis C virus replication by chloroquine targeting virus-associated autophagy. Journal of Gastroenterology. 2010;**45**:195-203. DOI: 10.1007/s00535-009-0132-9

[70] Qiu M, Chen Y, Chu Y, et al. Zinc ionophores pyrithione inhibits herpes simplex virus replication through interfering with proteasome function and NF-κB activation. Antiviral Research. 2013;**100**:44-53. DOI: 10.1016/j.antiviral.2013.07.001

[71] de Wilde AH, Jochmans D, Posthuma CC, et al. Screening of an FDA-approved compound library identifies four small-molecule inhibitors of Middle East respiratory syndrome coronavirus replication in cell culture. Antimicrobial Agents and Chemotherapy. 2014;**58**:4875-4884. DOI: 10.1128/AAC.03011-14

[72] Tsai WP, Nara PL, Kung HF, Oroszlan S. Inhibition of human immunodeficiency virus infectivity by chloroquine. AIDS Research and Human Retroviruses.

1990;**6**:481-489. DOI: 10.1089/aid.1990.6.481

[73] Romanelli F, Smith KM, Hoven AD. Chloroquine and hydroxychloroquine as inhibitors of human immunodeficiency virus (HIV-1) activity. Current Pharmaceutical Design. 2004;**10**:2643-2648. DOI: 10.2174/1381612043383791

[74] Li C, Zhu X, Ji X, et al. Chloroquine, a FDA-approved drug, prevents Zika virus infection and its associated congenital microcephaly in mice. eBioMedicine. 2017;**24**:189-194. DOI: 10.1016/j.ebiom.2017.09.034

[75] Yoshino S, Hara A, Sakakibara H, et al. Effect of quercetin and glucuronide metabolites on the monoamine oxidase-a reaction in mouse brain mitochondria. Nutrition. 2011;**27**:847-852. DOI: 10.1016/j.nut.2010.09.002

[76] Sakakibara H, Yoshino S, Kawai Y, Terao J. Antidepressant-like effect of onion (Allium cepa L.) powder in a rat behavioral model of depression. Bioscience, Biotechnology, and Biochemistry. 2008;**72**:94-100. DOI: 10.1271/bbb.70454

[77] Rojas P, Serrano-García N, Medina-Campos ON, et al. Antidepressant-like effect of a Ginkgo biloba extract (EGb761) in the mouse forced swimming test: Role of oxidative stress. Neurochemistry International. 2011;**59**:628-636. DOI: 10.1016/j.neuint.2011.05.007

[78] Bondi CO, Rodriguez G, Gould GG, et al. Chronic unpredictable stress induces a cognitive deficit and anxiety-like behavior in rats that is prevented by chronic antidepressant drug treatment. Neuropsychopharmacol Off Publ Am Coll Neuropsychopharmacol. 2008;**33**:320-331. DOI: 10.1038/sj.npp.1301410

[79] Gold PW. The organization of the stress system and its dysregulation in depressive illness. Molecular Psychiatry. 2015;**20**:32-47. DOI: 10.1038/mp.2014.163

[80] Wang J, Xu S, Chen X, et al. Antidepressant effect of EGCG through the inhibition of hippocampal neuroinflammation in chronic unpredictable mild stress-induced depression rat model. Journal of Functional Foods. 2020;**73**:104106. DOI: 10.1016/j.jff.2020.104106

[81] Hoang BX, Han B. A possible application of hinokitiol as a natural zinc ionophore and anti-infective agent for the prevention and treatment of COVID-19 and viral infections. Medical Hypotheses. 2020;**145**:110333. DOI: 10.1016/j.mehy.2020.110333

[82] Troyer EA et al. Are we facing a crashing wave of neuropsychiatric sequelae of COVID-19? Neuropsychiatric symptoms and potential immunologic mechanisms. Brain, Behavior, and Immunity. 2020;**87**:34-39. DOI: 10.1016/j.bbi.2020.04.027

[83] Kang L, Ma S, Chen M, et al. Impact on mental health and perceptions of psychological care among medical and nursing staff in Wuhan during the 2019 novel coronavirus disease outbreak: A cross-sectional study. Brain, Behavior, and Immunity. 2020;**87**:11-17. DOI: 10.1016/j.bbi.2020.03.028

[84] Lai J, Ma S, Wang Y, et al. Factors associated with mental health outcomes among health care workers exposed to coronavirus disease 2019. JAMA Network Open. 2020;**3**(3):e203976. DOI: 10.1001/jamanetworkopen.2020.3976

[85] Liu D, Baumeister RF, Zhou Y. Mental health outcomes of coronavirus infection survivors: A rapid meta-analysis. Journal of Psychiatric Research.

2021;**137**:542-553. DOI: 10.1016/j.jpsychires.2020.10.015

[86] Renaud-Charest O, Lui L, Eskander S, Ceban F, Ho R, Di Vincenzo JD, et al. Onset and frequency of depression in post-COVID-19 syndrome: A systematic review. Journal of Psychiatric Research. 2021;**144**:129-137. DOI: 10.1016/j.jpsychires.2021.09.054

[87] Jothimani D et al. COVID-19: Poor outcomes in patients with zinc deficiency. International Journal of Infectious Diseases : IJID : Official Publication of the International Society for Infectious Diseases. 2020;**100**:343-349. DOI: 10.1016/j.ijid.2020.09.014

[88] Ali N et al. Assessment of the role of zinc in the prevention of COVID-19 infections and mortality: A retrospective study in the Asian and European population. Journal of Medical Virology. 2021;**93**(7):4326-4333. DOI: 10.1002/jmv.26932

[89] Henry BM, Aggarwal G, Wong J, et al. Lactate dehydrogenase levels predict coronavirus disease 2019 (COVID-19) severity and mortality: A pooled analysis. The American Journal of Emergency Medicine. 2020;**38**(9):1722-1726. DOI: 10.1016/j.ajem.2020.05.073

[90] Amani R, Saeidi S, Nazari Z, Nematpour S. Correlation between dietary zinc intakes and its serum levels with depression scales in young female students. Biological Trace Element Research. 2010;**137**:150-158

[91] World Health Organization. The world health report 2002. Midwifery. 2003;**19**:72-73. DOI: 10.1054/midw.2002.0343

[92] Cereda G, Ciappolino V, Boscutti A, et al. Zinc as a neuroprotective nutrient for COVID-19-related neuropsychiatric manifestations: A literature review. Advances in Nutrition. 2022;**13**(1):66-79. DOI: 10.1093/advances/nmab110

[93] te Velthuis AJW, van den Worm SHE, Sims AC, Baric RS, Snijder EJ, van Hemert MJ. Zn2+ inhibits coronavirus and Arterivirus RNA polymerase activity In vitro and zinc Ionophores block the replication of these viruses in cell culture. PLoS Pathogens. 2010;**6**(11):e1001176. DOI: 10.1371/journal.ppat.1001176

[94] Carlucci PM, Ahuja T, Petrilli C, Rajagopalan H, Jones S, Rahimian J. Zinc sulfate in combination with a zinc ionophore may improve outcomes in hospitalized COVID-19 patients. Journal of Medical Microbiology. 2020;**69**(10):1228-1234. DOI: 10.1099/jmm.0.001250

Chapter 8

Perspective Chapter: Depression as a Disorder of Monoamine Axon Degeneration May Hold an Answer to Two Antidepressant Questions - Delayed Clinical Efficacy and Treatment-Resistant Depression

Shoji Nakamura

Abstract

It has long been known that the pathophysiology of depression is associated with a reduction in the brain concentrations of monoamines, that is, serotonin, noradrenaline, and dopamine. Although conventional antidepressant drugs increase monoamine contents immediately after their administration, it takes several weeks or more before their clinical efficacy becomes evident. The mechanism of the delayed onset of antidepressant effects remains elusive. Furthermore, over 30–50% of patients with depression show resistance to antidepressant drug treatment. Thus, two major questions remain to be resolved—(1) delayed clinical efficacy of antidepressant drugs, and (2) a large percentage of treatment-resistant depression. First, this review describes the evidence, obtained from animal and human studies, that similar to early-stage Parkinson's disease, depression is a neurodegenerative disease characterized by the degeneration of monoamine axons and the delayed clinical efficacy of antidepressants is due to their regenerative action on damaged monoamine axons. Moreover, the causes of treatment-resistant depression are discussed in relation to inflammation as a cause of neurodegeneration. This review provides new insights into not only the pathophysiology of depression but also the diagnosis and therapy of early stages of neurodegenerative diseases, such as Parkinson's disease and Alzheimer's disease.

Keywords: depression, parkinson's disease, antidepressant, treatment-resistant, omega-3 fatty acid, neurodegeneration, regeneration

1. Introduction

It has long been known that the pathophysiology of depression is associated with a reduction in the concentration of monoamines, that is, serotonin (5-HT), noradrenaline (NA), and dopamine (DA), in the brain [1, 2]. Conventional antidepressant drugs for clinical use increase monoamine contents immediately after their administration, whereas it takes several weeks or more before their clinical efficacy becomes evident. The delayed onset of action of antidepressants suggests that antidepressants exert their effects by inducing slowly occurring changes in the brain. Furthermore, over 30–50% of patients with depression show resistance to antidepressant drug treatment [3–5]. Thus, two major questions remain to be resolved—(1) How do the delayed clinical effects of antidepressant drugs occur, and (2) why does a large percentage of patients with depression show resistance to antidepressant treatment. This review article focuses on addressing these questions based on the evidence that depression is not a disease caused simply by the deficiency of neurotransmitters, but a neurodegenerative disease characterized by axonal degeneration of monoamine neurons without cell death [6–11].

2. Delayed onset of antidepressant effects

2.1 Antidepressants and monoamine axon regeneration/sprouting

Recent animal and human studies have demonstrated that depression is a neurodegenerative disease characterized by the degeneration of monoamine axons without cell death, and the delayed clinical efficacy of antidepressants is due to their regenerative action on damaged monoamine axons. In 1990, it was reported for the first time that antidepressants that increase the extracellular concentration of NA, such as desipramine, maprotiline, and mianserin, have the ability to induce regeneration of NA axons, but fluoxetine, a potent selective serotonin reuptake inhibitor (SSRI), does not [6, 7]. The regenerative effects of antidepressants on NA axons lesioned by 6-hydroxydopamine (6-OHDA) could be induced by antidepressant infusions in the rat cerebral cortex for more than 2 weeks but not for less than 1 week. Furthermore, the ability of antidepressants to induce axonal sprouting of 5-HT neurons has been demonstrated by systemic injections of antidepressants for 4 weeks daily in rats without damaging 5-HT axons [9]. In this study, fluoxetine and the 5-HT reuptake enhancer tianeptine, but not the NA reuptake inhibitor desipramine, increased the density of 5-HT axons in the cerebral cortex and some limbic forebrain areas. These findings indicate that antidepressants associated with 5-HT reuptake, but not NA reuptake, induce axonal sprouting of 5-HT neurons. Based on the sprouting or regenerative effects of antidepressants on NA and 5-HT axons, the axonal degeneration of monoamine neurons has been suggested to be involved in the pathophysiology of depression and antidepressants exert their action by inducing the regeneration of monoamine axons. In addition, it is suggested that the pathophysiology of depression includes NA-axon and/or 5-HT-axon degeneration, and NA- and 5-HT-specific antidepressants are effective in inducing NA and 5-HT axon regeneration, respectively.

2.2 Depression and monoamine axon degeneration

Further evidence has been provided using animal models of depression to show that axonal degeneration of monoamine neurons is involved in the pathophysiology of depression. The rat model of depression, which was developed by repeated exposure to forced walking stress for 2 weeks, showed depressive behaviors including prolonged inactivity, seclusion, aggression, motor retardation, lack of coupling behavior, fitful sleep, weight loss, and hypersensitivity to light and sound [12]. Subsequent studies have demonstrated that this stress-induced depression model reveals the degeneration of NA axons in the cerebral cortex [8]. In this depression model with NA axon degeneration, imipramine (intraperitoneal injections for 20 days) could induce regeneration of cortical NA axons and ameliorate the depression-like behaviors [8]. A most recent study showed that in a mouse model of poststroke depression with degeneration of NA- and 5-HT axons, chronic treatment with fluoxetine reversed depression-like behaviors and a loss of 5-HT axons, but not NA axons [11]. Furthermore, light deprivation was found to induce a loss of NA axons, but not 5-HT axons, in the frontal cortex and depression-like behaviors in rats, while desipramine improved the NA axon loss and depressive behaviors [10]. Postnatal isolation rearing, which induced depressive behavior in adolescent/young adult rats, reduced the density of 5-HT axons, but not NA axons, in the hippocampus and amygdala [13]. A recent study has shown that exposure to 1-bromopropane, an alternative to ozone-depleting solvents, which is known to induce depressive symptoms in a subset of people exposed to this chemical, induced the degeneration of NA axons, but not 5-HT axons, in the adult rat [14]. It has also been presented that repeated electroconvulsive shock that is most effective in the treatment of clinical depression promotes the regeneration of 5-HT axons of the rat hippocampus damaged by the 5-HT specific neurotoxin [15]. In the chronic social defeat stress model of depression with reduced 5-HT innervation in the hippocampal dentate gyrus (DG) and ventromedial prefrontal cortex (vmPFC) of mice, chronic deep brain stimulation of vmPFC reversed depression-like behavior and restored 5-HT innervation in the DG and vmPFC [16]. Further evidence for the involvement of the degeneration of monoamine axons in the pathophysiology of depression has been reported: Interferon-α, which is widely used for the treatment of cancers and viral illnesses, is known to frequently induce depressive symptoms [17], reduces the density of NA and 5-HT axons in the frontal cortex, hippocampus, and amygdala of rats [18]. Finally, human brain imaging studies have shown evidence that the degeneration of monoamine axons is associated with depressive symptoms [19–21]. In these studies, the density of axon terminals of monoamine neurons was measured by positron emission tomography using radiotracers of presynaptic monoamine transporters. Although scant in number and limited to Parkinson's diseases with depressive symptoms, the imaging studies have provided evidence to support the involvement of loss of monoamine axons in the occurrence of depressive symptoms. Importantly, a recent imaging study reported that depressed patients showing the improvement of depressive symptoms after cognitive behavioral therapy revealed an overall increase in cerebral 5-HT transporter availability, suggesting the occurrence of 5-HT axon regeneration/sprouting after depression treatment [22]. Furthermore, in depressed suicide victims, immunohistochemistry using an antibody to serotonin transporters showed a localized decrease in the density of 5-HT axons in the PFC [23].

All these studies support the view that depressive symptoms are caused by the loss of monoamine axons and antidepressants exert their effects by inducing the regeneration of monoamine axons. Thus, the delayed onset of antidepressant efficacy can be explained by the time required for the regeneration of monoamine axons.

3. Plausible causes of treatment-resistant depression

Based on the view that depression is a neurodegenerative disease, the possible causes of treatment-resistant depression are considered due to (1) mismatch of impaired monoamines and prescribed antidepressant drugs, (2) severe degeneration or cell death, (3) persistent inflammation, and (4) omega-3 fatty acid deficiency. Obviously, we cannot exclude other causes of treatment-resistant depression (**Figure 1**).

3.1 Mismatch of impaired monoamines and prescribed antidepressant drugs

One of the causes of treatment-resistant depression could be explained by the possibility that there are different types of depression whose pathophysiology differs in which monoamine is involved (5-HT, NA, DA, or two or more monoamines). The problem is that there are no objective diagnostic tools to differentiate which monoamine is involved in the pathophysiology of depressive symptoms of individual patients. In fact, as mentioned before, animal studies have suggested that there are various types of depression that differ in the monoamine(s) involved [10, 11, 13, 14, 18]. In clinical practice, SSRIs are most commonly prescribed as first-line antidepressant drugs without any distinct evidence that the depressive symptoms of patients are due to 5-HT deficiency. At present, it is difficult for clinicians to correctly administer antidepressant drugs to individual patients with depression. If patients with depression are not administered antidepressant drugs that are able to regenerate the particular monoamine axons that are damaged in their case, they may suffer from treatment-resistant depression.

3.2 Severe degeneration or cell death

Another likely cause of treatment-resistant depression may be attributable to the possibility that the degeneration of monoamine axons is not localized at axon terminals, but extends further from the terminals. In the most severe case, retrograde axonal degeneration may result in the degeneration of the neuron soma (cell death).

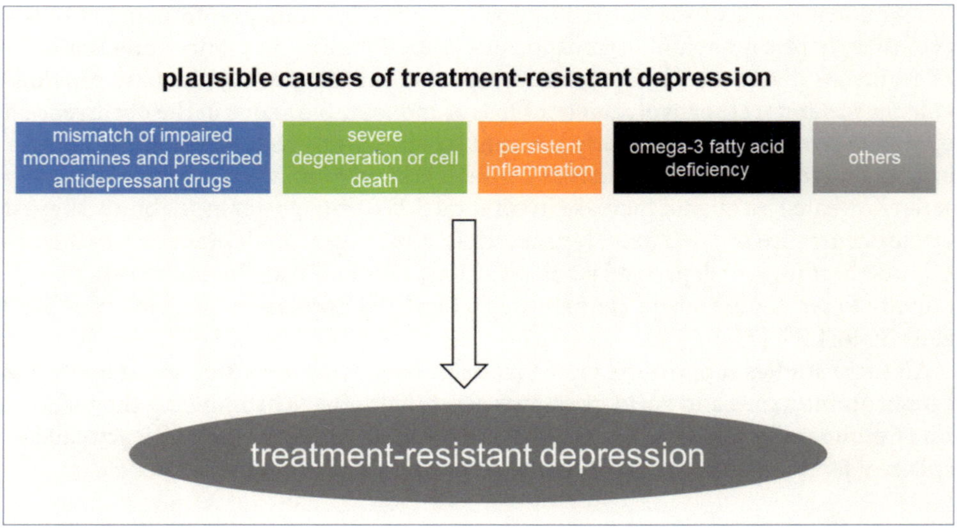

Figure 1.
Plausible causes of treatment-resistant depression. The causes of resistance to antidepressant drugs may be due to (1) mismatch of impaired monoamines and prescribed antidepressant drugs, (2) severe degeneration or cell death, (3) persistent inflammation, and (4) omega-3 fatty acid deficiency. Others may include deficiency of signaling pathways or molecules related to regeneration of monoamine axons.

In fact, a great loss of NA neurons in the locus coeruleus has been reported to be associated with depressive symptoms in patients without dementia as well as those with Alzheimer's disease or Parkinson's disease [24, 25]. A loss of 5-HT neurons in the raphe nucleus is also reported to be associated with depressive symptoms of patients with Parkinson's disease [26]. Depressive symptoms due to the loss of monoamine neurons can hardly be treated with the administration of conventional antidepressant drugs as well as electroconvulsive shock therapy. It is noted that at the early stages of Parkinson's disease and Alzheimer's disease the degeneration of the distal axons occurs first, and in the late stages, persistent axonal degeneration finally results in the degeneration of the neuron soma [27–29]. This implies that in neurodegenerative diseases such as Parkinson's disease and Alzheimer's disease, possibly including depression, the degeneration of the distal axons precedes the loss of the neuron soma. Postmortem and imaging studies have shown that in Parkinson's disease about 30% of DA neurons of the substantia nigra compacta (SNc) and about 50–70% of striatal DA axon terminals are lost by the time of motor symptom onset [30, 31]. The reason for making the distal axons more vulnerable to insults than the neuron soma can be explained by the fact that the distal portions of axons are most remote from the cell body that supplies proteins and chemicals required for the survival and growth of axons.

Whether distal axon degeneration is prone to cell death or not could be dependent on the length of axons from the neuron soma to the distal axon terminal and the morphological features of axon terminals (**Figure 2**). In Parkinson's disease, motor symptoms occur due to the degeneration of SNc DA neurons projecting to the dorsal striatum. Since the distance between the two brain regions is relatively short, retrograde axon degeneration of SNc DA neurons is considered to result in cell death more easily. In contrast, NA neurons of the locus coeruleus and 5-HT neurons of the raphe nucleus send their axons to long distances from the brainstem to the cerebral cortex [32], thus taking a long time to cause soma degeneration. On the other hand, it has been reported that DA neurons of the ventral tegmental area (VTA), which project their axons to the ventral striatum (nucleus accumbens) and are responsible for reward-related behavior, are involved in the pathophysiology of depression [33, 34]. Similar to SNc DA neurons, VTA DA neurons project relatively short axons to the nucleus accumbens. Although the axon length of both DA neurons is almost the same, however, DA neurons of the SNc are more prone to cell death in Parkinson's disease, compared to DA neurons of the VTA [35, 36]. A single-neuron tracing study demonstrated that a single DA neuron of the SNc forms highly overlapping innervation with extremely dense axonal arborizations in the dorsal striatum [37], while that of the VTA has much smaller axonal arbors in the ventral striatum (**Figure 2**) [27, 36]. A large and dense axonal arborization in the terminal field is considered to contribute to cell death of DA neurons of the SNc in Parkinson's disease [36]. Thus, in addition to axonal length, the spread and size of terminal axon arbors may play a pivotal role in vulnerability to neuronal cell death. It is also noted that because 5-HT, NA, and DA axons all have a great capacity to spontaneously regenerate or sprout in response to damage in the adult brain [38–41], the competition between degenerative and regenerative mechanisms may occur after axonal damage, finally resulting in either axonal regeneration or cell death.

3.3 Persistent inflammation

In recent years much evidence has been accumulating that inflammation is a key player in the pathogenesis of neurodegenerative diseases, such as Parkinson's disease

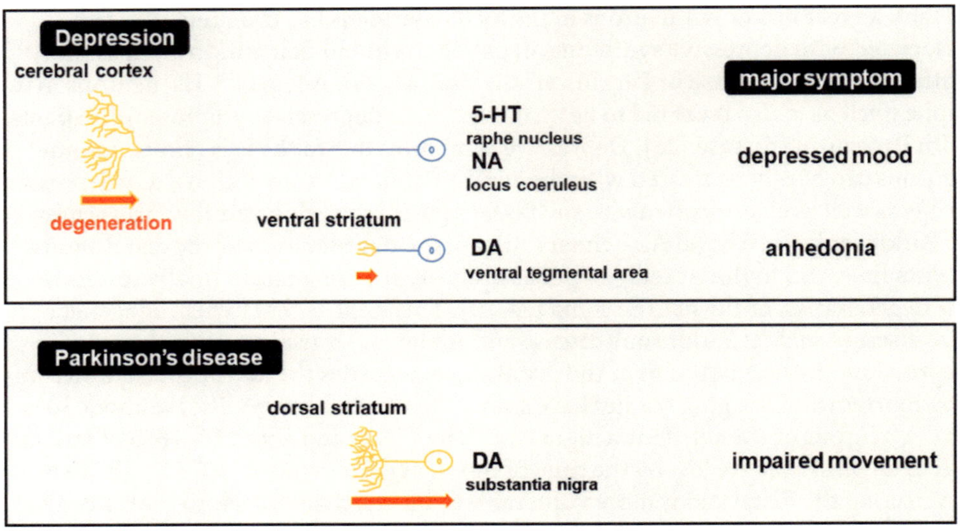

Figure 2.
Retrograde axonal degeneration and cell death of monoamine neurons depend on axonal length and morphological features of axon terminals. NA neurons of the locus coeruleus and 5-HT neurons of the raphe nucleus have long axons, rarely causing cell death, and depressive symptoms can occur predominantly due to axonal degeneration without cell death. In contrast, DA neurons of the VTA and SNc have relatively short axons. Although the axon length of both DA neurons is almost the same, DA neurons of the SNc are more prone to cell death in Parkinson's disease, compared to DA neurons of the VTA. A single DA neuron of the SNc forms highly overlapping innervation with extremely dense axonal arborizations, while that of the VTA has much smaller axonal arbors. A large and dense axonal arborization in the terminal field is considered to contribute to cell death of DA neurons of the SNc in Parkinson's disease. NA: Noradrenaline, 5-HT: Serotonin, DA: Dopamine, VTA: Ventral tegmental area, and SNc: Substantia nigra compacta.

and Alzheimer's disease [42, 43]. Many researchers also reported that inflammation plays an important role in the occurrence of depressive symptoms and is associated with treatment-resistant depression [4, 5, 44, 45]. A subset of patients with depression and animal models of depression revealed increased levels of pro-inflammatory cytokines in the periphery and brain, including IL-1β, IL-6, and TNF-α, and a variety of stresses including psychosocial stress could induce activation of key inflammatory pathways to elevate the serum levels of pro-inflammatory cytokines such as IL-6 [44–48]. Based on these findings, as mentioned previously, long-term repeated intraperitoneal injection of the pro-inflammatory cytokine interferon-α induces the degeneration of 5-HT and NA axons in the rat brain, though there is no apparent change in the number and shape of 5-HT and NA neuronal somata [18]. Accordingly, it is reasonable to assume that prolonged inflammation and persistent release of pro-inflammatory cytokines produce the degeneration of 5-HT and/or NA axons without cell death, resulting in the occurrence of depressive symptoms. If inflammation as a cause of the axonal degeneration of monoamine neurons persists without anti-inflammatory treatment during repeated administration of antidepressants, patients are likely to suffer from treatment-resistant depression.

3.4 Omega-3 fatty acid deficiency

Chronic treatment with antidepressants is reported to cause the downregulation of β-adrenergic receptors [49]. On the other hand, the denervation of cortical NA axons with the neurotoxin 6-OHDA causes upregulation (supersensitivity) in cortical β-adrenergic receptors [50]. As upregulation of β-adrenergic receptors is associated with NA axon degeneration, it is possible that downregulation of β-adrenergic receptors results from regeneration or sprouting of NA axons. If upregulation of β-adrenergic receptors occurs due to the degeneration of NA axons in the brains of patients with depression, antidepressants could normalize the sensitivity of β-adrenergic receptors by the downregulation following the regeneration of NA axons. Further studies have shown that downregulation of β-adrenergic receptors following repeated application of β-adrenergic agonists or chronic stress treatment is blocked by phospholipase A2 (PLA2) inhibitors, while this downregulation can be induced by the activation of PLA2 [51, 52]. Moreover, it has been demonstrated that PLA2 activation is involved in the downregulation of β-adrenergic receptors induced by chronic desipramine treatment [53]. A possible link between the downregulation of β-adrenergic receptors and the regeneration of NA axons raised the possibility that PLA2 is involved in the molecular mechanisms of the antidepressant-induced regeneration of NA axons. Based on these findings, the PLA2 inhibitor mepacrine or 4-bromphenacyl bromide could attenuate the regeneration of NA axons induced by desipramine, while the PLA2 activator melittin induced NA axon regeneration [54]. These findings suggested that the PLA2 signaling pathway is involved in the pathophysiology of depression.

PLA2 generates the omega-6 polyunsaturated fatty acid arachidonic acid (AA) and omega-3 polyunsaturated fatty acids eicosapentaenoic acid (EPA) and docosahexaenoic acid (DHA) by acting on membrane phospholipids. PLA2 enzymes are subdivided into several groups and among them, two groups of PLA2, cytosolic PLA2 (cPLA2) and calcium-independent PLA2 (iPLA2), play a major role in the release of AA, EPA, and DHA from the cell membrane [42, 55]. PLA2 and its products, omega-3 and omega-6 fatty acids, reveal the capacity to produce axon outgrowth of adult mouse sensory neurons *in vitro*, aged rat sensory neurons in culture, and cultured hippocampal and PC12 cells [56–58]. Importantly, acute administration of DHA is reported to induce sprouting of 5-HT axons as well as corticospinal axons in an adult rat model of spinal cord injury [59]. A recent study also reported that in the damaged cornea of the adult mouse, DHA induces axonal regeneration of trigeminal sensory nerves via the iPLA2 activity of the receptors of the neuroprotective molecule pigment epithelium-derived factor [60]. Furthermore, using iPLA2β-knockout mice, the impairment of iPLA2β was found to cause widespread degeneration of axons in the central and peripheral nervous systems, including nigrostriatal DA axons, although the changes were not observed in developing and young mice, but became evident in older mice [61, 62]. All these findings suggest that PLA2 and its products play a key role in the degeneration and regeneration of axons in the periphery and brain, including monoamine axons in the adult brain.

Recently, many reports have shown lower levels of EPA and/or DHA being associated with depression [63–66]. Animal studies demonstrated that administration of EPA and DHA had an antidepressant-like effect, reducing immobility in the forced swim test [67, 68]. Moreover, it has been reported that the antidepressant effect of maprotiline, an NA reuptake inhibitor, is mediated by DHA released by activation of iPLA2 in the mouse prefrontal cortex [69]. Notably important is that EPA and DHA are essential fatty acids and must be obtained from the diet. Consequently, if patients with depression do not get enough of these fatty acids from their diet during the administration of antidepressant drugs, they may suffer from treatment-resistant depression. Notably, in adolescents with SSRI-resistant depression who exhibited robust DHA deficits, DHA supplementation with fish oil increased DHA status and enhanced the antidepressant effects of SSRI [70].

4. Depression and neurodegenerative diseases

Depression is considered a neurodegenerative disease, such as Parkinson's disease and Alzheimer's disease. Parkinson's disease with the degeneration of DA neurons of the SNc related to motor function produces motor symptoms, while the degeneration of 5-HT and NA neurons related to mood regulation results in depressed mood and anxiety of patients with depression. In addition, the degeneration of DA neurons of the VTA may be associated with anhedonia in patients with depression. Nonspecific symptoms of depression, such as sleep problems, tiredness, and changes in appetite, may be attributable to the degeneration of 5-HT and NA axons, because loss of these monoamine axons, which are distributed to almost the entire brain, could likely produce a variety of symptoms. A major difference between depression and Parkinson's disease as well as Alzheimer's disease is that the neuropathology of depression is characterized predominantly by the degeneration of axons, while the neurodegenerative changes of Parkinson's disease and Alzheimer's disease include a great loss of the neuron cell somata. The depressive symptoms of patients with depression can occur due to axonal degeneration of monoamine neurons even without soma degeneration, whereas the motor symptoms of Parkinson's disease and cognitive impairment of Alzheimer's disease become evident after the occurrence of soma degeneration. This is well consistent with the fact that depression often precedes symptoms of neurodegenerative diseases, typically including Parkinson's disease and Alzheimer's disease [71, 72]. Thus, depression may be useful as a predictor of the future occurrence of neurodegenerative diseases characterized by cell death. In any case, detection of axonal degeneration before cell death is important for the treatment of Parkinson's disease and Alzheimer's disease. It is noted that DHA supplementation before the onset of dementia results in beneficial outcomes in patients with Alzheimer's disease [55, 73, 74]. Omega-3 supplementation, as a primary intervention, also reduces cognitive decline in patients with mild to moderate Alzheimer's disease [75]. These results suggest that in Alzheimer's disease omega-3 fatty acids reduce mild cognitive impairment by producing axonal regeneration before the occurrence of cell death.

5. Involvement of PLA2 signaling in antidepressants effects

As mentioned earlier, neuroinflammation is reported to play a key role in neurodegenerative changes of neurological diseases, such as Parkinson's disease and Alzheimer's disease. In addition, the possibility is also discussed that the degeneration of monoamine axons, which is considered to occur in patients with depression, may be due in part to neuroinflammation. In recent years much attention has been paid to the roles of the PLA2 signaling pathway in neuroinflammation in relation to neurodegenerative diseases. It has been reported that cPLA2 releases AA and EPA, while iPLA2 preferentially releases DHA. In addition, AA and its products, such as prostaglandins and leukotrienes, play a major role in pro-inflammatory responses, whereas DHA and EPA and their products, such as resolvins and protectins, are involved in anti-inflammatory responses [55, 76, 77]. Omega-3 fatty acids and their metabolites play a regulatory role in the transition from pro-inflammatory to anti-inflammatory phases by inhibiting pro-inflammatory signaling pathways [55]. Thus, the release of AA and its products in the brain induces inflammatory neuronal damage such as axonal degeneration, whereas omega-3 fatty acids and their metabolites exert anti-inflammatory actions to induce the resolution of inflammation and recovery, including the process of axonal regeneration (**Figure 3**).

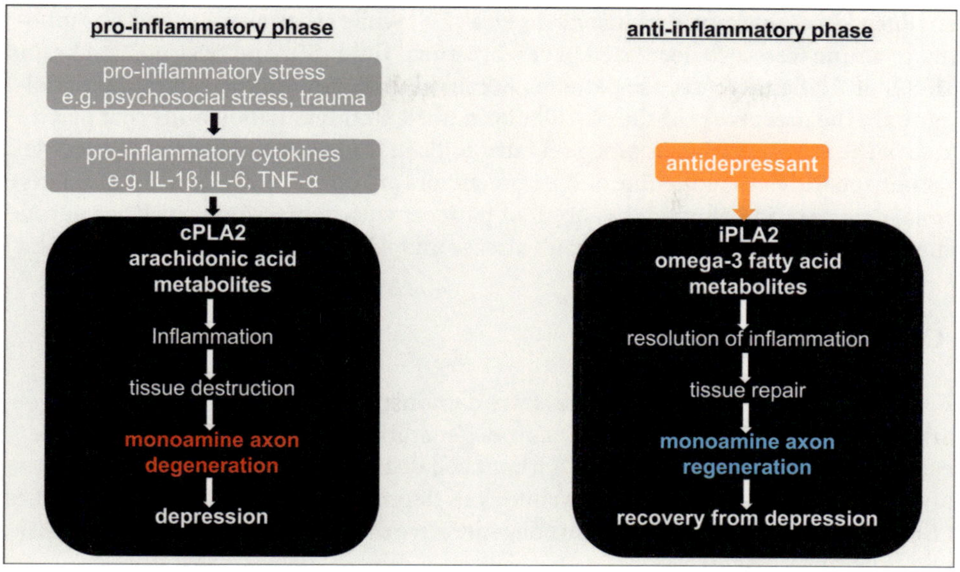

Figure 3.
A possible mechanism of degeneration and regeneration of monoamine axons related to pro-inflammatory and anti-inflammatory actions of PLA2. In the pro-inflammatory phase, cPLA2 and its pro-inflammatory metabolites cause the degeneration of monoamine axons, whereas iPLA2 and its anti-inflammatory metabolites (omega-3 fatty acids) play pivotal roles in inflammation-resolution and recovery by exerting anti-inflammatory and regenerative actions. There are distinct interactions between pro-inflammatory and anti-inflammatory signaling pathways. Antidepressants are considered to activate iPLA2 signaling pathway and induce anti-inflammatory response and the regeneration of monoamine axons through omega-3 fatty acids and their metabolites. PLA2: Phospholipase A2, cPLA2: Cytosolic phospholipase A2, iPLA2: Calcium-independent phospholipase A2.

Therefore, it is possible, at least in part, that antidepressants, which can activate iPLA2 signaling pathways, induce the axonal regeneration of monoamine neurons by anti-inflammatory and regenerative actions of omega-3 fatty acids and their metabolites.

6. Biomarkers for axonal degeneration

As noted in this review, many recent studies have clearly demonstrated that depression is a neurodegenerative disease and shares many similarities with well-known neurodegenerative diseases such as Parkinson's disease and Alzheimer's disease. Particularly, axonal degeneration is a common phenomenon that occurs at the early stages of Parkinson's disease and Alzheimer's disease, and possibly in depression. It is thus essential to devise new tools for the detection of axonal degeneration of affected neurons. If this is realized, Parkinson's disease and Alzheimer's disease at early stages, characterized by axonal degeneration without cell death, will be treatable with drugs with the ability to induce axonal regeneration. In depression, one of the promising and powerful tools for detecting monoamine axon degeneration is neuroimaging of monoamine axon terminals using radiotracers of transporters of each monoamine axon. Interestingly, a more recent study reported that plasma phosphoethanolamine is a reliable biomarker of depression because it was significantly decreased in patients with depression and inversely correlated with the severity of depressive symptoms, including depressed mood, loss of interest, and psychomotor retardation [78]. Similarly, plasma levels of ethanolamine and phosphatidylethanolamine were found to be reduced in early-stage Parkinson's disease [79], while ethanolamine and phosphoethanolamine were also decreased in cerebrospinal fluid [80] and postmortem brains [81, 82] of Alzheimer's disease patients. Because ethanolamine and phosphoethanolamine are the precursors of the phospholipid phosphatidylethanolamine that plays a role in the incorporation of omega-3 fatty acids in the cell membrane, it is possible that phosphatidylethanolamine and its precursors are one of the reliable biomarkers of axonal degeneration of at least a subset of patients with depression as well as neurodegenerative diseases such as Parkinson's disease and Alzheimer's disease.

7. Conclusion

Recent animal and human studies have demonstrated that similar to early-stage Parkinson's disease, depression is a neurodegenerative disease characterized by the degeneration of monoamine axons without cell death. This review may contribute not only to understanding the pathophysiology of depression but also to new approaches to the diagnosis and therapy of neurodegenerative diseases such as Parkinson's disease and Alzheimer's disease.

Acknowledgements

I would like to deeply thank Dr. James M Tepper, Distinguished Professor of Rutgers University-Newark, and Dr. Satoshi Kida, Professor of the University of Tokyo, for reviewing the manuscript and offering many helpful comments and suggestions.

Conflict of interest

The author declares no conflict of interest.

Abbreviations

AA	arachidonic acid
cPLA2	cytosolic phospholipase A2
DA	dopamine
DG	dentate gyrus
DHA	docosahexaenoic acid
EPA	eicosapentaenoic acid
5-HT	serotonin
iPLA2	calcium-independent phospholipase A2
NA	noradrenaline
6-OHDA	6-hydroxydopamine
PFC	prefrontal cortex
PLA2	phospholipase A2
SNc	substantia nigra compacta
SSRI	selective serotonin reuptake inhibitor
vmPFC	ventromedial prefrontal cortex
VTA	ventral tegmental area

Author details

Shoji Nakamura
Yamaguchi University Graduate School of Medicine, Ube, Yamaguchi, Japan

*Address all correspondence to: snaka@yic.ac.jp

References

[1] Schildkraut JJ. The catecholamine hypothesis of affective disorders: A review of supporting evidence. The American Journal of Psychiatry. 1965;**122**:509-522. DOI: 10.1176/ajp.122.5.509

[2] Coppen A. The biochemistry of affective disorders. The British Journal of Psychiatry. 1967;**113**:1237-1264. DOI: 10.1192/bjp.113.504.1237

[3] Krishnan V, Nestler EJ. The molecular neurobiology of depression. Nature. 2008;**455**:894-902. DOI: 10.1038/nature07455

[4] Hodes GE, Kana V, Menard C, Merad M, Russo SJ. Neuroimmune mechanisms of depression. Nature Neuroscience. 2015;**18**:1386-1393. DOI: 10.1038/nn.4113

[5] Feltes PK, Doorduin J, Klein HC, Juarez-Orozco LE, Dierckx RA, Moriguchi-Jeckel C, et al. Anti-inflammatory treatment for major depressive disorder: Implications for patients with an elevated immune profile and non-responders to standard antidepressant therapy. Journal of Psychopharmcology. 2017;**31**:1149-1165. DOI: 10.1177/0269881117711708

[6] Nakamura S. Antidepressants induce regeneration of catecholaminergic axon terminals in the rat cerebral cortex. Neuroscience Letters. 1990;**111**:64-68. DOI: 10.1016/0304-3940(90)90345-a

[7] Nakamura S. Effects of mianserin and fluoxetine on axonal regeneration of brain catecholamine neurons. Neuroreport. 1991;**2**:525-528. DOI: 10.1097/00001756-199109000-00007

[8] Kitayama I, Yaga T, Kayahara T, Nakano K, Murase S, Otani M, et al. Long-term stress degenerates, but imipramine regenerates, noradrenergic axons in the rat cerebral cortex. Biological Psychiatry. 1997;**42**:687-696. DOI: 10.1016/s0006-3223(96)00502-1

[9] Zhou L, Huang KX, Kecojevic A, Welsh AM, Koliatsos VE. Evidence that serotonin reuptake modulators increase the density of serotonin innervation in the forebrain. Journal of Neurochemistry. 2006;**96**:396-406. DOI: 10.1111/j.1471-4159.2005.03562.x

[10] González MM, Aston-Jones G. Light deprivation damages monoamine neurons and produces a depressive behavioral phenotype in rats. Proceedings of the National Academy of Sciences of the United States of America. 2008;**105**:4898-4903. DOI: 10.1073/pnas.0703615105

[11] Zahrai A, Vahid-Ansari F, Daigle M, Albert PR. Fluoxetine-induced recovery of serotonin and norepinephrine projections in a mouse model of post-stroke depression. Translational Psychiatry. 2020;**10**:334. DOI: 10.1038/s41398-020-01008-9

[12] Hatotani N, Nomura J, Inoue K, Kitayama I. Psychoendocrine model of depression. Psychoneuroendocrinology. 1979;**4**:155-172. DOI: 10.1016/0306-4530(79)90029-5

[13] Kuramochi M, Nakamura S. Effects of postnatal isolation rearing and antidepressant treatment on the density of serotonergic and noradrenergic axons and depressive behavior in rats. Neuroscience. 2009;**163**:448-455. DOI: 10.1016/j.neuroscience.2009.06.017

[14] Mohideen SS, Ichihara G, Ichihara S, Nakamura S. Exposure to 1-bromopropane causes degeneration of noradrenergic axons in the rat brain. Toxicology. 2011;**285**:67-71. DOI: 10.1016/j.tox.2011.04.005

[15] Madhav TR, Pei Q, Grahame-Smith DG, Zetterstrom TS. Repeated electroconvulsive shock promotes the sprouting of serotonergic axons in the lesioned rat hippocampus. Neuroscience. 2000;**97**:677-683. DOI: 10.1016/s0306-4522(00)00083-x

[16] Veerakumar A, Challis C, Gupta P, Da J, Upadhyay A, Beck SG, et al. Antidepressant-like effects of cortical deep brain stimulation coincide with pro-neuroplastic adaptations of serotonin systems. Biological Psychiatry. 2014;**76**:203-212. DOI: 10.1016/j.biopsych.2013.12.009

[17] Raison CL, Capuron L, Miller AH. Cytokines sing the blues: Inflammation and the pathogenesis of depression. Trends in Immunology. 2006;**27**:24-31. DOI: 10.1016/j.it.2005.11.006

[18] Ishikawa J, Ishikawa A, Nakamura S. Interferon-α reduces the density of monoaminergic axons in the rat brain. Neuroreport. 2007;**18**:137-140. DOI: 10.1097/WNR.0b013e328010231a

[19] Remy P, Doder M, Lees A, Turjanski N, Brooks D. Depression in Parkinson's disease: Loss of dopamine and noradrenaline innervation in the limbic system. Brain. 2005;**128**:1314-1322. DOI: 10.1093/brain/awh445

[20] Maillet A, Krack P, Lhommée E, Météreau E, Klinger H, Favre E, et al. The prominent role of serotonergic degeneration in apathy, anxiety and depression in de novo Parkinson's disease. Brain. 2016;**139**:2486-2502. DOI: 10.1093/brain/aww162

[21] Grosch J, Winkler J, Kohl Z. Early degeneration of both dopaminergic and serotonergic axons—Common mechanism in Parkinson's disease. Frontiers in Cellular Neuroscience. 2016;**10**:293-300. DOI: 10.3389/fncel.2016.00293

[22] Svensson JE, Svanborg C, Plavén-Sigray P, Kaldo V, Halldin C, Schain M, et al. Serotonin transporter availability increases in patients recovering from a depressive episode. Translational Psychiatry. 2021;**11**:264. DOI: 10.1038/s41398-021-01376-w

[23] Austin MC, Whitehead RE, Edgar CL, Janosky JE, Lewis DA. Localized decrease in serotonin transporter-immunoreactive axons in the prefrontal cortex of depressed subjects committing suicide. Neuroscience. 2002;**114**:807-815. DOI: 10.1016/s0306-4522(02)00289-0

[24] Chan-Palay V, Asan E. Quantitation of catecholamine neurons in the locus coeruleus in human brains of normal young and older adults and in depression. The Journal of Comparative Neurology. 1989;**287**:357-372. DOI: 10.1002/cne.902870307

[25] Chan-Palay V, Asan E. Alterations in catecholamine neurons of the locus coeruleus in senile dementia of the Alzheimer type and in Parkinson's disease with and without dementia and depression. The Journal of Comparative Neurology. 1989;**287**:373-392. DOI: 10.1002/cne.902870308

[26] Paulus W, Jellinger K. The neuropathologic basis of different clinical subgroups of Parkinson's disease. Journal of Neuropathology and Experimental Neurology. 1991;**50**:743-755. DOI: 10.1097/00005072-199111000-00006

[27] Tagliaferro P, Burke RE. Retrograde axonal degeneration in Parkinson

disease. Journal of Parkinson's Disease. 2016;**6**:1-15. DOI: 10.3233/JPD-150769

[28] Salvadores N, Sanhueza M, Manque P, Court FA. Axonal degeneration during aging and its functional role in neurodegenerative disorders. Frontiers in Neuroscience. 2017;**11**:451-472. DOI: 10.3389/fnins.2017.00451

[29] Kneynsberg A, Combs B, Christensen K, Morfini G, Kanaan NM. Axonal degeneration in tauopathies: Disease relevance and underlying mechanisms. Frontiers in Neuroscience. 2017;**11**:572-586. DOI: 10.3389/fnins.2017.00572

[30] Nandhagopal R, McKeown MJ, Stoessl AJ. Functional imaging in Parkinson disease. Neurology. 2008;**70**:1478-1488. DOI: 10.1212/01.wnl.0000310432.92489.90

[31] Cheng HC, Ulane CM, Burke RE. Clinical progression in Parkinson disease and the neurobiology of axons. Annals of Neurology. 2010;**67**:715-725. DOI: 10.1002/ana.21995

[32] Ungerstedt U. Stereotaxic mapping of the monoamine pathways in the rat brain. Acta Physiologica Scandinavica. Supplementum. 1971;**367**:1-48. DOI: 10.1111/j.1365-201x

[33] Furlanetti LL, Coenen VA, Döbrössy MD. Ventral tegmental area dopaminergic lesion-induced depressive phenotype in the rat is reversed by deep brain stimulation of the medial forebrain bundle. Behavioural Brain Research. 2016;**299**:132-140. DOI: 10.1016/j.bbr.2015.11.036

[34] Nobili A, Latagliata EC, Viscomi MT, Cavallucci V, Cutuli D, Giacovazzo G, et al. Dopamine neuronal loss contributes to memory and reward dysfunction in a model of Alzheimer's disease. Nature Communications. 2017;**8**:14727. DOI: 10.1038/ncomms14727

[35] Damier P, Hirsch EC, Agid Y, Graybiel AM. The substantia nigra of the human brain. II. Patterns of loss of dopamine-containing neurons in Parkinson's disease. Brain. 1999; **122**:1437-1448. DOI: 10.1093/brain/122.8.1437

[36] Bolam JP, Pissadaki EK. Living on the edge with too many mouths to feed: Why dopamine neurons die. Movement Disorders. 2012;**27**:1478-1483. DOI: 10.1002/mds.25135

[37] Matsuda W, Furuta T, Nakamura KC, Hioki H, Fujiyama F, Arai R, et al. Single nigrostriatal dopaminergic neurons form widely spread and highly dense axonal arborizations in the neostriatum. The Journal of Neuroscience. 2009; **29**:444-453. DOI: 10.1523/JNEUROSCI.4029-08.2009

[38] Fritschy JM, Grzanna R. Restoration of ascending noradrenergic projections by residual locus coeruleus neurons: Compensatory response to neurotoxin-induced cell death in the adult rat brain. The Journal of Comparative Neurology. 1992;**321**:421-441. DOI: 10.1002/cne.903210309

[39] Finkelstein DI, Stanic D, Parish CL, Thomas D, Dickson K, Horne MK. Axonal sprouting following lesions of the rat substantia nigra. Neuroscience. 2000;**97**:99-112. DOI: 10.1016/s0306-4522(00)00009-9

[40] Liu Y, Nakamura S. Stress-induced plasticity of monoamine axons. Frontiers in Bioscience. 2006;**11**:1794-1801. DOI: 10.2741/1923

[41] Jin Y, Dougherty SE, Wood K, Sun L, Cudmore RH, Abdalla A, et al.

Regrowth of serotonin axons in the adult mouse brain following injury. Neuron. 2016;**91**:748-762. DOI: 10.1016/j.neuron.2016.07.024

[42] Farooqui AA, Ong WY, Horrocks LA. Inhibitors of brain phospholipase A2 activity: Their neuropharmacological effects and therapeutic importance for the treatment of neurologic disorders. Pharmacological Reviews. 2006;**58**:591-620. DOI: 10.1124/pr.58.3.7

[43] Stephenson J, Nutma E, van der Valk P, Amor S. Inflammation in CNS neurodegenerative diseases. Immunology. 2018;**154**:204-219. DOI: 10.1111/imm.12922

[44] Miller AH, Raison CL. The role of inflammation in depression: From evolutionary imperative to modern treatment target. Nature Reviews Immunology. 2016;**16**:22-34. DOI: 10.1038/nri.2015.5

[45] Pfau ML, Menard C, Russo SJ. Inflammatory mediators in mood disorders: Therapeutic opportunities. Annual Review of Pharmacology and Toxicology. 2018;**58**:411-428. DOI: 10.1146/annurev-pharmtox-010617-052823

[46] Bierhaus A, Wolf J, Andrassy M, Rohleder N, Humpert PM, Petrov D, et al. A mechanism converting psychosocial stress into mononuclear cell activation. Proceedings of the National Academy of Sciences of the United States of America. 2003;**100**:1920-1925. DOI: 10.1073/pnas.0438019100

[47] Dunn AJ, Swiergiel AH, de Beaurepaire R. Cytokines as mediators of depression: What can we learn from animal studies? Neuroscience & Biobehavioral Reviews. 2005;**29**:891-909. DOI: 10.1016/j.neubiorev.2005.03.023

[48] Pace TW, Mletzko TC, Alagbe O, Musselman DL, Nemeroff CB, Miller AH, et al. Increased stress-induced inflammatory responses in male patients with major depression and increased early life stress. The American Journal of Psychiatry. 2006;**163**:1630-1633. DOI: 10.1176/ajp.2006.163.9.1630

[49] Banerjee SP, Kung LS, Riggi SJ, Chanda SK. Development of β-adrenergic receptor subsensitivity by antidepressants. Nature. 1977;**268**:455-456. DOI: 10.1038/268455a0

[50] Sporn JR, Harden TK, Wolfe BB, Molinoff PB. β-adrenergic receptor involvement in 6-hydroxydopamine-induced supersensitivity in rat cerebral cortex. Science. 1976;**194**:624-626. DOI: 10.1126/science.10626

[51] Hirata F, Axelrod J. Phospholipid methylation and biological signal transmission. Science. 1980;**209**:1082-1090. DOI: 10.1126/science.6157192

[52] Torda T, Yamaguchi I, Hirata F, Kopin IJ, Axelrod J. Quinacrine-blocked desensitization of adrenoceptors after immobilization stress or repeated injection of isoproterenol in rats. The Journal of Pharmacology and Experimental Therapeutics. 1981;**216**:334-338

[53] Manji HK, Chen GA, Bitran JA, Potter WZ. Down-regulation of beta receptors by desipramine in vitro involves PKC/phospholipase A2. Psychopharmacology Bulletin. 1991;**27**:247-253

[54] Nakamura S. Involvement of phospholipase A2 in axonal regeneration of brain noradrenergic neurones. Neuroreport. 1993, 1993;**4**:371-374. DOI: 10.1097/00001756-199304000-00007

[55] Layé S, Nadjar A, Joffre C, Bazinet RP. Anti-inflammatory effects

of omega-3 fatty acids in the brain: Physiological mechanisms and relevance to pharmacology. Pharmacological Reviews. 2018;**70**:12-38. DOI: 10.1124/pr.117.014092

[56] Hornfelt M, Ekström PA, Edström A. Involvement of axonal phospholipase A2 activity in the outgrowth of adult mouse sensory axons in vitro. Neuroscience. 1999;**91**:1539-1547. DOI: 10.1016/s0306-4522(98)00684-8

[57] Darios F, Davletov B. Omega-3 and omega-6 fatty acids stimulate cell membrane expansion by acting on syntaxin 3. Nature. 2006;**440**:813-817. DOI: 10.1038/nature04598

[58] Robson LG, Dyall S, Sidloff D, Michael-Titus AT. Omega-3 polyunsaturated fatty acids increase the neurite outgrowth of rat sensory neurones throughout development and in aged animals. Neurobiology of Aging. 2010;**31**:678-687. DOI: 10.1016/j.neurobiolaging.2008.05.027

[59] Liu ZH, Yip PK, Adams L, Davies M, Lee JW, Michael GJ, et al. A single bolus of docosahexaenoic acid promotes neuroplastic changes in the innervation of spinal cord interneurons and motor neurons and improves functional recovery after spinal cord injury. The Journal of Neuroscience. 2015;**35**:12733-12752. DOI: 10.1523/JNEUROSCI.0605-15.2015

[60] Pham TL, He J, Kakazu AH, Jun B, Bazan NG, Bazan HEP. Defining a mechanistic link between pigment epithelium-derived factor, docosahexaenoic acid, and corneal nerve regeneration. The Journal of Biological Chemistry. 2017;**292**:18486-18499. DOI: 10.1074/jbc.M117.801472

[61] Shinzawa K, Sumi H, Ikawa M, Matsuoka Y, Okabe M, Sakoda S, et al. Neuroaxonal dystrophy caused by group VIA phospholipase A2 deficiency in mice: A model of human neurodegenerative disease. The Journal of Neuroscience. 2008;**28**:2212-2220. DOI: 10.1523/JNEUROSCI.4354-07.2008

[62] Beck G, Shinzawa K, Hayakawa H, Baba K, Sumi-Akamaru H, Tsujimoto Y, et al. Progressive axonal degeneration of nigrostriatal dopaminergic neurons in calcium-independent phospholipase A2β knockout mice. PLoS One. 2016;**11**:e0153789. DOI: 10.1371/journal.pone.0153789

[63] McNamara RK, Hahn CG, Jandacek R, Rider T, Tso P, Stanford KE, et al. Selective deficits in the omega-3 fatty acid docosahexaenoic acid in the postmortem orbitofrontal cortex of patients with major depressive disorder. Biological Psychiatry. 2007;**62**:17-24. DOI: 10.1016/j.biopsych.2006.08.026

[64] Su K, Huang S, Peng C, Lai H, Huang C, Chen Y, et al. Phospholipase A2 and cyclooxygenase 2 genes influence the risk of interferon-α–induced depression by regulating polyunsaturated fatty acids levels. Biological Psychiatry. 2010;**67**:550-557. DOI: 10.1016/j.biopsych.2009.11.005

[65] Rapaport MH, Nierenberg AA, Schettler PJ, Kinkead B, Cardoos A, Walker R, et al. Inflammation as a predictive biomarker for response to omega-3 fatty acids in major depressive disorder: A proof-of-concept study. Molecular Psychiatry. 2016;**21**:71-79. DOI: 10.1038/mp.2015.22

[66] Guu T-W, Mischoulon D, Sarris J, Hibbeln J, McNamara RK, Hamazaki K, et al. International society for nutritional psychiatry research practice guidelines for omega-3 fatty acids in the treatment of major depressive disorder. Psychotherapy and Psychosomatics.

2019;**88**:263-273. DOI: 10.1159/000502652

[67] Carlezon WA Jr, Mague SD, Parow AM, Stoll AL, Cohen BM, Renshaw PF. Antidepressant-like effects of uridine and omega-3 fatty acids are potentiated by combined treatment in rats. Biological Psychiatry. 2005;**57**:343-350. DOI: 10.1016/j.biopsych.2004.11.038

[68] Huang SY, Yang HT, Chiu CC, Pariante CM, Su KP. Omega-3 fatty acids on the forced-swimming test. Journal of Psychiatric Research. 2008;**42**:58-63. DOI: 10.1016/j.jpsychires.2006.09.004

[69] Lee LH, Tan CH, Shui G, Wenk MR, Ong WY. Role of prefrontal cortical calcium independent phospholipase A2 in antidepressant-like effect of maprotiline. The International Journal of Neuropsychopharmacology. 2011;**11**:1-12. DOI: 10.1017/S1461145711001234

[70] McNamara RK, Strimpfel J, Jandacek R, Rider T, Tso P, Welge JA, et al. Detection and treatment of long-chain omega-3 fatty acid deficiency in adolescents with SSRI-resistant major depressive disorder. PharmaNutrition. 2014;**2**:38-46. DOI: 10.1016/j.phanu.2014.02.002

[71] Speck CE, Kukull WA, Brenner DE, Bowen JD, McCormick WC, Teri L, et al. History of depression as a risk factor for Alzheimer's disease. Epidemiology. 1995;**6**:366-369. DOI: 10.1097/00001648-199507000-00006

[72] Schuurman AG, van den Akker M, Ensinck KT, Metsemakers JF, Knottnerus JA, Leentjens AF, et al. Increased risk of Parkinson's disease after depression: A retrospective cohort study. Neurology. 2002;**58**:1501-1504. DOI: 10.1212/wnl.58.10.1501

[73] Cardoso C, Afonso C, Bandarra NM. Dietary DHA and health: Cognitive function ageing. Nutrition Research Reviews. 2016;**29**:281-294. DOI: 10.1017/S0954422416000184

[74] Yassine HN, Braskie MN, Mack WJ, Castor KJ, Fonteh AN, Schneider LS, et al. Association of docosahexaenoic acid supplementation with Alzheimer disease stage in apolipoprotein E ε4 carriers: A review. JAMA Neurology. 2017;**74**:339-347. DOI: 10.1001/jamaneurol.2016.4899

[75] Freund-Levi Y, Eriksdotter-Jönhagen M, Cederholm T, Basun H, Faxén-Irving G, Garlind A, et al. Omega-3 fatty acid treatment in 174 patients with mild to moderate Alzheimer disease: OmegAD study: A randomized double-blind trial. Archives of Neurology. 2006;**63**:1402-1408. DOI: 10.1001/archneur.63.10.1402

[76] Green JT, Orr SK, Bazinet RP. The emerging role of group VI calcium-independent phospholipase A2 in releasing docosahexaenoic acid from brain phospholipids. Journal of Lipid Research. 2008;**49**:939-944. DOI: 10.1194/jlr.R700017-JLR200

[77] Su KP. Biological mechanism of antidepressant effect of omega-3 fatty acids: How does fish oil act as a 'mind-body interface'? Neuro-Signals. 2009;**17**:144-152. DOI: 10.1159/000198167

[78] Kawamura N, Shinoda K, Sato H, Sasaki K, Suzuki M, Yamaki K, et al. Plasma metabolome analysis of patients with major depressive disorder. Psychiatry and Clinical Neurosciences. 2018;**72**:349-361. DOI: 10.1111/pcn.12638

[79] Stoessel D, Schulte C, Teixeira dos Santos MC, Scheller D, Rebollo-Mesa I, Deuschle C, et al. Promising metabolite profiles in the plasma and CSF of early clinical Parkinson's disease. Frontiers in

Aging Neuroscience. 2018;**10**:1. DOI: 10.3389/fnagi.2018.00051

[80] Molina JA, Jiménez-Jiménez FJ, Vargas C, Gómez P, de Bustos F, Ortí-Pareja M, et al. Cerebrospinal fluid levels of non-neurotransmitter amino acids in patients with Alzheimer's disease. Journal of Neural Transmission (Vienna). 1998;**105**:279-286. DOI: 10.1007/s007020050057

[81] Ellison DW, Beal MF, Martin JB. Phosphoethanolamine and ethanolamine are decreased in Alzheimer's disease and Huntington's disease. Brain Research. 1987;**417**:389-392. DOI: 10.1016/0006-8993(87)90471-9

[82] Nitsch RM, Blusztajn JK, Pittas AG, Slack BE, Growdon JH, Wurtman RJ. Evidence for a membrane defect in Alzheimer disease brain. Proceedings of the National Academy of Sciences of the United States of America. 1992;**89**: 1671-1675. DOI: 10.1073/pnas.89.5.1671

Section 2

Mid- and Long-Term Sequelae of COVID-19: Clinical Conditions and Proposed Approaches

Chapter 9

Chronic Mild Stress and COVID-19 Sequelae

Dragana Komnenov

Abstract

Although COVID-19 clinical presentation primarily involves the respiratory system causing bilateral pneumonia, it is becoming increasingly recognized that COVID-19 is in fact a systemic disease. Neurological presentations have been reported in patients with both mild and severe COVID-19 symptoms. As such, elderly individuals are at a significantly higher risk of developing severe COVID-19 as well as neurocognitive consequences due to the presence of comorbidities associated with aging and the direct consequences of infection. Several neurological disorders that have been described in the literature include insomnia, depression, anxiety, post-traumatic stress disorder and cognitive insufficiencies. The potential underlying mechanisms are still incompletely understood but are likely multifaceted, involving both direct neurotrophic effect of SARS-CoV-2 and the indirect consequences related to social isolation in long intensive care units, the use of mechanical ventilation and sedation and the resultant brain hypoxia, systemic inflammation and secondary effects of medications used in treatment of COVID-19. Furthermore, neuro-cardiovascular adaptations resulting from the chronic stress and depression milieu of COVID-19 is expected to contribute negatively to the cardiovascular health of the survivors. It is thus imperative to implement a rigorous monitoring program for COVID-19 survivors, particularly among the elderly population, to assess potential neuro-cognitive and cardiovascular deteriorations.

Keywords: COVID-19, neuroinflammation, chronic stress, depression, cardiovascular disease

1. Introduction

Since the unfolding of COVID-19 pandemic starting in early 2020 it has become increasingly apparent that the disease has evolved from primarily affecting the respiratory system to being a systemic disease. A common manifestation of the latter involves the neurologic system, ranging from headache and myalgia to neuroinflammation and encephalopathies. Additionally, neuropsychiatric manifestations such as anxiety, stress, depression and post-traumatic stress disorder (PTSD) have been reported [1–4]. Another common manifestation affects the cardiovascular system, with pathologies ranging from pericarditis, myocarditis, right-hearted dysfunction, enodothelialitis and prothrombotic state (as reviewed in [5]). Any potential long-term effects of these disorders are yet to manifest in the coming months and years. Based on the available data, the interactions among chronic mild stress, neurological consequences and cardiovascular manifestations due to COVID-19 pandemic are likely to contribute to a significant public health problem worldwide. These interactions are explored below throughout the chapter.

Stress, depression and anxiety are being recognized as risk factors for the development of cardiovascular disease (CVD). COVID-19 pandemic has induced many stressors on everyday life, including fear of infection, lack of social interactions due to quarantine, helplessness due to inevitability, loss of income, misinformation spread mostly by social media, and food and household item shortage. Furthermore, the viral infection itself can cause detriment to the cardiovascular system via cerebrovascular ischemia, coagulopathy and endothelial dysfunction. Therefore, both individuals who become infected and those who do not, but are exposed to the chronic mild stress (CMS) of COVID-19 pandemic may be at risk of developing neurologic and cardiovascular consequences (please see a model in **Figure 1**). In any event, the stressors of the pandemic can be modeled by the CMS rodent model of depression. The CMS paradigm is typically conducted for 4 weeks and consists of the exposure of rodents to mild stressors such as exposure to strobe light and white noise, acute withdrawal of water, damp bedding and social isolation [6–9]. This procedure causes depression as evidenced by anhedonia (in rodents manifested as reduced 1–2% sucrose solution consumption and spontaneous wheel running), circadian rhythm disturbances and demeanor. This rodent model of human depression was used extensively to demonstrate the cardiovascular dysfunction following 4 weeks of exposure to the mild stressors, characterized by increased mean arterial pressure and sympathetic nervous system activity and decreased heart rate variability [6, 7, 9]. One study found that the 4 week period of stress exposure followed by 4 week period of stress reduction (i.e. no exposure to stressors) recovered the behavioral manifestations of depressions, such as sucrose consumption and spontaneous wheel running, but did not result in the reversal of the cardiovascular dysfunction measured by heart rate variability [9]. Such long term effects of stress exposure, as is seen in the COVID-19 pandemic, could therefore be detrimental in the post-pandemic era, highlighting the importance of cardiovascular health monitoring in all individuals.

2. Cognitive and neuropsychiatric manifestations of COVID-19

Pandemics are considered to be one of the most devastating disaster types, since they have global consequences that particularly affect mental health. Although not of pandemic proportions, previous outbreaks of viral infections involving coronaviruses, SARS (SARS-CoV) and MERS (MERS-CoV), and other viruses such as Ebola and Zika, provided valuable insights into the potential devastating effects on mental health status [10, 11].

Multiple reports and meta-analyses described that most common neuropsychiatric manifestations of COVID-19 are insomnia, depression and anxiety, PTSD, and various psychoses. In terms of prevalence, almost one quarter (22.5%) of those infected were found to have experienced some neurological and/or psychiatric episodes among 40,469 patients of whom majority was in the United States [3]. Subsequent studies from Europe reported similar outcomes [12–14]. Critically ill

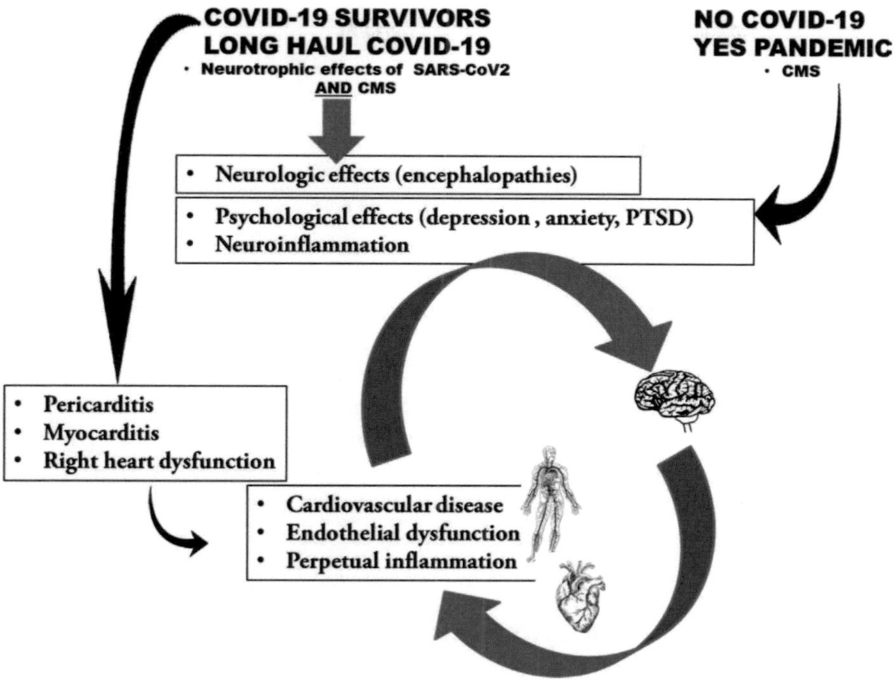

Figure 1.
Direct and indirect effects of COVID-19 on the central nervous and cardiovascular systems. Individuals who became infected with SARS-CoV2 virus could experience neurologic and cardiovascular dysfunction due to the direct neurotrophic effects of the virus as well as indirectly, via experiencing chronic stress associated with the pandemic (i.e. loss of loved ones, loss of income, lack of exercise, poor nutrition etc.). Individual who evaded infection, although spared from the direct effects of the virus, are also at an increased risk of developing neuropsychiatric and cardiovascular diseases via experiencing chronic stress associated with the pandemic. Therefore, those who survived COVID-19 and those who never got the disease but lived through the pandemic should be monitored both for mental health and cardiovascular health changes in the years to come.

individuals who required intensive care unit (ICU) admissions are particularly at risk of developing cognitive and neuropsychiatric manifestations, due to sedation, intubation, presence of comorbidities and older age [15–19]. One study from France reported that in a small cohort of 45 patients, 15 of them reported cognitive disturbances in form of dysexecutive syndrome (dysregulated movement patterns and lack of attention) at discharge from ICU [14]. Furthermore, almost half of them presented with confusion upon admission that was accompanied by brain hypoperfusion in several individuals revealed after brain imaging [14]. Depressive symptoms were also prevalent among individuals who recovered from COVID-19 in China [20–22]. Moreover, immune system suppression was evidenced in those with depressive symptoms indicated by increased white blood cell count and pro-inflammatory markers [21].

The impact of COVID-19 on one's neuropsychological well-being can be a direct result of SARS-CoV2 viral infection of the central nervous system (CNS) and/or an indirect result of endured psychological stress due to the devastating elements of the pandemic, such as fear of infection, social isolation, loss of income etc. The characteristic, mechanisms and implications of the first are detailed below throughout Section 2 of this Chapter, and those of the latter are elaborated on in Section 3 of this Chapter.

2.1 Mechanisms of cognitive and neuropsychiatric sequelae of COVID-19

Initially in early 2020, it was speculated but not confirmed that SARS-CoV2 is indeed a neurotrophic virus [23]. Shortly thereafter, the first case of viral encephalitis was reported in May of 2020 [24], making it obvious that the virus is capable of invading the CNS. Similar to other coronaviruses, SARS-CoV1 and MERS-CoV, SARS-CoV2 infection can cause CNS issues that range from mild such as loss of taste and smell (ageusia and anosmia, respectively), headache and dizziness, to very serious such as stroke, seizures, loss of balance and mental status alterations [25]. These consequences could result from: (i) the direct infection of neuronal cells by the virus, (ii) immune system dysregulation, (iii) autoimmunity resulting from the infection itself and/or (iv) any combination of the above three [26]. In addition to the direct invasion of neuronal cells, a secondary systemic mechanism could also be at play. This mechanism involves acute respiratory distress syndrome (ARDS). ARDS is accompanied by hypoxemia, oxidative stress and uremia resulting from multi-organ failure, including the cardiovascular system derangements and such complications could lead to encephalopathy. Immune system dysregulation may involve the cytokine storm and subsequent breakdown of the blood brain barrier (BBB) allowing entry of SARS-CoV2 into the CNS. This model is further supported by the fact that the virus binds ACE2 receptor that is present on capillary endothelium, thus leading to BBB damage and entry of the virus into the CNS [27]. Furthermore, immune system involvement could occur at the level of toll like receptors (TLRs), of which there are 10 identified members in humans, numbered 1–10 [28]. In particular, TLR 7/8 is recruited in response to single stranded RNA viruses, such as SARS-CoV2, leading to the production of pro-inflammatory mediators such as interleukin (IL)-1, IL-6, tumor necrosis factor alpha and interferon gamma [29]. Uncontrolled production of the pro-inflammatory mediators may lead to cytokine storm which causes ARDS, leading to encephalopathy secondary to an inflammatory response [30]. In another model, it was suggested that SRAS-CoV2 may operate similar to HIV in that HIV causes encephalopathy via a mixed approach: both directly via neuronal cell invasion and indirectly via the above discussed inflammatory mechanisms [26].

2.2 Potential long-term neuro-psychiatric effects: long haul COVID-19

The syndrome of persistent symptoms associated with COVID-19 that extend beyond the period of initial infection was originally termed long haul (LH) COVID-19 by a patient [31], the features of which have been identified in individuals irrespective of the initial illness severity [32]. One characteristic of LH COVID-19 is that the symptoms may either persist past the 3–4 week mark and/or new symptoms may develop after the 3–4 week mark. In fact, the National Institute for Health and Care Excellence has defined the LH or post-COVID-19 syndrome as "signs and symptoms that develop during or after an infection consistent with COVID-19, continue for more than 12 weeks (3 months) and are not explained by an alternative diagnosis" [33]. LH COVID-19 appears in the literature under several synonyms: post-COVID-19 condition (WHO defined), post-acute COVID-19 syndrome (PACS) [34] and post-acute sequelae of COVID-19 [32].

Neurological symptoms discussed above may contribute individually or synergistically to the persistence of neurological pathophysiology past the acute phase. The loss of BBB integrity and neuroinflammation [35–37], coupled with coagulopathy and the development of micro-emboli in the CNS [38, 39] may lead to the progression of LH COVID-19. Additionally, factors associated with hospital stay (i.e. intubation, mechanical ventilation and the use of sedatives) may further exacerbate the clinical course in those with severe acute symptoms. Neuro-psychiatric features of LH COVID-19 are likely related to prolonged stress associated with the pandemic and loss of family members/friends [40].

A recently published meta-analysis aimed to evaluate the neurological and neuropsychiatric features of LH COVID-19 in three cohorts: outpatient (community), non-ICU hospitalized an ICU hospitalized and at two different time points: 3–6 months and past the 6 month mark after the initial infection [41]. Primary outcomes included neurologic and psychiatric symptoms. Neurologic symptoms included: anosmia, dysgeusia, headache, cognitive dysfunction, fatigue, chronic fatigue syndrome, post exertional malaise, pain, peripheral nervous system symptoms. Neuropsychological symptoms included: anxiety, depression, sleep disturbances and/or insomnia and PTSD. A total number of full text articles screened were 80, and 18 studies, including 10,530 patients met the inclusion criteria. The most frequent neurological symptom of LH COVID-19 was fatigue (37%), followed by brain fog (32%), sleep disturbances (31%) and memory issues (28%). The prevalence of these symptoms tended to be higher in non-hospitalized individuals. Similarly, the neuropsychiatric symptoms of anxiety (31%) and depression (27%) were higher in the community cohort compared to the hospitalized patients (6% and 12%, respectively). Additionally, the neuropsychiatric symptoms substantially increased from mid-term follow-up to long term follow-up (i.e. past 6 months), suggesting that LH COVID-19 patients may experience increasing neuropsychiatric burden well past the initial infection. It is however not known when and whether it tapers off. On the other hand, the neurological symptoms in this cohort appear to progress from mid- to long-term highlighting that this may be the critical period of LH COVID-19 during which patients should be screen for neurological pathophysiological events and represents the critical therapeutic window. Other large retrospective cohort studies reported similar timelines [40, 42]. This may be explained by the chronic aspect of neuro-inflammation that ensues secondary to initial infection, leading to neuronal loss in that critical time period.

Taken together, the existing large cohort studies [40, 42] and meta-analyses [41] indicate that neurological and neuropsychiatric symptoms are a common feature of LH COVID-19, with specific symptoms occurring in as much as a third of the individuals who were infected with SARS-CoV2. Future research should be directed towards identifying the therapeutic strategies during the critical window, which appears to be 3–6 months post-acute illness, in an effort to decrease neuroinflammation, restore the blood brain barrier and prevent neuronal loss.

3. Chronic stress associated with COVID-19: multifaceted attack on the cardiovascular system

The cardiovascular system is one of the direct targets of SARS-CoV2 made possible by the viral entry into the cells via ACE2 receptors expressed on endothelial cells and cardiomyocytes. The myocardial injury associated with the acute COVID-19 illness has been well documented [43–46]. The responsible mechanisms include direct cytotoxicity [47] and/or dysregulation of the renin angiotensin system (RAS) [33] and the immune response [33, 34]. The initial insights into myocardial injury came from autopsy studies which reported the presence of SARS-CoV2 pools located not in the cardiomyocytes but rather in interstitial cells and resident macrophages [48].

Perseverance of these viral reservoirs is still debatable and potentially insidious as they could play an important role in myocardial and vascular sequel in LH COVID-19. Furthermore, psychological or mental stress-related consequences of the COVID-19 pandemic are expected to contribute to the rising cases of cardiovascular disease. The link between mental stress and coronary artery disease, atrial fibrillation and stroke has been reported in various studies [49–52]. A large multicenter, multinational study, INTERHEART, reported after adjustment for covariates a more than 2-fold increase in the risk of myocardial infarction as a consequence of mental stress [53]. Although the long-term implications of COVID-19 pandemic on cardiovascular health are yet to be realized, previous work done in this area foreshadows a significant uptick of CVD globally, and independently of other comorbidities.

3.1 Chronic stress-associated effects on the central nervous and the cardiovascular systems

In order to study stress as a risk factor, a proper definition must be set in place. The first distinction that must be made is between the stressor and the response of an individual to that stressor (i.e. how well they can cope with it). A stressor is not necessarily perilous *per se*, neither physiologically or psychologically, as there are many stressors that contribute to desirable outcomes. Much like physical exercise represents a stressor that leads to improved cardiovascular and musculoskeletal health, some psychological stress increases readiness and attention resulting in better outcomes in scholarly activities or sporting competitions. It is when individuals have unique perceptions of the stress and their inability to cope with it that creates a favorable milieu for psychological disturbance and new onset CVD. In fact, different personality types have been reported to be more susceptible to CVD as a consequence of mental stress, including Type A (hostile and angry outlook) [54] and Type D (tendency for pessimism and social inhibition) personalities [55]. Given that the COVID-19 pandemic has brought groups of stressors globally, the impact on psychological and cardiovascular well-being remains to be described.

The CMS rodent model is perhaps the most used in studying mental stress that humans endure and has the highest constructive, face and predicative validity [56]. It consists of exposing the animals to a series of mild, yet unpredictable stressors for at least 4 weeks. One could argue that this is a high-fidelity model of the pattern of stressful events that people experienced consistently during the COVID-19 pandemic, and in that view the data generated in CMS rats may necessitate a closer examination in terms of the CVD comorbidities after the chronic stress to inform future treatment strategies. Namely, the data has shown that rodents exposed to CMS develop depressive-like symptoms and behaviors with adverse cardiovascular symptoms including reduced heart rate variability, elevated resting heart rate, reduced baroreceptor function and increased sympathetic nervous system activity [6–8, 57]. The sympathetic drive has been shown to be mediated at least in part by the paraventricular nucleus (PVN), and via the vasopressinergic system rather than oxytocin [7, 8]. The CMS rats have also been shown to have increased expression of vasopressin receptors V1a and V1b in the PVN and that the simultaneous inhibition of both V1a and V1b receptors produced maximal inhibition of the neurocardiovascular responses to the exogenous vasopressin administration [7].

Stress can be categorized as acute, lasting seconds to weeks, and chronic, in the months to years range. COVID-19 pandemic-associated stress thus falls into the latter category, and further can be described as CMS. Chronic stressors associated with work and life related issues, such as injustice, effort-reward imbalance, marital stress at home, lack of life partnership, financial stress have all been shown to increase the risk of CVD [58–61]. Studies in humans have relied on measuring several parameters of the cardiovascular system function to assess the impact of mental stress, including cardiovascular reactivity, levels of catecholamines and inflammatory markers, heart and brain imaging, Holter monitoring and measures of endothelial function with flow-mediated dilatation [62–65]. It has been suggested that it is not the cardiac function but rather the vasculature, endothelium in particular, where the mental stress translates into CVD. Studies done in monkeys where they were exposed to a novel social environment showed increased endothelial damage in the thoracic aorta and coronary arteries [66]. Other studies in mice reported that both acute and chronic stress reduce the expression of nitric oxide synthase [67, 68], which is responsible for the synthesis of the vasodilatory molecule nitric oxide, leading to endothelial dysfunction. Stimulation of the sympathetic nervous system further increases local norepinephrine production and increase in the expression of adhesion molecules on the endothelium, and cytokine and chemokine production by macrophages and vascular smooth muscle cells. These feed forward cycles ultimately lead to leukocyte adhesion, vascular inflammation, atherosclerotic plaques instability, precipitating a cardiovascular event. Therefore, it is apparent that CMS endured during COVID-19 pandemic may cause similar vascular and endothelial dysfunction in humans as was shown in the above-described animal CMS models.

Chronic mild stress that individuals worldwide have endured during the COVID-19 pandemic has put them at a higher risk of developing anxiety and depression [69]. Lockdown policies instituted across the world resulted in isolation from human contact, worsening dementia and anxiety in individuals in long-term care facilities, exacerbation of conflict due to confinement and fear and confusion resulting from continuous bombardment with reporting information on all media, many of which were unreliable. Additionally, physical activity decreased partly due to the closure of fitness facilities as well as the lack of motivation and fear of SARS-CoV2 infection when leaving outside to obtain exercise. Some of the examples of reduced physical activity can be appreciated from the data from 30 million Fitbit activity tracker users, which showed a significant reduction in daily step counts by as much as 38% in Spain [70]. Similar data was obtained from analyzing step count trends from the app Argus in almost half a million users- a mean reduction in activity by 27.4% [71]. Some implied outcomes from these reductions in daily activity include exacerbation of hypertension. Several cross sectional studies indicated that reductions in step counts led to an increase of systolic blood pressure (SBP) of up to 7 mmHg [72, 73] and an increase of 4.5 mmHg for every additional hour of sitting every day [74]. Other behaviors during the pandemic that could have deleterious effects on blood pressure management include increase in body weight [75], increased sodium and decreased potassium intake [76, 77] which is particularly detrimental in the western countries where dietary intake of sodium is already high [78–81], and increase in alcohol consumption [82–84].

Most notably, CMS associated with the pandemic is expected to have adverse consequences on BP in both normotensive and hypertensive individuals. Although no study to date has reported direct associations related to COVID-19, published data indicate that chronic stress leads to an increase in the sympathetic drive as assessed with norepinephrine levels, changes in heart rate as well as via direct neurography [85–88]. Published clinical evidence repeatedly shows that depressed patients are at a higher risk of developing CVD which persists for a decade following the initial onset of depression [89–91]. This relationship is not unipolar, as patients with CVD have been shown to develop depressive symptoms [90–93]. Some of the mechanisms explaining the co-occurrence of depression and CVD include neuroinflammation [94] and autonomic dysfunction [95], but they are by no means an exhaustive list (**Figure 1**).

Important knowledge has been gleaned from reliable, validated rodent models of CMS [96], which are still utilized to tease apart the mechanistic links between CVD and stress/depression. Importantly, the new and ongoing investigations have been focusing on explaining the difference in vulnerability of individual animals to stress-associated CVD development [97–100], much like occurs in humans. Rodents exhibit two distinct coping styles when exposed to stress: [1] the proactive coping, which is characterized by more offensive, aggressive and impulsive behavior; and [2] and reactive coping, which is characterized by more cautious and fearful behavior [99, 101]. In addition to the behavioral differences, physiologically the two differ as well, where the proactive (active) copers exhibit heightened sympathetic activity and low HPA axis reactivity and the reactive (passive) copers show the opposite trends [99, 102]. The passive coping rats were also shown to have persistently elevated levels of pro-inflammatory cytokine IL-1β and oxidative stress [103], and it is thus plausible that neuroinflammation is at the intersection of depressive symptoms and CVD.

The sex-based dichotomy in the prevalence and severity of depression has been well-characterized [104, 105]. Furthermore, the efficacy of antidepressant pharmacotherapeutic agents also differs between men and women [106, 107]. Likewise, women are more likely to develop CVD that co-occurs with depression [108]. A growing body of evidence has emerged indicating that COVID-19 pandemic has increased the incidence of depression, with the meta-analysis of 12 community-based studies worldwide highlighting a prevalence of depression of 25% [109], with female gender emerging as a significant risk factor [110–112]. One study reported that women under 50 persist more devastating symptoms such as fatigue, myalgia, brain fog and fatigue after being hospitalized for COVID-19 [113]. Animal model studies of CMS that address this disparity in males and females are scarce, and some have shown differences in behavioral and hormonal profiles. Anhedonia associated with depressive-like state in CMS rodents is typically measured by an intake of 1–2% sucrose solution, and has been found to be more pronounced in females than in males [114]. The same study found no differences in the corticosterone levels however, indicating similar stress hormonal profiles. These findings are the extend of our understanding of sex-based differences in CVD susceptibility as a function of chronic stress thus representing a large gap in knowledge that future preclinical studies should address. Developing treatments that will target both the depressive symptomatology and the cardiovascular pathology, while also being titratable, will be of utmost importance since there may be a difference in the magnitude of effects caused by chronic stress associated with the pandemic between women than men.

3.2 Long haul COVID-19: emerging effects on the brain, heart and vasculature

During the acute phase of SARS-CoV2 infection, the viral entry into the CNS can be accomplished either directly or indirectly (via neuroinflammation) [115]. The direct viral entry, as mentioned previously, can occur via the olfactory [116] or terminal cranial nerves [117]. ACE2 expression has been recognized on endothelial cells, pericytes and astrocytes, allowing the viral invasion of the CNS via compromised BBB. Alternatively or even additionally, the virus could traverse the microvascular endothelial cells, as has been shown [118]. Consequently, the BBB leakage would allow the influx of the circulating pro-inflammatory cytokines, chemokines and mediators, further perpetuating neuroinflammation. *In vitro* studies also described the capabilities of SARS-CoV2 to initiate activation of astrocytes and microglia via its structural protein subunit (S1) [119]. This has been confirmed in autopsy studies of COVID-19 patients showing enlarged astrocytes and activated microglia [37]. Under normal physiological conditions, astrocytes play a crucial role in neurotransmission, as they control the synthesis of most essential neurotransmitters glutamate and GABA [120]. Additionally, astrocytes are involved in maintenance of synaptic plasticity via reuptake and recycling of neurotransmitters [121]. Under inflammatory conditions (i.e. SARS-CoV2 infection) astrocytes become reactive, which disrupts the glutamatergic balance, leading to excess extracellular glutamate contributing to dysfunction in both the CNS [58] and the cardiovascular systems [122]. Reactive astrocytosis is further supported by microglia via the NFkB pathway [123]. In the absence of the mechanisms that will shut down reactive astrocytosis (i.e. during COVID-19) the process could lead to the formation of astrocytic scars and in the long term neuronal death and neurodegeneration. Data describing the contribution of reactive astrocytosis in LH COVID-19 is lacking. One study so far has been published that measured plasma biomarkers of CNS injury in 100 COVID-19 survivors in Sweden. The biomarkers included nuerofilament light chain, glial fibrillary acidic protein (GFAP) and differentiation factor 15. In the acute phase, patients with severe symptoms had elevated neurfilament light chain compared to both age-matched controls and mild and moderate COVID-19, as well as higher GFAP than controls. However, after the median follow up of 225 days all CNS injury markers normalized and were indistinguishable from those found in healthy controls [124]. Since emerging data are pointing towards increased neuropathological manifestations one-year out compared to 6 months out [7], more studies are urgently needed to explain the mechanistic details and thus inform appropriate therapeutic strategies.

Data from the prospective post-acute follow up studies focusing on cardiac events have been more abundant in the literature compared to those on the CNS abnormalities. Several large (n > 400) observational studies are still ongoing in 2022. Transthoracic echocardiography and cardiac magnetic resonance are the gold standard techniques used in the diagnosis of cardiac pathologies [125, 126]. The vast majority of the studies have reported the presence of pericarditis, right ventricular dysfunction and myocardial infarctions [127–133]. Persistent myocarditis was reported in a cohort of 100 patients [127], while in another study of healthcare workers matched for comorbidities and severity of infection showed no difference in cardiac abnormalities 6 months post-infection [128]. Studies in athletes [129–132] were undertaken within 1–2 months of infection, and the prevalence of myocarditis is generally considered to be low (0–3%), albeit studies beyond the 2 month mark are lacking. Echocardiographic studies have consistently reported right heart abnormalities [133–135] while the left systolic function is significantly less impaired [133, 136], even in patients with severe acute symptomatology. On the other hand, perhaps the emerging trend that will have to be closely monitored in LH COVID-19 is the diastolic dysfunction, as it was shown to be common in up to 60% of hospitalized patients [137]. It is thus plausible to speculate that the pathologic changes in diastology could manifest during LH COVID-19, given the time lapse from the initial infection. In terms of vasculature, one angiography study reported an association between vascular inflammation caused by the variant B1.1.7 (WHO label Alpha) and increased mortality risk [138]. Although multiple studies have been published so far that have highlighted or implied the development of cardiovascular pathologies in LH COVID-19, one common denominator of limitations in most of them is that the comparator groups were either healthy individuals or individuals unmatched for comorbidities. Perhaps the most important consideration should be the lack of pre-COVID cardiac imaging studies, which makes it difficult to discern whether the pathologies observed were due to COVID-19 or other comorbidities, or perhaps both. Nevertheless, given the non-invasive nature of echocardiography, it likely behooves the cardiac clinicians to implement cardiac imaging in LH COVID-19 given the evidence from prospective studies and the available therapeutics for ensuing cardiac pathologies.

The concerning aspect of the known and implied consequences of COVID-19 discussed above and LH COVID-19 is that these pathological processes do not exist in isolation and ultimately lead to multisystem dysfunction. A multi-organ magnetic resonance imaging study on a small cohort of recovered COVID-19 patients and matched controls revealed some level of abnormalities in the lung (60%), heart (26%), liver (10%), kidneys (29%) and brain (11%) [18]. Recovery from multisystem damage has been shown to be impeded by the persistent pro-inflammatory state [139] as well as endothelial dysfunction [140–142] and perpetual prothrombotic state [143]. These studies highlight the importance of approaching treatment strategies from the multisystem perspective rather than treating isolated pathologies. For example, anti-thrombotic therapy may be beneficial for individuals who present with the prothrombotic phenotype and have persistent inflammation in their LH COVID-19 phase.

4. Conclusions

According to the above discussed evidence and implications, the potential neurologic and cardiovascular consequences (**Figure 1**), coupled with the ensuing healthcare burden of COVID-19 necessitate a careful crafting of the clinical approach in the coming months and years. Both individuals who survived the infection and those who survived the pandemic without becoming infected with SARS-CoV2 (but were exposed to CMS) are at an appreciable risk of developing neurogenic and neuropsychiatric disturbances (**Figure 1**), and thus mental health checks for virtually all individuals on an ongoing basis are warranted. Furthermore, female gender may add another layer of risk for developing depression and CVD as a consequence of pandemic-associated CMS exposure. Studies conducted so far underscore the utility of echocardiography in revealing COVID-19-associated pericarditis, myocarditis and right heart dysfunction. Furthermore, resolution of inflammation should be at the forefront of treatment strategies, since prolonged inflammatory state is associated with poorer outcomes and LH COVID-19 symptomatology. Ultimately, clinical vigilance in monitoring individuals' mental and cardiovascular health will be of utmost importance in the post-pandemic years and research strategies aimed at mitigating the defunct mechanisms at the intersection of neurological and cardiovascular pathologies are merited.

Author details

Dragana Komnenov
Wayne State University School of Medicine, Detroit, MI, United States of America

*Address all correspondence to: dkomneno@med.wayne.edu

References

[1] Rogers JP, Chesney E, Oliver D, Pollak TA, McGuire P, Fusar-Poli P, et al. Psychiatric and neuropsychiatric presentations associated with severe coronavirus infections: A systematic review and meta-analysis with comparison to the COVID-19 pandemic. Lancet Psychiatry. 2020;7(7):611-627. DOI: 10.1016/S2215-0366(20)30203-0

[2] Liguori C, Pierantozzi M, Spanetta M, Sarmati L, Cesta N, Iannetta M, et al. Subjective neurological symptoms frequently occur in patients with SARS-CoV2 infection. Brain, Behavior, and Immunity. 2020;**88**:11-16. DOI: 10.1016/j.bbi.2020.05.037

[3] Nalleballe K, Reddy Onteddu S, Sharma R, Dandu V, Brown A, Jasti M, et al. Spectrum of neuropsychiatric manifestations in COVID-19. Brain, Behavior, and Immunity. 2020;**88**:71-74. DOI: 10.1016/j.bbi.2020.06.020

[4] Dinakaran D, Manjunatha N, Naveen Kumar C, Suresh BM. Neuropsychiatric aspects of COVID-19 pandemic: A selective review. Asian Journal of Psychiatry. 2020;**53**:102188. DOI: 10.1016/j.ajp.2020.102188

[5] Raman B, Bluemke DA, Luscher TF, Neubauer S. Long COVID: Post-acute sequelae of COVID-19 with a cardiovascular focus. European Heart Journal. 2022;**43**(11):1157-1172. DOI: 10.1093/eurheartj/ehac031

[6] Grippo AJ, Moffitt JA, Johnson AK. Evaluation of baroreceptor reflex function in the chronic mild stress rodent model of depression. Psychosomatic Medicine. 2008;**70**(4):435-443. DOI: 10.1097/PSY.0b013e31816ff7dd

[7] Komnenov D, Quaal H, Rossi NF. V-1a and V-1b vasopressin receptors within the paraventricular nucleus contribute to hypertension in male rats exposed to chronic mild unpredictable stress. American Journal of Physiology-Regulatory, Integrative and Comparative Physiology. 2021;**320**(3):R213-RR25. DOI: 10.1152/ajpregu.00245.2020

[8] Das S, Komnenov D, Newhouse L, Rishi AK, Rossi NF. Paraventricular nucleus V1a receptor knockdown blunts neurocardiovascular responses to acute stress in male rats after chronic mild unpredictable stress. Physiology & Behavior. 2022;**253**:113867. DOI: 10.1016/j.physbeh.2022.113867

[9] Grippo AJ, Beltz TG, Johnson AK. Behavioral and cardiovascular changes in the chronic mild stress model of depression. Physiology & Behavior. 2003;**78**(4-5):703-710. DOI: 10.1016/s0031-9384(03)00050-7

[10] Esterwood E, Saeed SA. Past epidemics, natural disasters, COVID19, and mental health: Learning from history as we Deal with the present and prepare for the future. Psychiatric Quarterly. 2020;**91**(4):1121-1133. DOI: 10.1007/s11126-020-09808-4

[11] Morganstein JC, Fullerton CS, Ursano RJ, Donato D, Holloway HC. Pandemics: Health Care Emergencies. Textbook of Disaster Psychiatry. 2nd ed. Cambridge, UK: Cambridge University Press; 2017. pp. 270-284. DOI: 10.1017/9781316481424

[12] Varatharaj A, Thomas N, Ellul MA, Davies NWS, Pollak TA, Tenorio EL, et al. Neurological and neuropsychiatric complications of COVID-19 in 153 patients: A UK-wide surveillance study. Lancet Psychiatry. 2020;7(10):875-882. DOI: 10.1016/S2215-0366(20)30287-X

[13] Parra A, Juanes A, Losada CP, Alvarez-Sesmero S, Santana VD, Marti I, et al. Psychotic symptoms in COVID-19 patients. A retrospective descriptive study. Psychiatry Research. 2020;**291**:113254. DOI: 10.1016/j.psychres.2020.113254

[14] Helms J, Meziani F. Neurologic features in severe SARS-CoV-2 infection. New England Journal of Medicine. 2020;**382**(23):2268-2270. DOI: 10.1056/NEJMc2008597

[15] Taquet M, Luciano S, Geddes JR, Harrison PJ. Bidirectional associations between COVID-19 and psychiatric disorder: Retrospective cohort studies of 62 354 COVID-19 cases in the USA. Lancet Psychiatry. 2020;**8**(1):E1-EE. DOI: 10.1016/S2215-0366(20)30462-4

[16] Kremer S, Lersy F, Anheim M, Merdji H, Schenck M, Oesterle H, et al. Neurologic and neuroimaging findings in patients with COVID-19 a retrospective multicenter study. Neurology. 2020;**95**(13):E1868-E1E82. DOI: 10.1212/Wnl.0000000000010112

[17] Pezzini A, Padovani A. Lifting the mask on neurological manifestations of COVID-19. Nature Reviews. Neurology. 2020;**16**(11):636-644. DOI: 10.1038/s41582-020-0398-3

[18] Raman B, Cassar MP, Tunnicliffe EM, Filippini N, Griffanti L, Alfaro-Almagro F, et al. Medium-term effects of SARS-CoV-2 infection on multiple vital organs, exercise capacity, cognition, quality of life and mental health, post-hospital discharge. Eclinicalmedicine. 2021;**31**. DOI: 10.1016/j.eclinm.2020.100683

[19] Cipriani G, Di Fiorino M. Access to care for dementia patients suffering from COVID-19. American Journal of Geriatric Psychiatry. 2020;**28**(7):796-797

[20] Cai X, Hu XP, Ekumi IO, Wang JC, An YW, Li ZW, et al. Psychological distress and its correlates among COVID-19 survivors during early convalescence across age groups. American Journal of Geriatric Psychiatry. 2020;**28**(10):1030-1039. DOI: 10.1016/j.jagp.2020.07.003

[21] Yuan B, Li WX, Liu HQ, Cai X, Song S, Zhao J, et al. Correlation between immune response and self-reported depression during convalescence from COVID-19. Brain Behavior and Immunity. 2020;**88**:39-43. DOI: 10.1016/j.bbi.2020.05.062

[22] Zhang J, Lu HP, Zeng HP, Zhang SN, Du QF, Jiang TY, et al. The differential psychological distress of populations affected by the COVID-19 pandemic. Brain Behavior and Immunity. 2020;**87**:49-50. DOI: 10.1016/j.bbi.2020.04.031

[23] Kabbani N, Olds JL. Does COVID19 infect the brain? If so, smokers might be at a higher risk. Molecular Pharmacology. 2020;**97**(5):351-353. DOI: 10.1124/molpharm.120.000014

[24] Moriguchi T, Harii N, Goto J, Harada D, Sugawara H, Takamino J, et al. A first case of meningitis/encephalitis associated with SARS-Coronavirus-2. International Journal of Infectious Diseases. 2020;**94**:55-58. DOI: 10.1016/j.ijid.2020.03.062

[25] Mirfazeli FS, Sarabi-Jamab A, Jahanbakhshi A, Kordi A, Javadnia P, Shariat SV, et al. Neuropsychiatric manifestations of COVID-19 can be clustered in three distinct symptom categories. Scientific Reports. 2020;**10**(1). DOI: 10.1038/s41598-020-78050-6

[26] Troyer EA, Kohn JN, Hong SZ. Are we facing a crashing wave of neuropsychiatric sequelae of COVID-19?

Neuropsychiatric symptoms and potential immunologic mechanisms. Brain Behavior and Immunity. 2020;**87**:34-39. DOI: 10.1016/j.bbi.2020.04.027

[27] Baig AM, Khaleeq A, Ali U, Syeda H. Evidence of the COVID-19 virus targeting the CNS: Tissue distribution, host-virus interaction, and proposed neurotropic mechanisms. ACS Chemical Neuroscience. 2020;**11**(7):995-998. DOI: 10.1021/acschemneuro.0c00122

[28] Onofrio L, Caraglia M, Facchini G, Margherita V, De Placido S, Buonerba C. Toll-like receptors and COVID-19: A two-faced story with an exciting ending. Future Science OA. 2020;**6**(8). DOI: 10.2144/fsoa-2020-0091

[29] van Vuren EJ, Steyn SF, Brink CB, Moller M, Viljoen FP, Harvey BH. The neuropsychiatric manifestations of COVID-19: Interactions with psychiatric illness and pharmacological treatment. Biomedicine & Pharmacotherapy. 2021;**135**. DOI: 10.1016/j.biopha.2020.111200

[30] Wang YX, Wang YY, Chen Y, Qin QS. Unique epidemiological and clinical features of the emerging 2019 novel coronavirus pneumonia (COVID-19) implicate special control measures. Journal of Medical Virology. 2020;**92**(6):568-576. DOI: 10.1002/jmv.25748

[31] Long COVID: Let patients help define long-lasting COVID symptoms. Nature. 2020;**586**(7828):170. DOI: 10.1038/d41586-020-02796-2

[32] Al-Aly Z, Xie Y, Bowe B. High-dimensional characterization of post-acute sequelae of COVID-19. Nature. 2021;**594**(7862):259-264. DOI: 10.1038/s41586-021-03553-9

[33] Shah W, Hillman T, Playford ED, Hishmeh L. Managing the long term effects of covid-19: Summary of NICE, SIGN, and RCGP rapid guideline. BMJ: British Medical Journal. 2021;**372**. DOI: 10.1136/bmj.n136

[34] Nalbandian A, Sehgal K, Gupta A, Madhavan MV, McGroder C, Stevens JS, et al. Post-acute COVID-19 syndrome. Nature Medicine. 2021;**27**(4):601-615. DOI: 10.1038/s41591-021-01283-z

[35] Buzhdygan TP, DeOre BJ, Baldwin-Leclair A, Bullock TA, McGary HM, Khan JA, et al. The SARS-CoV-2 spike protein alters barrier function in 2D static and 3D microfluidic in-vitro models of the human blood-brain barrier. Neurobiology of Disease. 2020;**146**. DOI: 10.1016/j.nbd.2020.105131

[36] Crook H, Raza S, Nowell J, Young M, Edison P. Long covid-mechanisms, risk factors, and management. BMJ: British Medical Journal. 2021;**374**. DOI: 10.1136/bmj.n1648

[37] Perl DP, Folkerth RD, Nath A. Microvascular injury in the brains of patients with Covid-19. New England Journal of Medicine. 2021;**384**(5):481-483. DOI: 10.1056/NEJMc2033369

[38] Dixon L, McNamara C, Gaur P, Mallon D, Coughlan C, Tona F, et al. Cerebral microhaemorrhage in COVID-19: A critical illness related phenomenon? Stroke and Vascular Neurology. 2020;**5**(4):315-322. DOI: 10.1136/svn-2020-000652

[39] Sawlani V, Scotton S, Nader K, Jen JP, Patel M, Gokani K, et al. COVID-19-related intracranial imaging findings: A large single-centre experience. Clinical Radiology. 2021;**76**(2):108-116. DOI: 10.1016/j.crad.2020.09.002

[40] Taquet M, Geddes JR, Husain M, Luciano S, Harrison PJ. 6-month neurological and psychiatric outcomes in 236 379 survivors of COVID-19: A retrospective cohort study using electronic health records. Lancet Psychiatry. 2021;**8**(5):416-427. DOI: 10.1016/S2215-0366(21)00084-5

[41] Premraj L, Kannapadi NV, Briggs J, Seal SM, Battaglini D, Fanning J, et al. Mid and long-term neurological and neuropsychiatric manifestations of post-COVID-19 syndrome: A meta-analysis. Journal of the Neurological Sciences. 2022;**434**. DOI: 10.1016/j.jns.2022.120162

[42] Estiri H, Strasser ZH, Brat GA, Semenov YR, Patel CJ, Murphy SN, et al. Evolving phenotypes of non-hospitalized patients that indicate long COVID. BMC Medicine. 2021;**19**(1). DOI: 10.1186/s12916-021-02115-0

[43] Lala A, Johnson KW, Januzzi JL, Russak AJ, Paranjpe I, Richter F, et al. Prevalence and impact of myocardial injury in patients hospitalized with COVID-19 infection. Journal of the American College of Cardiology. 2020;**76**(5):533-546. DOI: 10.1016/j.jacc.2020.06.007

[44] Shi S, Qin M, Shen B, Cai Y, Liu T, Yang F, et al. Association of cardiac injury with mortality in hospitalized patients with COVID-19 in Wuhan, China. JAMA Cardiology. 2020;**5**(7):802-810. DOI: 10.1001/jamacardio.2020.0950

[45] Shi S, Qin M, Cai Y, Liu T, Shen B, Yang F, et al. Characteristics and clinical significance of myocardial injury in patients with severe coronavirus disease 2019. European Heart Journal. 2020;**41**(22):2070-2079. DOI: 10.1093/eurheartj/ehaa408

[46] Wang D, Hu B, Hu C, Zhu F, Liu X, Zhang J, et al. Clinical characteristics of 138 hospitalized patients with 2019 novel coronavirus-infected pneumonia in Wuhan, China. JAMA. 2020;**323**(11):1061-1069. DOI: 10.1001/jama.2020.1585

[47] Dong E, Du H, Gardner L. An interactive web-based dashboard to track COVID-19 in real time. The Lancet Infectious Diseases. 2020;**20**(5):533-534. DOI: 10.1016/S1473-3099(20)30120-1

[48] Kawakami R, Sakamoto A, Kawai K, Gianatti A, Pellegrini D, Nasr A, et al. Pathological evidence for SARS-CoV-2 as a cause of myocarditis JACC review topic of the week. Journal of the American College of Cardiology. 2021;**77**(3):314-325. DOI: 10.1016/j.jacc.2020.11.031

[49] Dragano N, Siegrist J, Nyberg ST, Lunau T, Fransson EI, Alfredsson L, et al. Effort-reward imbalance at work and incident coronary heart disease a multicohort study of 90,164 individuals. Epidemiology. 2017;**28**(4):619-626. DOI: 10.1097/Ede.0000000000000666

[50] Huang YL, Xu SX, Hua JH, Zhu DJ, Liu CH, Hu YZ, et al. Association between job strain and risk of incident stroke a meta-analysis. Neurology. 2015;**85**(19):1648-1654. DOI: 10.1212/Wnl.0000000000002098

[51] Kivimaki M, Kawachi I. Work stress as a risk factor for cardiovascular disease. Current Cardiology Reports. 2015;**17**(9). DOI: 10.1007/s11886-015-0630-8

[52] Kivimaki M, Jokela M, Nyberg ST, Singh-Manoux A, Fransson EI, Alfredsson L, et al. Long working hours and risk of coronary heart disease and stroke: A systematic review and meta-analysis of published and unpublished data for 603 838 individuals. Lancet. 2015;**386**(10005):1739-1746. DOI: 10.1016/S0140-6736(15)60295-1

[53] Rosengren A, Hawken S, Ounpuu S, Sliwa K, Zubaid M, Almahmeed WA, et al. Association of psychosocial risk factors with risk of acute myocardial infarction in 11119 cases and 13 648 controls from 52 countries (the INTERHEART study): Case-control study. Lancet. 2004;**364**(9438):953-962. DOI: 10.1016/S0140-6736(04)17019-0

[54] Chida Y, Steptoe A. The association of anger and hostility with future coronary heart disease a meta-analytic review of prospective evidence. Journal of the American College of Cardiology. 2009;**53**(11):936-946. DOI: 10.1016/j.jacc.2008.11.044

[55] Grande G, Romppel M, Barth J. Association between type D personality and prognosis in patients with cardiovascular diseases: A systematic review and meta-analysis. Annals of Behavioral Medicine. 2012;**43**(3):299-310. DOI: 10.1007/s12160-011-9339-0

[56] Willner P. Chronic mild stress (CMS) revisited: Consistency and behavioural-neurobiological concordance in the effects of CMS. Neuropsychobiology. 2005;**52**(2):90-110. DOI: 10.1159/000087097

[57] Bouzinova EV, Moller-Nielsen N, Boedtkjer DB, Broegger T, Wiborg O, Aalkjaer C, et al. Chronic mild stress-induced depression-like symptoms in rats and abnormalities in catecholamine uptake in small arteries. Psychosomatic Medicine. 2012;**74**(3):278-287. DOI: 10.1097/PSY.0b013e31824c40a9

[58] Sara JD, Prasad M, Eleid MF, Zhang M, Widmer RJ, Lerman A. Association between work-related stress and coronary heart disease: A review of prospective studies through the job strain, effort-reward balance, and organizational justice models. Journal of the American Heart Association. 2018;**7**(9):e008073. DOI: 10.1161/JAHA.117.008073

[59] Orth-Gomer K, Wamala SP, Horsten M, Schenck-Gustafsson K, Schneiderman N, Mittleman MA. Marital stress worsens prognosis in women with coronary heart disease—the Stockholm female coronary risk study. JAMA—Journal of the American Medical Association. 2000;**284**(23):3008-3014. DOI: 10.1001/jama.284.23.3008

[60] Albert MA, Durazo EM, Slopen N, Zaslavsky AM, Buring JE, Silva T, et al. Cumulative psychological stress and cardiovascular disease risk in middle aged and older women: Rationale, design, and baseline characteristics. American Heart Journal. 2017;**192**:1-12. DOI: 10.1016/j.ahj.2017.06.012

[61] Carlsson AC, Starrin B, Gigante B, Leander K, Hellenius ML, de Faire U. Financial stress in late adulthood and diverse risks of incident cardiovascular disease and all-cause mortality in women and men. BMC Public Health. 2014;**14**. DOI: 10.1186/1471-2458-14-17

[62] Widmer RJ, Prasad M, Gomaa M, Sara JDS, Reriani MK, Lerman LO, et al. Vascular reactivity to mental stress is associated with poor cardiovascular disease outcomes in females following acute coronary syndrome. Coronary Artery Disease. 2020;**31**(3):300-305. DOI: 10.1097/Mca.0000000000000831

[63] Bandodkar AJ, Wang J. Non-invasive wearable electrochemical sensors: A review. Trends in Biotechnology. 2014;**32**(7):363-371. DOI: 10.1016/j.tibtech.2014.04.005

[64] Mitchell JS, Lowe TE, Ingram JR. Rapid ultrasensitive measurement of salivary cortisol using nano-linker chemistry coupled with surface plasmon resonance detection. The Analyst.

2009;**134**(2):380-386. DOI: 10.1039/b817083p

[65] Rozanski A, Bairey CN, Krantz DS, Friedman J, Resser KJ, Morell M, et al. Mental stress and the induction of silent myocardial ischemia in patients with coronary-artery disease. New England Journal of Medicine. 1988;**318**(16):1005-1012. DOI: 10.1056/Nejm198804213181601

[66] Strawn WB, Bondjers G, Kaplan JR, Manuck SB, Schwenke DC, Hansson GK, et al. Endothelial dysfunction in response to psychosocial stress in monkeys. Circulation Research. 1991;**68**(5):1270-1279. DOI: 10.1161/01.Res.68.5.1270

[67] Custodis F, Gertz K, Balkaya M, Prinz V, Mathar I, Stamm C, et al. Heart rate contributes to the vascular effects of chronic mental stress effects on endothelial function and ischemic brain injury in mice. Stroke. 2011;**42**(6):1742-1749. DOI: 10.1161/Strokeaha.110.598607

[68] Chung IM, Kim YM, Yoo MH, Shin MK, Kim CK, Suh SH. Immobilization stress induces endothelial dysfunction by oxidative stress via the activation of the angiotensin II/its type I receptor pathway. Atherosclerosis. 2010;**213**(1):109-114. DOI: 10.1016/j.atherosclerosis.2010.08.052

[69] Brooks SK, Webster RK, Smith LE, Woodland L, Wessely S, Greenberg N, et al. The psychological impact of quarantine and how to reduce it: Rapid review of the evidence. Lancet. 2020;**395**(10227):912-920. DOI: 10.1016/S0140-6736(20)30460-8

[70] Kreutz R, Dobrowolski P, Prejbisz A, Algharably EAEH, Bilo G, Creutzig F, et al. Lifestyle, psychological, socioeconomic and environmental factors and their impact on hypertension during the coronavirus disease 2019 pandemic. Journal of Hypertension. 2021;**39**(6):1077-1089. DOI: 10.1097/Hjh.0000000000002770

[71] Tison GH, Avram R, Kuhar P, Abreau S, Marcus GM, Pletcher MJ, et al. Worldwide effect of COVID-19 on physical activity: A descriptive study. Annals of Internal Medicine. 2020;**173**(9):767. DOI: 10.7326/M20-2665

[72] Menai M, Brouard B, Vegreville M, Chieh A, Schmidt N, Oppert JM, et al. Cross-sectional and longitudinal associations of objectively-measured physical activity on blood pressure: Evaluation in 37 countries. Health Promotion Perspectives. 2017;**7**(4):190-196. DOI: 10.15171/hpp.2017.34

[73] Zucatti ATN, de Paula TP, Viana LV, DallAgnol R, Cureau FV, Azevedo MJ, et al. Low levels of usual physical activity are associated with higher 24 h blood pressure in type 2 diabetes mellitus in a cross-sectional study. Journal Diabetes Research. 2017;**2017**:6232674. DOI: 10.1155/2017/6232674

[74] Maasakkers CM, de Heus RAA, Thijssen DHJ, Melis RJF, Gardiner PA, Claassen J. Objectively-measured activity patterns are associated with home blood pressure in memory clinic patients. Journal of Alzheimer's Disease. 2020;**74**(2):691-697. DOI: 10.3233/JAD-191310

[75] Sidor A, Rzymski P. Dietary choices and habits during COVID-19 lockdown: Experience from Poland. Nutrients. 2020;**12**(6). DOI: 10.3390/nu12061657

[76] Yilmaz C, Gokmen V. Neuroactive compounds in foods: Occurrence, mechanism and potential health effects. Food Research International. 2020;**128**:108744. DOI: 10.1016/j.foodres.2019.108744

[77] Rodriguez-Martin BC, Meule A. Food craving: New contributions on its assessment, moderators, and consequences. Frontiers in Psychology. 2015;**6**:21. DOI: 10.3389/fpsyg.2015.00021

[78] Aburto NJ, Hanson S, Gutierrez H, Hooper L, Elliott P, Cappuccio FP. Effect of increased potassium intake on cardiovascular risk factors and disease: Systematic review and meta-analyses. BMJ. 2013;**346**:f1378. DOI: 10.1136/bmj.f1378

[79] Adler AJ, Taylor F, Martin N, Gottlieb S, Taylor RS, Ebrahim S. Reduced dietary salt for the prevention of cardiovascular disease. Cochrane Database of Systematic Reviews. 2014;(12):CD009217. DOI: 10.1002/14651858.CD009217.pub3

[80] Binia A, Jaeger J, Hu Y, Singh A, Zimmermann D. Daily potassium intake and sodium-to-potassium ratio in the reduction of blood pressure: A meta-analysis of randomized controlled trials. Journal of Hypertension. 2015;**33**(8):1509-1520. DOI: 10.1097/HJH.0000000000000611

[81] He FJ, MacGregor GA. Fortnightly review: Beneficial effects of potassium. BMJ. 2001;**323**(7311):497-501. DOI: 10.1136/bmj.323.7311.497

[82] Hamer M, Kivimaki M, Gale CR, Batty GD. Lifestyle risk factors, inflammatory mechanisms, and COVID-19 hospitalization: A community-based cohort study of 387,109 adults in UK. Brain, Behavior, and Immunity. 2020;**87**:184-187. DOI: 10.1016/j.bbi.2020.05.059

[83] Colbert S, Wilkinson C, Thornton L, Richmond R. COVID-19 and alcohol in Australia: Industry changes and public health impacts. Drug and Alcohol Review. 2020;**39**(5):435-440. DOI: 10.1111/dar.13092

[84] The lancet gastroenterology H. drinking alone: COVID-19, lockdown, and alcohol-related harm. Lancet Gastroenterología y Hepatología. 2020;**5**(7):625. DOI: 10.1016/S2468-1253(20)30159-X

[85] Mancia G, Grassi G, Pomidossi G, Gregorini L, Bertinieri G, Parati G, et al. Effects of blood-pressure measurement by the doctor on patients blood-pressure and heart-rate. Lancet. 1983;**2**(8352):695-698

[86] Grassi G, Turri C, Vailati S, Dell'Oro R, Mancia G. Muscle and skin sympathetic nerve traffic during the "white-coat" effect. Circulation. 1999;**100**(3):222-225. DOI: 10.1161/01.Cir.100.3.222

[87] Esler M, Eikelis N, Schlaich M, Lambert G, Alvarenga M, Dawood T, et al. Chronic mental stress is a cause of essential hypertension: Presence of biological markers of stress. Clinical and Experimental Pharmacology and Physiology. 2008;**35**(4):498-502. DOI: 10.1111/j.1440-1681.2008.04904.x

[88] Esler M, Eikelis N, Schlaich M, Lambert G, Alvarenga M, Kaye D, et al. Human sympathetic nerve biology parallel influences of stress and epigenetics in essential hypertension and panic disorder. Annals of the New York Academy of Sciences. 2008;**1148**:338-348. DOI: 10.1196/annals.1410.064

[89] Ford DE, Mead LA, Chang PP, Cooper-Patrick L, Wang NY, Klag MJ. Depression is a risk factor for coronary artery disease in men—The precursors study. Archives of Internal Medicine. 1998;**158**(13):1422-1426. DOI: 10.1001/archinte.158.13.1422

[90] Cohen BE, Edmondson D, Kronish IM. State of the art review: Depression, stress, anxiety, and cardiovascular disease. American Journal of Hypertension. 2015;**28**(11):1295-1302. DOI: 10.1093/ajh/hpv047

[91] Hare DL, Toukhsati SR, Johansson P, Jaarsma T. Depression and cardiovascular disease: A clinical review. European Heart Journal. 2014;**35**(21):1365-1372. DOI: 10.1093/eurheartj/eht462

[92] Whooley MA, de Jonge P, Vittinghoff E, Otte C, Moos R, Carney RM, et al. Depressive symptoms, health behaviors, and risk of cardiovascular events in patients with coronary heart disease. Journal of the American Medical Association. 2008;**300**(20):2379-2388. DOI: 10.1001/jama.2008.711

[93] Wu JR, Frazier SK, Rayens MK, Lennie TA, Chung ML, Moser DK. Medication adherence, social support, and event-free survival in patients with heart failure. Health Psychology. 2013;**32**(6):637-646. DOI: 10.1037/a0028527

[94] Slavich GM, Irwin MR. From stress to inflammation and major depressive disorder: A social signal transduction theory of depression. Psychological Bulletin. 2014;**140**(3):774-815. DOI: 10.1037/a0035302

[95] Sgoifo A, Carnevali L, Alfonso Mde L, Amore M. Autonomic dysfunction and heart rate variability in depression. Stress. 2015;**18**(3):343-352. DOI: 10.3109/10253890.2015.1045868

[96] Carnevali L, Montano N, Statello R, Sgoifo A. Rodent models of depression-cardiovascular comorbidity: Bridging the known to the new. Neuroscience and Biobehavioral Reviews. 2017;**76**(Pt A):144-153. DOI: 10.1016/j.neubiorev.2016.11.006

[97] Armario A, Nadal R. Individual differences and the characterization of animal models of psychopathology: A strong challenge and a good opportunity. Frontiers in Pharmacology. 2013;**4**:137. DOI: 10.3389/fphar.2013.00137

[98] de Boer SF, Buwalda B, Koolhaas JM. Untangling the neurobiology of coping styles in rodents: Towards neural mechanisms underlying individual differences in disease susceptibility. Neuroscience and Biobehavioral Reviews. 2017;**74**(Pt B):401-422. DOI: 10.1016/j.neubiorev.2016.07.008

[99] Koolhaas JM, Korte SM, De Boer SF, Van Der Vegt BJ, Van Reenen CG, Hopster H, et al. Coping styles in animals: Current status in behavior and stress-physiology. Neuroscience and Biobehavioral Reviews. 1999;**23**(7):925-935. DOI: 10.1016/s0149-7634(99)00026-3

[100] Krishnan V, Han MH, Graham DL, Berton O, Renthal W, Russo SJ, et al. Molecular adaptations underlying susceptibility and resistance to social defeat in brain reward regions. Cell. 2007;**131**(2):391-404. DOI: 10.1016/j.cell.2007.09.018

[101] Coppens CM, de Boer SF, Koolhaas JM. Coping styles and behavioural flexibility: Towards underlying mechanisms. Philosophical Transactions of the Royal Society of London. Series B, Biological Sciences. 2010;**365**(1560):4021-4028. DOI: 10.1098/rstb.2010.0217

[102] Wood SK. Individual differences in the neurobiology of social stress: Implications for depression-cardiovascular disease comorbidity. Current Neuropharmacology. 2014;**12**(2):205-211. DOI: 10.2174/1570159X11666131120224413

[103] Wood CS, Valentino RJ, Wood SK. Individual differences in the locus coeruleus-norepinephrine system: Relevance to stress-induced cardiovascular vulnerability. Physiology & Behavior. 2017;**172**:40-48. DOI: 10.1016/j.physbeh.2016.07.008

[104] Hyde JS, Mezulis AH. Gender differences in depression: Biological, affective, cognitive, and sociocultural factors. Harvard Review of Psychiatry. 2020;**28**(1):4-13. DOI: 10.1097/Hrp.0000000000000230

[105] Kuehner C. Why is depression more common among women than among men? Lancet Psychiatry. 2017;**4**(2):146-158. DOI: 10.1016/S2215-0366(16)30263-2

[106] Marcus SM, Flynn HA, Blow F, Barry K. A screening study of antidepressant treatment rates and mood symptoms in pregnancy. Archives of Women's Mental Health. 2005;**8**(1):25-27. DOI: 10.1007/s00737-005-0072-1

[107] Sloan DM, Kornstein SG. Gender differences in depression and response to antidepressant treatment. The Psychiatric Clinics of North America. 2003;**26**(3):581-594. DOI: 10.1016/s0193-953x(03)00044-3

[108] Moller-Leimkuhler AM. Gender differences in cardiovascular disease and comorbid depression. Dialogues in Clinical Neuroscience. 2007;**9**(1): 71-83

[109] Bueno-Notivol J, Gracia-Garcia P, Olaya B, Lasheras I, Lopez-Anton R, Santabarbara J. Prevalence of depression during the COVID-19 outbreak: A meta-analysis of community-based studies. International Journal of Clinical and Health Psychology. 2021;**21**(1). DOI: 10.1016/j.ijchp.2020.07.007

[110] Sriharan A, Ratnapalan S, Tricco AC, Lupea D, Ayala AP, Pang H, et al. Occupational stress, burnout, and depression in women in healthcare during COVID-19 pandemic: Rapid scoping review. Frontiers in Global Women's Health. 2020;**1**:596690. DOI: 10.3389/fgwh.2020.596690

[111] Almeida M, Shrestha AD, Stojanac D, Miller LJ. The impact of the COVID-19 pandemic on women's mental health. Archives of Women's Mental Health. 2020;**23**(6):741-748. DOI: 10.1007/s00737-020-01092-2

[112] Solomou I, Constantinidou F. Prevalence and predictors of anxiety and depression symptoms during the COVID-19 pandemic and compliance with precautionary measures: Age and sex matter. International Journal of Environmental Research and Public Health. 2020;**17**(14). DOI: 10.3390/ijerph17144924

[113] Torjesen I. Covid-19: Middle aged women face greater risk of debilitating long term symptoms. BMJ. 2021;**372**:n829. DOI: 10.1136/bmj.n829

[114] Page GG, Opp MR, Kozachik SL. Sex differences in sleep, anhedonia, and HPA axis activity in a rat model of chronic social defeat. Neurobiology of Stress. 2016;**3**:105-113. DOI: 10.1016/j.ynstr.2016.03.002

[115] Heneka MT, Golenbock D, Latz E, Morgan D, Brown R. Immediate and long-term consequences of COVID-19 infections for the development of neurological disease. Alzheimer's Research & Therapy. 2020;**12**(1):69. DOI: 10.1186/s13195-020-00640-3

[116] Meinhardt J, Radke J, Dittmayer C, Franz J, Thomas C, Mothes R, et al. Olfactory transmucosal SARS-CoV-2 invasion as a port of central nervous

system entry in individuals with COVID-19. Nature Neuroscience. 2021;**24**(2):168-175. DOI: 10.1038/s41593-020-00758-5

[117] Bilinska K, von Bartheld CS, Butowt R. Expression of the ACE2 virus entry protein in the nervus terminalis reveals the potential for an alternative route to brain infection in COVID-19. Frontiers in Cellular Neuroscience. 2021;**15**. DOI: 10.3389/fncel.2021.674123

[118] Zhang L, Zhou L, Bao LL, Liu JN, Zhu H, Lv Q, et al. SARS-CoV-2 crosses the blood-brain barrier accompanied with basement membrane disruption without tight junctions alteration. Signal Transduction and Targeted Therapy. 2021;**6**(1). DOI: 10.1038/s41392-021-00719-9

[119] Frank MG, Nguyen KH, Ball JB, Hopkins S, Kelley T, Baratta MV, et al. SARS-CoV-2 spike S1 subunit induces neuroinflammatory, microglial and behavioral sickness responses: Evidence of PAMP-like properties. Brain Behavior and Immunity. 2022;**100**:267-277. DOI: 10.1016/j.bbi.2021.12.007

[120] Schousboe A. Metabolic signaling in the brain and the role of astrocytes in control of glutamate and GABA neurotransmission. Neuroscience Letters. 2019;**689**:11-13. DOI: 10.1016/j.neulet.2018.01.038

[121] De Pitta M, Brunel N, Volterra A. Astrocytes: Orchestrating synaptic plasticity? Neuroscience. 2016;**323**:43-61. DOI: 10.1016/j.neuroscience.2015.04.001

[122] Matott MP, Kline DD, Hasser EM. Glial EAAT2 regulation of extracellular nTS glutamate critically controls neuronal activity and cardiorespiratory reflexes. Journal of Physiology London. 2017;**595**(17):6045-6063. DOI: 10.1113/Jp274620

[123] Villarreal A, Vidos C, Busso MM, Cieri MB, Ramos AJ. Pathological neuroinflammatory conversion of reactive astrocytes is induced by microglia and involves chromatin remodeling. Frontiers in Pharmacology. 2021;**12**. DOI: 10.3389/fphar.2021.689346

[124] Kanberg N, Simren J, Eden A, Andersson LM, Nilsson S, Ashton NJ, et al. Neurochemical signs of astrocytic and neuronal injury in acute COVID-19 normalizes during long-term follow-up. Ebiomedicine. 2021;**70**. DOI: 10.1016/j.ebiom.2021.103512

[125] Flachskampf FA. Cardiac imaging to evaluate left ventricular diastolic function. JACC: Cardiovascular Imaging. 2015;**8**(9):1072-1093

[126] Pennell DJ. Cardiovascular magnetic resonance. Circulation. 2010;**121**(5):692-705. DOI: 10.1161/Circulationaha.108.811547

[127] Puntmann VO, Carerj ML, Wieters I, Fahim M, Arendt C, Hoffmann J, et al. Outcomes of cardiovascular magnetic resonance imaging in patients recently recovered from coronavirus disease 2019 (COVID-19). JAMA Cardiology. 2020;**5**(11):1265-1273. DOI: 10.1001/jamacardio.2020.3557

[128] Joy G, Artico J, Kurdi H, Seraphim A, Lau C, Thornton GD, et al. Prospective case-control study of cardiovascular abnormalities 6 months following mild COVID-19 in healthcare workers. JACC: Cardiovascular Imaging. 2021;**14**(11):2155-2166. DOI: 10.1016/j.jcmg.2021.04.011

[129] Vago H, Szabo L, Dohy Z, Merkely B. Cardiac magnetic resonance findings in patients recovered from COVID-19 initial experiences in elite athletes. JACC: Cardiovascular Imaging.

2021;**14**(6):1279-1281. DOI: 10.1016/j.jcmg.2020.11.014

[130] Daniels CJ, Rajpal S, Greenshields JT, Rosenthal GL, Chung EH, Terrin M, et al. Prevalence of clinical and subclinical myocarditis in competitive athletes with recent SARS-CoV-2 infection results from the big ten COVID-19 cardiac registry. JAMA Cardiology. 2021;**6**(9):1078-1087. DOI: 10.1001/jamacardio.2021.2065

[131] Martinez MW, Tucker AM, Bloom OJ, Green G, DiFiori JP, Solomon G, et al. Prevalence of inflammatory heart disease among professional athletes with prior COVID-19 infection who received systematic return-to-play cardiac screening. JAMA Cardiology. 2021;**6**(7):745-752. DOI: 10.1001/jamacardio.2021.0565

[132] Moulson N, Petek BJ, Drezner JA, Harmon KG, Kliethermes SA, Patel MR, et al. SARS-CoV-2 cardiac involvement in Young competitive athletes. Circulation. 2021;**144**(4):256-266. DOI: 10.1161/Circulationaha.121.054824

[133] Moody WE, Liu BY, Mahmoud-Elsayed HM, Senior J, Lalla SS, Khan-Kheil AM, et al. Persisting adverse ventricular Remodeling in COVID-19 survivors: A longitudinal echocardiographic study. Journal of the American Society of Echocardiography. 2021;**34**(5):562-566. DOI: 10.1016/j.echo.2021.01.020

[134] Argulian E, Sud K, Vogel B, Bohra C, Garg VP, Talebi S, et al. Right ventricular dilation in hospitalized patients with COVID-19 infection. JACC: Cardiovascular Imaging. 2020;**13**(11):2459-2461. DOI: 10.1016/j.jcmg.2020.05.010

[135] Kim J, Volodarskiy A, Sultana R, Pollie MP, Yum B, Nambiar L, et al. Prognostic utility of right ventricular remodeling over conventional risk stratification in patients with COVID-19. Journal of the American College of Cardiology. 2020;**76**(17):1965-1977. DOI: 10.1016/j.jacc.2020.08.066

[136] Kotecha T, Knight DS, Razvi Y, Kumar K, Vimalesvaran K, Thornton G, et al. Patterns of myocardial injury in recovered troponin-positive COVID-19 patients assessed by cardiovascular magnetic resonance. European Heart Journal. 2021;**42**(19):1866-1878. DOI: 10.1093/eurheartj/ehab075

[137] Sonnweber T, Sahanic S, Pizzini A, Luger A, Schwabl C, Sonnweber B, et al. Cardiopulmonary recovery after COVID-19: An observational prospective multicentre trial. The European Respiratory Journal. 2021;**57**(4). DOI: 10.1183/13993003.03481-2020

[138] Kotanidis CP, Xie C, Adlam D, Rodrigues JC, Siddique M, Lockstone H, et al. Radiotranscriptomic analysis of perivascular adipose tissue quantifies vascular inflammation in Covid-19 from routine Ct angiograms: Stratification of "new Uk variant" infection and prediction of in-hospital outcomes. Heart. 2021;**107**:A177-A1A8. DOI: 10.1136/heartjnl-2021-BCS.238

[139] Evans RA, McAuley H, Harrison EM, Shikotra A, Singapuri A, Sereno M, et al. Physical, cognitive, and mental health impacts of COVID-19 after hospitalisation (PHOSP-COVID): A UK multicentre, prospective cohort study. Lancet Respiratory Medicine. 2021;**9**(11):1275-1287. DOI: 10.1016/S2213-2600(21)00383-0

[140] Fogarty H, Townsend L, Morrin H, Ahmad A, Comerford C, Karampini E, et al. Persistent endotheliopathy in the pathogenesis of long COVID syndrome. Journal of Thrombosis and Haemostasis.

2021;**19**(10):2546-2553. DOI: 10.1111/jth.15490

[141] Chioh FWJ, Fong SW, Young BE, Wu KX, Siau A, Krishnan S, et al. Convalescent COVID-19 patients are susceptible to endothelial dysfunction due to persistent immune activation. eLife. 2021;**10**:e64909. DOI: 10.7554/eLife.64909

[142] Gavriilaki E, Eftychidis I, Papassotiriou I. Update on endothelial dysfunction in COVID-19: Severe disease, long COVID-19 and pediatric characteristics. Journal of Laboratory Medicine. 2021;**45**(6):293-302. DOI: 10.1515/labmed-2021-0134

[143] Ho FK, Man KKC, Toshner M, Church C, Celis-Morales C, Wong ICK, et al. Thromboembolic risk in hospitalized and nonhospitalized COVID-19 patients: A self-controlled case series analysis of a nationwide cohort. Mayo Clinic Proceedings. 2021;**96**(10):2587-2597. DOI: 10.1016/j.mayocp.2021.07.002

Chapter 10

Mental Health Impact of Post-Infection Fatigue

Mary Olamide Akinwola, Adesola Oyinkansola Abiodun and Yusuff Tunde Gbonjubola

Abstract

Post-infective fatigue is a major long-lasting complication of COVID-19. Among long COVID-19 survivors, the persistent fatigues experienced have had a significant impact on their physical health and mental health. Post-infective fatigue has been described as a loss of energy and a feeling of heaviness. Likewise, more evidence has highlighted the mental health component of fatigue triggered by subjectively minor physical and cognitive activities. These bouts of fatigue are commonly associated with mental health issues such as anxiety, depression, and sleep disorders. Ultimately, these mental health problems affect the quality of life of survivors. Although necessary public health efforts were directed at controlling the spread of COVID-19 and treating physical symptoms, it is crucial to backtrack, to develop inclusive mental health services for individuals plagued by post-COVID-19 fatigue.

Keywords: fatigue, long COVID-19, anxiety, depression, sleep disorders

1. Introduction

Since the COVID-19 pandemic hit, we have continued to experience an aftershock beyond acute symptoms of the virus. In December 2019, an acute respiratory disease from Wuhan, China spread rapidly across the globe [1]. It was soon identified as the novel coronavirus which was named severe acute respiratory syndrome coronavirus-2 (SARS-CoV-2) [1]. On March 11, 2020, the disease was declared a pandemic by the World Health Organization [2]. The mode of transmission of this virus is usually from human to human commonly through air droplets, and this feature was responsible for its rapid and progressive outbreak [3]. As of May 1, 2022, 513 million people have been infected by the virus with 6.23 million deaths globally [3].

As a respiratory disease, the COVID-19 virus primarily affects the respiratory system [4]. Although other organs are involved, lower respiratory tract infection symptoms such as fever, dry cough, and dyspnea were commonly reported [4]. Other symptoms such as headache, dizziness, generalized weakness, vomiting, and diarrhea were also observed [4]. Like the virus, it was noted that the respiratory symptoms of COVID-19 could progress rapidly [5]. As such, the symptoms could vary from minimal to significant hypoxia with acute respiratory distress syndrome (ARDS) [5]. In addition to the progressive nature of the virus, the short duration for the onset of symptoms was an added disadvantage to the nature of COVID-19. In earlier reports, the time of onset of symptoms to development of ARDS-related hypoxia may be as short as 9 days [6]. Typically, these symptoms can prove to be fatal. Although mechanisms have been placed to ensure acute response and control the spread of the virus, some survivors still experience distress long after management [7]. Therefore, the management of COVID-19 from the acute phase may be the beginning of a long path to full recovery. Months following hospitalization and acute care, some symptoms still persist in the post-COVID-19 phase [8].

Post-Covid-19, also known as, long COVID is used to describe the persistence of symptoms, weeks or months after an acute infection of Covid-19 irrespective of the viral status [8]. This state can be continuous, relapsing or remitting in nature. Post-COVID-19 can be divided into two stages depending on the duration of symptoms. The first is post-acute COVID-19 where symptoms are more than 3 weeks but less than 12 weeks and the other, chronic COVID-19 where symptoms continue beyond 12 weeks [8, 9]. The commonly reported symptoms include fatigue, dyspnea, joint pain, chest pain, cough, skin rashes, palpitations, headache, diarrhea, and paresthesia [8]. Of these symptoms, post-infective fatigue is the most persistent and debilitating [10].

Post-infective fatigue syndrome (PIFS) is a persistent, severe fatigue after an infection that cannot be explained by other medical or psychiatric conditions, which has been present for at least 6 months and significantly affects daily functioning [11]. After the onset of COVID-19, prevalence rates of fatigue persisting for months ranged from 9% to 58% [11]. It is observed that an increasing number of previously fit young people continue to have persistent fatigue months after mild cases of COVID-19 [9, 12]. Although it is currently established in some post-COVID-19 individuals, PIFS is not unique to coronavirus [12]. According to Rudroff et al. [7], it is noticed that patients treated for viral infections may sustain functional limitations over long periods. Hence, in comparison to COVID-19, patients with severe acute respiratory syndrome (SARS) had similar symptoms and persistent fatigue that was observed months and years beyond the initial infection [7]. Following the SARS epidemic, the health outcomes of recovered patients were observed 3 months, 6 months, and 12 months after hospital discharge, the findings reported that 64% had fatigue at 3 months, 54% at 6 months, and 60% at 12 months [13]. It was also discovered that chronic fatigue was related to sleeping difficulties [13]. Other studies also reported that patients experienced myalgia, joint pain, and depressive symptoms in addition to their fatigue [14]. In addition to SARS, studies have reported a similar trend of persistent fatigue with influenza virus, Ebola virus, and West Nile virus months after they have recovered [11, 13]. There has also been a recognized link between viral symptoms and fatigue [15]. Anecdotal reports suggest that patients who do not recover fully from COVID-19 experience some lingering symptoms of fatigue. Likewise, studies suggest that COVID-19 has had an exacerbating effect among those with chronic fatigue syndrome [13].

Mental health symptoms such as depression and anxiety are identified to be related to post-COVID-19 [16, 17]. Studies support that there is an established link between fatigue and mental health problems [18]. Hence, among long-COVID patients or post-COVID-19 individuals, these symptoms were found present. Mental health disorders such as depression, anxiety, post-traumatic stress disorder, and sleep disorders were found to occur with the chronic and debilitating nature of the fatigue [19]. According to the DSM-V, these disorders are characteristically mental health disorders. Overall, these mental disorders, in addition to the physical impact of fatigue, result in a decline in the quality of life of individuals [20]. In COVID-19, since the public health focus was on safety and survival, the mental health issue has been widely overlooked [21]. A proper and proactive approach to the prevention and management of the mental disorders associated with post-COVID fatigue is necessary to improve the individual's quality of life long after the onset of the disease.

2. Pathophysiology of post-COVID-19 fatigue

Typically, across various infections, symptoms of fatigue persist long after the onset of the disease [18]. Although the characteristics of chronic fatigue commonly associated with post-infectious diseases such as post-COVID-19 remain controversial, the manifestations remain similar to other post-infectious diseases irrespective of the pathogen. According to Poenaru et al. [17], the proposed mechanism of chronic fatigue in post-infection is likely multifactorial.

2.1 Immune/inflammatory mechanisms

In post-infectious fatigue, the immune system appears to be impacted by the pathogen [13]. The process remains unclear and can involve multiple pathways. A proposed mechanism is that during acute infection by the COVID-19 virus, tissue damage is sustained which results in the activation of auto-reactive bystander cells and molecular mimicry [16]. For example, in patients with severe COVID-19, there has been a substantial production of anti-nuclear antibodies. Also, rheumatic factor was detected among such individuals suggesting that there is increased activation of auto-reactive B-cells [16]. However, in chronic fatigue syndromes, antibodies that work against muscarinic and adrenergic receptors have been the syndrome but no auto-antibody has been linked to chronic antibodies [16].

Another mechanism purports that the deregulation of cytokine networks may play a role in chronic fatigue [8, 22]. A study on encephalitis detected those increased levels of pro-inflammatory cytokines were observed from the acute phase and remained consistently elevated 30 days post-infection within the central nervous system [16, 17]. However, evidence found no significant association between cytokine levels and chronic fatigue. Better still, new evidence suggested that cytokine signaling was more significant [16].

2.2 Mitochondrial function

Within the muscle tissue, alterations in mitochondrial structure, metabolism, and energy production may be associated with chronic fatigue [8, 11, 17]. Mitochondrial degeneration, pleomorphic features, and structural abnormalities were found in muscles of individuals diagnosed with post-viral symptoms [16]. From the onset of symptoms, mitochondrial enzymes are involved in the inflammatory and anti-oxidant pathways due to their involvement in peripheral vasodilation and autonomic regulation of the cardiovascular system [16]. This mechanism has not been evidence enough to link post-infectious chronic fatigue with mitochondrial dysfunction [8]. Also, a clear logical way to explain the pathway of lasting mitochondrial abnormalities among post-infectious individuals is also lacking [8].

2.3 Central nervous system involvement

Mental health symptoms such as sleep disorders and post-anxiety stress disorders commonly with chronic fatigue may reflect impairment of the central nervous system [21].

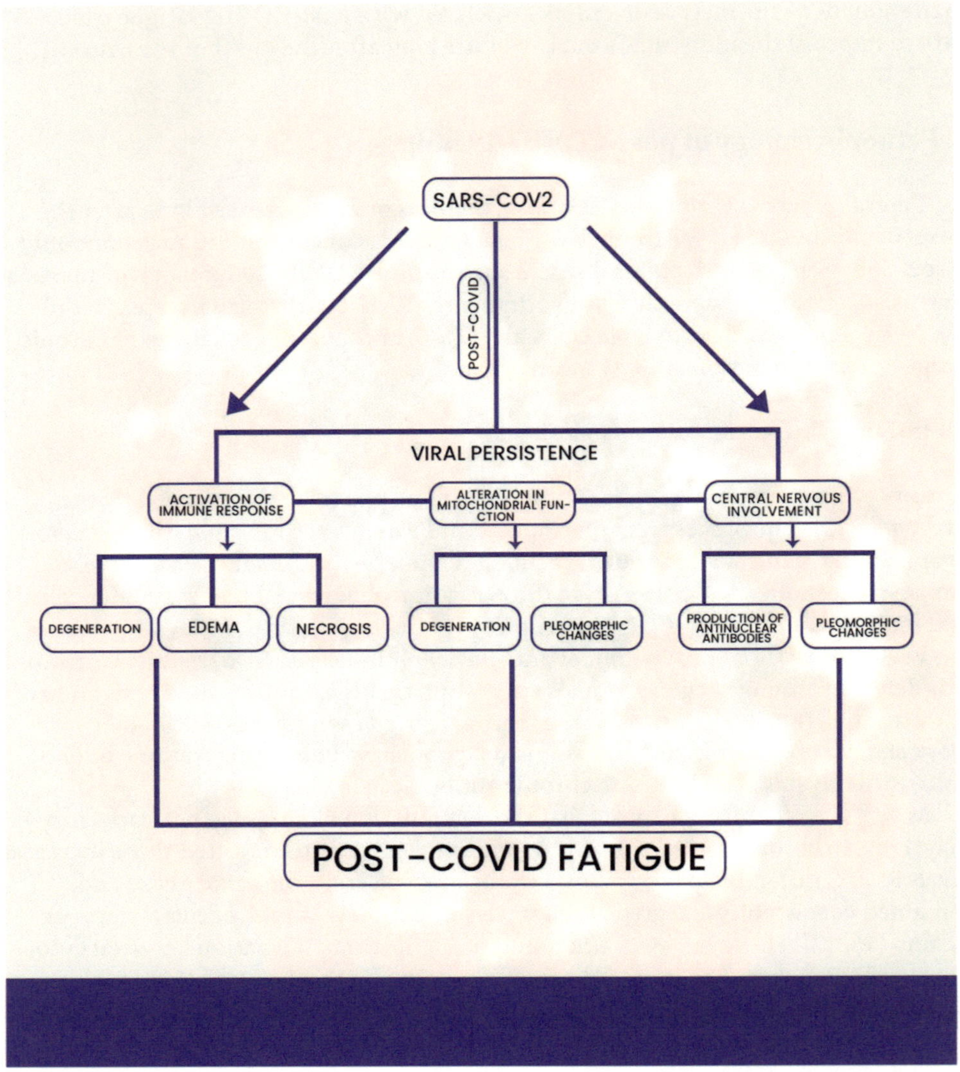

Figure 1.
The pathophysiology of post-COVID fatigue.

Many viruses, including coronaviruses, have been shown to cause damage to the CNS tissue [11, 21]. For example, SARS-CoV1, as well as COVID-19, has been associated with edema, neuronal degeneration, demyelination, and necrosis resulting in an increased risk for cerebral ischemic events. In addition, a high proportion of rapid eye movements and alpha electroencephalographic sleep disorders were found among SARS survivors who had chronic fatigue [16]. This is a common mechanism behind sleep disorders in post-infectious fatigue. Although this mechanism has been defined, the causal relationship between the infection, altered CNS structure, and chronic fatigue still remain unclear (**Figure 1**) [16].

3. Effects of post-COVID 19 fatigue on mental health

There is an inconsequential effect of post-COVID-19 fatigue on the mental health of survivors [22]. Several factors such as reduced physical functioning, and social and economic issues that may trigger fatigue may subsequently cause mental health issues [22]. The history of pre-existing mental health problems may also aggravate the mental health issues activated by fatigue [21]. Mental health problems such as depression, anxiety, post-traumatic stress disorder, and sleep disorders are commonly related to symptoms of post-COVID-19 [23]. However, among people who have developed post-COVID-19 fatigue, the mental health problems are usually co-occurring and potentially codependent on post-COVID-19 fatigue [24]. A study on neuropsychological and neurophysiological correlates of fatigue in post-covid-19 patients supports that there was no significant correlation between apathy, depression, and fatigue. Although they were found to co-exist in post-COVID patients, they were not associated [25]. There is a paucity of literature on the direct impact of fatigue on mental health disorders. However, the effects on mental health were mainly a result of biological, psychosocial, and economic factors [25]. Reduced physical activity, which is an outcome of the chronic nature of post-COVID-19 fatigue influences the onset of or exacerbation of mental health problems [26]. Likewise, the mental component of fatigue, such as reduced motivation can influence developing mental health disorders [27].

4. Factors affecting the mental health impact of post-COVID fatigue

The mental health impact of post-COVID fatigue is typically a co-existing component of fatigue. However, contributing factors responsible for their onset or aggravation exists [7]. They include:

a. Biological factors: Serotonin and Dopamine play major roles in the mental/psychological aspects of fatigue. Among COVID-19 patients, COVID-19 may be transported via the olfactory bulb to the forebrain, which has a substantial amount of dopamine and serotonin [7]. This may alter the levels of dopamine and serotonin responsible for controlling moods and other affect [7]. These changes in the brain may be responsible for mental effects such as anxiety and depression among post-COVID-19 individuals [7].

b. Task dependent factors: this includes changes in fatigue that are dependent on the tasks performed. Fatigue is commonly triggered by specific cognitive or motor tasks performed [7]. The extent of the task persons, especially one that over-exerts the individual may trigger or aggravate the mental effects of the fatigue [7].

c. Environmental factors: This refers to how the environment affects the COVID-19 survivors from the acute phase and throughout the process of recovery [7]. For example, the financial implications of the pandemic or management, self-isolation, lockdown, and social isolation may contribute negatively to the individuals' mental capacity. It has been reported by some earlier authors that the financial loss as a result of Covid-19, was associated with depression [7]. Therefore, the environmental and societal effects of the pandemic may be largely responsible for mental effects such as anxiety, depression, and post-traumatic stress disorders among post-COVID fatigued individuals [7].

d. Physical and Mental capacity: Initial physical capacity, that is, the prior state of well-being can be a contributing factor to the physical as well as the mental component of post-COVID fatigue [7]. In addition, an initial mental orientation about COVID-19, resulting in individuals' experiencing anxiety and distress can lead to and aggravate the levels of fatigue [25]. In such cases, pre-existing medical conditions should also be considered as primary or supplementary causes of the mental effects of fatigue. Conditions such as cardiovascular diseases, diabetes, and chronic kidney disease may cause these populations to be affected by the persistent effects of fatigue in comparison to people with no co-morbid conditions [7].

5. Management of mental health issues related to post-COVID fatigue

Depression, anxiety and stress are common mental health issues that have been identified in COVID survivors [28]. While these mental health conditions may not be directly linked to post-COVID fatigue, they commonly co-exist in the study population. These mental health disorders have been reported to be effectively managed using a combination of psychological and pharmacological treatment methods [29].

In the management of people with depression, literature suggests psychotherapy by psychologists or psychiatrists, as the first line of management [29]. This includes behavioral activation (helping the individual to identify and adopt new routines that could motivate or make them happy); and guide them in the process of identifying the major problems responsible for the health status, as well as self-developing solutions to these problems [30, 31]. Self-help materials can also be provided for these individuals to guide and foster the development of healthy behaviors [29].

Furthermore, it is important that healthcare professionals monitor these individuals during the process of healing, to ensure that they achieve their set goals [32]. Considering the residual fatigue post-COVID, it is important that the gradual return to activities is stressed. This will help them slowly adjust to the energy demand of activities, while this keeping their goals in mind. A sudden return to strenuous activities (which may be top on their list) may be very difficult, if not impossible for some of them to achieve. If not properly managed, this may demoralize the patient further, or in extreme cases lead to a sequela of other events. In cases where the symptoms persist or reoccur after psychological intervention, antidepressants are prescribed [33]. Cleare et al. [34] suggests that people who suffer from severe depression should undergo both psychological and pharmacologic management from the onset to achieve the best treatment outcomes.

While healthcare professionals await comprehensive research and reports on how to manage patients with long-COVID symptoms, it is imperative that we continue to use the available methods such as cognitive behavioral therapy (CBT), and peer support to management patients who suffer from mental health conditions due to the COVID experience [34]. People who report symptoms of anxiety should be asked about the exact reason or source of worry. Management of their condition should begin by addressing these worries. It is also important to educate patients on making treatment goals. Using these goals as a guide in helping patients during psychotherapy sessions, to ensure return to activity. Patients should be asked to make a list of activities they would like to return to. These activities should then be ranked based on the level of anxiety they cause the client. The healthcare professional should then advice the client to gradually commence their 'return to activity' with activities that worry them the least.

In addition, pharmacological means have proven to be effective in the management of anxiety in this population. Class of medications such as selective serotonin reuptake inhibitors, serotonin norepinephrine reuptake inhibitors, tricyclic antidepressants, benzodiazepenes, and gabapentinoids, among others have been successfully used in the management of anxiety [35]. Beyond the psychopharmacological treatment protocols, other conservative management techniques such as acupuncture, meditation, yoga, and exercise have been equally reported to be effective in managing anxiety in this population [35]. Exercises will steadily help to improve endurance, boost mood and improve immunity. Hence, I recommend exercises as an effective method of treating mental health issues in people with post-COVID fatigue.

Overall, due to the dearth of information on evidence-based techniques in managing mental health conditions in people suffering from long-COVID symptoms, mental health and rehabilitation experts have resorted to using the generally accepted methods to manage these conditions. So far, these are the best available approaches to help improve the quality of life of these individuals. However, it is necessary to view the patient holistically and take other symptoms (such as the co-existing fatigue) that the patients report into cognizance. This way, health care outcomes will be optimized. It is recommended that more mental health experts should carry out research to explore the effectiveness of various protocols in the management of mental health issues that are associated with post-COVID fatigue.

6. Consequences of neglecting the mental health impact of post-COVID fatigue

There is an overall decline in the quality of life of individuals as a result of a neglect of the mental health component of post-COVID 19 fatigue [36]. Commonly, the public health strategies focused on controlling the spread of and reducing the acute symptoms accompanying the virus [37]. These strategies have ranged from proper pharmacological management to the dissemination of COVID-19 vaccines [38]. However, as studies begin to report the symptoms of post-COVID-19 fatigue, the mental health impact is repeatedly highlighted [39, 40]. More often, post-COVID-19 fatigue and mental health effects such as sleep disorders, anxiety and depression, and post-traumatic stress disorders are co-occurring and sometimes associated with physical components [39, 40]. Therefore, when mental health becomes repeatedly overlooked, the overall quality of life of the individuals declines [36, 41]. For example, the mental health disorder may aggravate the physical component of fatigue, resulting in muscle weakness and reduction in cognition. This neglect can also have a disproportionate impact on other mental health consequences such as suicide [42]. In the United States of America, during the 2 months of lockdown, more suicides caused by mental health disorders were recorded than COVID-19 deaths. Likewise, poor coping mechanisms such as drug and alcohol abuse can be taken up to alleviate the mental health effects [43]. With these debilitating consequences, it is important that strategies are put in place to alleviate them.

7. Beyond the surge: strategies to address the mental health impact of post-COVID fatigue

Chronic fatigue experienced by some individuals who recovered from the COVID-19 infection may be a menace to its victims. It exposes people to new vulnerabilities that significantly impact their mental health status. Considering the widespread of the corona virus in the last two (2) years, it is imperative that its mental health effects are checked promptly to prevent an overwhelming surge in the prevalence of global mental health dysfunction.

Despite a surge in the mental health issues following the first few months of the pandemic, the World Health Organization (2020) reported a marked reduction in the delivery of and accessibility to mental health services. Nonetheless, mental health experts came up with new ways of rendering efficient mental health services to individuals who need it. By mid-2020, many developed nations had established the use of digital health means to deliver mental health care [44, 45]. Chew et al. [35] reported the effective use of digital health methods such as cloud-based big data systems, artificial intelligence (AI)–based chatbots, online health communities (OHCs), and telehealth platforms in mental healthcare delivery.

In 2020, the National Institute for Health and Care Excellence (NICE) [46] proposed the empowerment of individuals to return to the community fully and take charge of their own management with the help of a multidisciplinary rehabilitation team. Healthcare practitioners have identified the need for psychologists and physicians to collaborate to ensure the successful management mental health issues due to long-COVID [47]. A psychologist, Hardin reported the lack of an absolute treatment (surgery, or medication) that would instantly relieve the mental health symptoms experienced by survivors of the COVID-19 diseases [47]. She however opined that early intervention and provision of realistic advice to help patients manage their feelings during this period, may significantly impact the efficacy of treatment. Aiyegbusi et al. [48] suggested routine mental health screening as a part of the follow-up treatment for people suffering from post-COVID fatigue and other long-COVID syndromes. This will help healthcare providers to promptly identify individuals who are at risk and commence management early [48].

8. Conclusion

Summarily, post-COVID fatigue is a potentially debilitating condition that may negatively impact the quality of life of individuals. Although available evidence suggests that mental health conditions such as depression and anxiety that exist in individuals with long-COVID is not directly linked to chronic fatigue experienced by some members of this group, they often co-exist. This implies that the status of one may impact the other on the long run, hence, the need for them to both be managed effectively. Healthcare practitioners have worked tirelessly in the last few years to come up with efficient and effective methods to deliver mental health care to individuals who require them. However, the body of knowledge will be greatly improved if more research is done to explore this aspect of health care.

Author details

Mary Olamide Akinwola[1], Adesola Oyinkansola Abiodun[2]
and Yusuff Tunde Gbonjubola[3]*

1 College of Medicine, University of Ibadan, Nigeria

2 Pearl Essence Physiotherapy Clinic, Ibadan, Nigeria

3 Centre for Early Development, Learning and Care, Ibadan, Nigeria

*Address all correspondence to: gbonjubola4mercy@gmail.com

References

[1] Yuki K, Fujiogi M, Koutsogiannaki S. COVID-19 pathophysiology: A review. Clinical Immunology (Orlando, Fla.). 2020;**215**:108427

[2] Cucinotta D, Vanelli M. WHO declares COVID-19 a pandemic. Acta bio-medica: Atenei Parmensis. 2020;**91**(1):157-160

[3] Our World in Data. 2022. Available from: https://ourworldindata.org/explorers/coronavirus-data-explorer. [Accessed: May 1, 2022]

[4] Alizadehsani R, Alizadeh Sani Z, Behjati M, Roshanzamir Z, Hussain S, Abedini N, et al. Risk factors prediction, clinical outcomes, and mortality in COVID-19 patients. Journal of Medical Virology. 2021;**93**(4):2307-2320

[5] Maveddat A, Mallah H, Rao S, Ali K, Sherali S, Nugent K. Severe acute respiratory distress syndrome secondary to coronavirus 2 (SARS-CoV-2). The International Journal of Occupational and Environmental Medicine. 2020;**11**(4):157

[6] Lin SH, Zhao YS, Zhou DX, Zhou FC, Xu F. Coronavirus disease 2019 (COVID-19): Cytokine storms, hyper-inflammatory phenotypes, and acute respiratory distress syndrome. Genes & Diseases. 2020;**7**(4):520-527

[7] Rudroff T, Fietsam AC, Deters JR, Bryant AD, Kamholz J. Post-COVID-19 fatigue: Potential contributing factors. Brain Sciences. 2020;**10**(12):1012

[8] Raveendran AV, Jayadevan R, Sashidharan S. Long COVID: an overview. Diabetes & Metabolic Syndrome: Clinical Research & Reviews. 2021;**15**(3):869-875

[9] Fernández-de-Las-Peñas C, Palacios-Ceña D, Gómez-Mayordomo V, Cuadrado ML, Florencio LL. Defining post-COVID symptoms (post-acute COVID, long COVID, persistent post-COVID): An integrative classification. International Journal of Environmental Research and Public Health. 2021; **18**(5):2621

[10] Smith A. Post-viral fatigue: Implications for long COVID. Asian Journal of Research in Infectious Diseases. 2021;**6**(1):17-23

[11] Vink-Niese A. Could cognitive behavioral therapy be an effective treatment for long COVID and post COVID-19 fatigue syndrome? Lessons from the Qure Study for Q-Fever Fatigue Syndrome. Healthcare (Basel Switzerland). 2020;**8**(4):552

[12] Verveen A, Müller F, Lloyd A, Moss-Morris R, Omland T, Penninx B, et al. A research agenda for post-COVID-19 fatigue. Journal of Psychosomatic Research. 2022;**154**:110726

[13] El Sayed S, Shokry D, Gomaa SM. Post-COVID-19 fatigue and anhedonia: A cross-sectional study and their correlation to post-recovery period. Neuropsychopharmacology Reports. 2021;**41**(1):50-55

[14] Islam MF, Cotler J, Jason LA. Post-viral fatigue and COVID-19: Lessons from past epidemics. Fatigue: Biomedicine, Health & Behavior. 2020;**8**(2):61-69

[15] Kamal M, Abo Omirah M, Hussein A, Saeed H. Assessment and characterization of post-COVID-19 manifestations. International Journal of Clinical Practice. 2021;**75**(3):e13746

[16] Townsend L, Dyer AH, Jones K, Dunne J, Mooney A, Gaffney F, et al. Persistent fatigue following SARS-CoV-2 infection is common and independent of severity of initial infection. Plos One. 2020;**15**(11):e0240784

[17] Poenaru S, Abdallah SJ, Corrales-Medina V, Cowan J. COVID-19 and post-infectious myalgic encephalomyelitis/chronic fatigue syndrome: A narrative review. Therapeutic Advances in Infectious Disease. 2021;**8**

[18] Zawadka-Kunikowska M, Zalewski P, Newton JL. The similarities between Long-haul COVID-19 and Myalgic Encephalomyelitis/Chronic Fatigue Syndrome (ME/CFS). Medical Research Journal. 2021;**6**(1):77-78

[19] Rupp I, Boshuizen HC, Jacobi CE, Dinant HJ, van den Bos GA. Impact of fatigue on health-related quality of life in rheumatoid arthritis. Arthritis Care & Research. 2004;**51**(4):578-585

[20] Simani L, Ramezani M, Darazam I. A, Sagharichi M, Aalipour M. A, Ghorbani F, Pakdaman H. Prevalence and correlates of chronic fatigue syndrome and post-traumatic stress disorder after the outbreak of the COVID-19. Journal of Neurovirology, 2021;**27**(1):154-159

[21] ShanbehzadehS,TavahomiM,ZanjariN, Ebrahimi-Takamjani I, Amiri-Arimi S. Physical and mental health complications post-COVID-19: Scoping review. Journal of Psychosomatic Research. 2021;**147**:110525

[22] Zürcher SJ, Banzer C, Adamus C, Lehmann AI, Richter D, Kerksieck P. Post-viral mental health sequelae in infected persons associated with COVID-19 and previous epidemics and pandemics: Systematic review and meta-analysis of prevalence estimates. Journal of Infection and Public Health. 2022;**S1876-0341**(22):00090-00099

[23] Low RN, Low RJ, Akrami A. A cytokine-based model for the pathophysiology of long COVID symptoms. OSF Preprints. 2020. DOI: 10.31219/osf.io/7gcnv

[24] Vollbracht C, Kraft K. Feasibility of vitamin C in the treatment of post viral fatigue with focus on long COVID, based on a systematic review of IV Vitamin C on fatigue. Nutrients. 2021;**13**(4):1154

[25] Mardani M. Post COVID syndrome. Archives of Clinical Infectious Diseases. 2020;**15**(2):e108819

[26] Rudroff T, Workman CD, Bryant AD. Potential factors that contribute to post-COVID-19 fatigue in women. Brain Sciences. 2022;**12**(5):556

[27] Tabacof L, Tosto-Mancuso J, Wood J, Cortes M, Kontorovich A, McCarthy D, et al. Post-acute COVID-19 syndrome negatively impacts physical function, cognitive function, health-related quality of life, and participation. American Journal of Physical Medicine & Rehabilitation. 2022;**101**(1):48

[28] Kathirvel N. Post COVID-19 pandemic mental health challenges. Asian Journal of Psychiatry. 2020;**53**:102430. DOI: 10.1016/j.ajp.2020.102430

[29] Abas MA. Combining active ingredients to treat depression in the wake of COVID-19. The Lancet Psychiatry. 2021;**93**(3):190-191

[30] Ekers D, Webster L, Van Straten A, Cuijpers P, Richards D, Gilbody S. Behavioural activation for depression; an update of meta-analysis of effectiveness and subgroup analysis. PLoS One. 2014;**9**:e100100

[31] Wampold BE. How important are the common factors in psychotherapy?

An update. World Psychiatry. 2015; **14**:270-277

[32] Hides L, Carroll S, Lubman DL, Baker A. Brief motivational interviewing for depression and anxiety. In: Bennett-Levy J, Richards D, Farrand P, editors. Oxford Guide to Low Intensity CBT Interventions. USA: Oxford University Press; 2010. pp. 177-186

[33] Dunlop BW. Evidence-based applications of combination psychotherapy and pharmacotherapy for depression. Focus American Psychiatric Association Publishing. 2016;**14**:156-173

[34] Cleare A, Pariante CM, Young AH, et al. Evidence-based guidelines for treating depressive disorders with antidepressants: A revision of the 2008 British Association for Psychopharmacology guidelines. Journal of Psychopharmacology. 2015;**29**:459-525

[35] Uzunova G, Pallanti S, Hollander E. Presentation and management of anxiety in individuals with acute symptomatic or asymptomatic COVID-19 infection, and in the post-COVID-19 recovery phase. International Journal of Psychiatry in Clinical Practice. 2021;**25**(2):115-131

[36] Byrne A, Barber R, Lim CH. Impact of the COVID-19 pandemic–A mental health service perspective. Progress in Neurology and Psychiatry. 2021;**25**(2):27-33

[37] Ortelli P, Ferrazzoli D, Sebastianelli L, Engl M, Romanello R, Nardone R, et al. Neuropsychological and neurophysiological correlates of fatigue in post-acute patients with neurological manifestations of COVID-19: Insights into a challenging symptom. Journal of the Neurological Sciences. 2021;**420**:117271

[38] Bil JS, Buława B, Świerzawski J. Mental health and the city in the post-COVID-19 era. Sustainability. 2021;**13**(14):7533

[39] Adhikari SP, Meng S, Wu YJ, Mao YP, Ye RX, Wang QZ, et al. Epidemiology, causes, clinical manifestation and diagnosis, prevention and control of coronavirus disease (COVID-19) during the early outbreak period: A scoping review. Infectious Diseases of Poverty. 2020;**9**(1):1-12

[40] Chen X, Huang H, Ju J, Sun R, Zhang J. Impact of vaccination on the COVID-19 pandemic in US states. Scientific Reports. 2022;**12**(1):1-10

[41] Rao S, Benzouak T, Gunpat S, Burns RJ, Tahir TA, Jolles S, et al. Fatigue symptoms associated with COVID-19 in convalescent or recovered COVID-19 patients; a systematic review and meta-analysis. Annals of Behavioral Medicine. 2022;**56**(3):219-234

[42] Morgul E, Bener A, Atak M, Akyel S, Aktaş S, Jordan TR. COVID-19 pandemic and psychological fatigue in Turkey. International Journal of Social Psychiatry. 2021;**67**(2):128-135

[43] Vieira CM, Franco OH, Restrepo CG, Abel T. COVID-19: The forgotten priorities of the pandemic. Maturitas. 2020;**136**:38-41

[44] World Health Organization. The Impact of COVID-19 on Mental, Neurological and Substance Use Services: Results of a Rapid Assessment. Geneva: World Health Organization

[45] Gratzer D, Torous J, Lam RW, Patten SB, Kutcher S, Chan S, et al. Our digital moment: Innovations and opportunities in digital mental

health care. Canadian Journal of Psychiatry. Revue canadienne de psychiatrie. 2021;**66**(1):5-8. DOI: 10.1177/0706743720937833

[46] Kai CAM, Ryan O, Hsien-Hsien L, Rajendram M, Grisan KV, Verma SK, et al. Digital health solutions for mental health disorders during COVID-19. Frontiers in Psychiatry. 2020;**11**

[47] Schreiber M. Treating patients with long COVID. American Psychological Association. 2021;**52**(5)

[48] Aiyegbusi OL, Hughes SE, Turner G, et al. Symptoms, complications and management of long COVID: A review. Journal of the Royal Society of Medicine. 2021;**114**(9):428-442. DOI: 10.1177/01410768211032850

Chapter 11

Prevalence of Various Psychological Disorders during the COVID-19 Pandemic

Robabe Khalili and Leila Karimi

Abstract

As a global threat, the COVID-19 pandemic is a challenge to psychological resilience. The aim was to determine the prevalence of various psychological disorders during the COVID-19 pandemic. This is a systematic review. Studies using different combinations of keywords COVID-19, SARS-COV, pandemic, psychological disorders, mental health and, psychological consequences were retrieved from different scientific databases Elsevier, Pubmed, Science Direct, Scopus, Web of Science. These studies were published from December 1, 2019, to May 30, 2020. Twenty-eight studies out of 410 retrieved articles were evaluated and analyzed for data extraction. The analysis of studies revealed that the different types of psychological disorders like stress, anxiety, depression, post-traumatic stress disorder, mental distress, schizophrenia, sleep disorders and sleep disturbances, vicarious traumatization, and internet addiction on moderate to severe in public and medical personnel were recorded during COVID-19 crisis. The frontline health care workers were more depressed, anxious, insomniac, and mentally disturbed. Women were more vulnerable to psychological disorders and sleep problems. Young people were more likely to experience generalized anxiety disorder and mental distress. COVID-19 has led to high prevalence and a wide range of psychological disorders in society. It is essential to provide psychological assistance and training strategies to deal with a variety of these psychological disorders.

Keywords: psychological disorders, pandemic, COVID-19, SARS-COV, systematic review

1. Introduction

Coronavirus Disease 2019 [COVID-19] appeared in Wuhan, China in December 2019 and spread rapidly throughout the country and then the world, so today we are facing a pandemic [1]. From 15 April 2020 to 21 July 2022, a number of 571,833,637 Covid-19 patients were identified in the world, of which 6,396,439 deaths due to the virus occurred [2]. So far, this virus has caused 108,721,646 total infected cases and 1,499,042 total deaths in the USA. The most cases and mortality of 212,621,751 and 1,868,908 respectively, occurred after this pandemic in Europe. Also, in Asia, there have been 165,724,865 total cases and 1,444,347 total deaths due to this virus [2].

The ambiguous nature of the disease and its unfamiliarity, as well as the implementation of quarantine measures that were strictly applied in some countries, such as China, to keep a large number of people in isolation, increased the burden of the disease and affected many aspects of their lives. It has caused widespread psychological problems such as panic disorder, anxiety, and depression along with physical problems [3]. Sirati Nir mentions according to Wang & et al "Anxiety caused by the fear of being in the community causes people not to enter shopping centers, students do not enter educational centers, and workers and tourists do not enter work and leisure institutions, and these cases lead to feelings of reduced independence and stress and worries about income and security occupations and other issues have led to psychological problems, with governments in China, Singapore, and Australia expressing concern about the psychological side effects of Covid-19, and the long-term effects of this isolation and fear in society are considered serious threats to mental health" [4].

Psychiatric disorders are highly prevalent in medical illnesses. According to world health organization (WHO) figures, at least 52 million people worldwide suffer from severe mental illness and 150 million from severe mental disorders [5]. A mental disorder is a behavioral and psychological pattern that occurs in a person and is associated with a functional disorder caused by a biological disorder [social, psychological, genetic, physical, or chemical] [6]. In addition to the suffering and limitations that it creates for the individual, mental illness causes discrimination in social and professional activities due to the stigma of mental illness and thus imposes a heavy financial burden on society and the individual [7]. In a systematic review, it was reported that the quality of life of communities that suffer from Covid-19 is greatly reduced due to social distance [8].

Also, epidemic outbreaks can cause significant psychological stress that may lead to adverse effects on the quality of life and overall mental health of employees, which emphasizes the need to establish psychological support programs for medical workers during infectious disease outbreaks. It has been suggested that social support may be a powerful strategy to reduce the negative consequences of mental status faced by medical workers during infectious disease epidemics [9, 10]. In research on previous epidemics in recent years, a wide range of psychosocial effects on individuals at the individual, community, and Internationally reported at the time of the outbreak of infection [11]; so the flu outbreak, about 3–10% of the general public were concerned about being infected with the virus and the disease [12]. In the study of the Ebola outbreak, a wide range of psychosocial effects on individuals during the outbreak of infection were reported at the individual, national and international levels, and at the individual level, individuals seeking high fears of illness or death, feeling weak. They had experienced disability and social stigma [11]. Closing schools and businesses increased the negative emotions that people experienced. For example, during the outbreak of SARS, significant psychological effects were reported, especially in younger people than in older people [13, 14].

2. The importance of the issue

Because the coronavirus COVID-19 is a public health emergency of international concern, it poses a challenge to psychological resilience. According to the evidence ordinary people, patients, staff, and family members of patients and health workers are exposed to the psychological damage caused by the epidemic of the virus.

Understanding the mental state of people exposed to psychological disorders can help professionals to provide targeted psychological interventions to improve the patient's mental health. Also, it is necessary to provide evidence-based strategies to policymakers in any community to reduce the adverse psychological effects and psychiatric symptoms during an epidemic, which can lead to restrictive measures to control and alleviate psychological problems following or during the COVID-19 epidemic [15]. Due to the onset of the Covid-19 epidemic in China, evidence-based assessments and mental health interventions for patients and health care staff are relatively rare [16]. Therefore, conducting a systematic study by reviewing and combining all related documents can create a more complete picture of the dimensions of this problem in society. Coronavirus infection has been performed worldwide and has looked for symptoms such as depression, anxiety, insomnia and anxiety and potential risk factors associated with it, and can therefore provide a clear basis for intervention and implementation of mental health intervention policies for confronting this challenge efficiently and effectively.

3. Investigation's method

This study was conducted by systematic review. To access articles related to various types of psychological disorders in the face of the coronavirus covid-19 epidemic, articles published in databases such as Elsevier, Pubmed, Science Direct, Scopus, Web of Science, and Google Scholar search engines were used to search for articles using systematic search with the keywords Psychiatric consequences, Psychological disorder, Mental health problem, COVID-19, Outbreak in the period from 1 December to 30 May 2020. In addition, the reference list of the obtained articles was examined to identify the articles that were not obtained using the above methods. An initial search found 410 articles and then according to the title and abstract of articles and several levels and removal of unrelated and duplicate articles, finally 28 articles were included in the study for extraction and evaluation (**Figure 1**). Inclusion criteria included: main articles and studies on psychological disorders in the face of the Covid-19 coronavirus epidemic. Unknown reports from gray literature, book

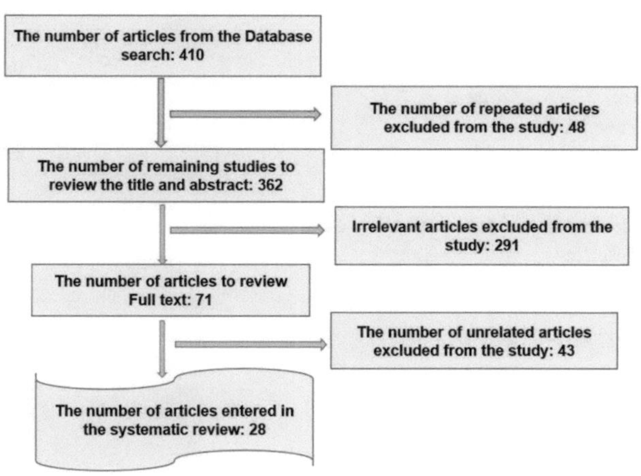

Figure 1.
The process of investigation, screening, and selection of articles.

chapters, personal views, letters to the editor, historical articles, and non-scientific articles were excluded from this study. A screening tool for the quality of articles to select relevant articles PRISMA checklist was used. After collecting the relevant information was read by one of the authors and the most important points were summarized. The information was recorded in the standard format and then registered as a validity summary.

4. Finding

Table 1 shows a summary of information from 28 evaluated articles on the prevalence of various psychological disorders in the face of the Corona Covid-19 pandemic. The items listed in **Table 1** include the author and year of study, purpose, location, tools used, number of samples, population, study method, and related results. Based on **Table 1**, the types of psychological disorders following coronavirus can be categorized in different studies. All studies on the Covid-19 crisis in six countries, China, Iran, Iraq, India, Mexico, and the United Kingdom, were performed using standard tools using quantitative and qualitative methods. Of course, only a qualitative study was conducted in Iran [36]. Studies have been done only

Author/year	Aim	Instrument	Population/ sample size	Study design	Conclusion
Qiu & et al. 2020 [17]	A nationwide survey of psychological distress among Chinese people in the COVID-19 epidemic/ Hong Kong, Macau and Taiwan	Leveraging the Siuvo Intelligent Psychological Assessment Platform, the COVID-19 Peritraumatic Distress Index (CPDI)	Isolated people in House/52,730	Cross -sectional	35% of the study population had (stress, anxiety, and depression). Women, and the age group 18-30 years; had a higher level of psychological distress.
Yang & et al. 2020 [15]	Analysis of psychological state and clinical psychological intervention model of patients with COVID-19	Hamilton depression scale (HAMD) and Hamilton anxiety scale (HAMA)	Patients (113) and healthy people (30)/143	Experimental	The anxiety and depression score of patients admitted with Covid - 19 was higher than volunteers. After Psychological intervention dramatically anxiety and depression subsided.
Lai & et al. 2020 [16]	Factors Associated With Mental Health Outcomes Among Health Care Workers Exposed to Coronavirus Disease 2019	Chinese versions of Patient Health Questionnaire, Generalized Anxiety Disorder scale, Insomnia Severity Index, and the 22-item Impact of Event Scale–Revised.	Nurse (764) and doctor (493)/1257	Cross -sectional	Severity of depressive symptoms; Anxiety and insomnia and psychological distress in 41.5% of medical staff on the front line Treatment at Wuhan hospitals Were higher than the others.

Author/year	Aim	Instrument	Population/ sample size	Study design	Conclusion
Zhang & et al. 2020 [18]	Health, distress, and life satisfaction of people one-month into COVID-19 outbreak in China.	On the eight dimensions of health (SF12), distress (K6), and life satisfaction	Adult citizen/369	Cross -sectional	Those who quit their jobs due to the corona epidemic Had lower health and life satisfaction scores and had more psychological distress.
Wang & et al. 2020 [4]	Immediate Psychological Responses and Associated Factors during the Initial Stage of the 2019 Coronavirus Disease (COVID-19) Epidemic among the General Population in China	Event Scale-Revis Depression, Anxiety and Stress Scale (DASS-21)ed. (IES-R)	Adult citizen/1210	Cross -sectional	53.8% moderate to severe psychological disorders they had. 16.5% depression, 28.8% Anxiety, and 1.8% moderate to severe stress they had. Poor personal health status Wearing a mask and hand washing) with higher levels He was associated with psychological disorders.
Huang & Zhao 2020 [19]	Generalized anxiety disorder, depressive symptoms and sleep quality during COVID-19 epidemic in China	General anxiety disorder (GHQ), Pittsburg Sleep Quality Index (PSQI), Center for Epidemiologic Scale-Depression (CES-D)	Health care worker and non Health care worker/603	Cross -sectional	34% of generalized anxiety, 18% of depression, and 18.1% reported sleep disorders. Persons with Younger Depression and more widespread anxiety And medical staff also had sleep disorders Showed more.
Ying & et al. 2020 [20]	Mental health status among family members of health care workers in Ningbo, China during the Coronavirus Disease 2019 (COVID -19) outbreak	Chinese version of Patient Health Questionnaire-9 (PHQ-9) and the Chinese version of Generalized Anxiety Disorder-7(GAD-7)	Family of health care worker/822	Cross -sectional	33.7% reported generalized anxiety disorder and 3.29% reported depression. Family members who came in direct contact with suspected or positive Covid-19 cases were more prone to widespread anxiety.
Liu & et al. 2020 [21]	Online mental health services in China during the COVID-19 outbreak.	The Hospital, Anxiety and Depression scale – Anxiety (HASD-A)	Health care worker/patients/ students/General population/72 health screenings in 31 province	Cross -sectional	50.7% anxiety; 36.1% had insomnia and 73.43% had stress related to the symptoms of the disease.

Author/year	Aim	Instrument	Population/ sample size	Study design	Conclusion
Kwok & et al. 2020 [22]	Social Responses During the Early Stage of the COVID-19	The Hospital, Anxiety and Depression scale - Anxiety (HASD-A)	General population/1715	Cross-sectional	The majority (97%) were concerned about the prevalence of Covid-19, and 98% had a slight disturbance in their daily activities. Also, their anxiety score was on average abnormal.
Jiang & et al. 2020 [23]	Psychological Impact and Coping Strategies of Frontline Medical Staff in Hunan Between January and March 2020 During the Outbreak of Coronavirus Disease 2019 (COVID-19) in Hubei, China.	Researcher based Questionnaire (5 sections)	doctors, nurses, and other hospital staff/534	Cross-sectional observational study	The COVID-19 outbreak in Hubei resulted in increased stress for medical staff in adjacent Hunan province. Continued acknowledgment of the medical staff by hospital management and the government, provision of infection control guidelines, specialized equipment, and facilities for the management of COVID-19 infection should be recognized as factors that may encourage medical staff to work during future epidemics.
Dai & et al. 2020 [24]	Psychological impact of the coronavirus disease 2019 (COVID-19) outbreak on healthcare workers in China.	General Health Questionnaire	Healthcare workers/4357	Cross-sectional study	Among the front-line staff at Wuhan Hospitals who were isolated and family members and co-workers had affected, there was a 39 percent psychological distress.
Liu & et al. 2020 [25]	Prevalence and predictors of PTSS during COVID-19 Outbreak in China's Hardest-hit Areas: Gender differences matter	PTSD Checklist for DSM-5, the Pittsburgh Sleep Quality Index (PSQI0), (PCL-5)	Residents of cities in crisis/285	Cross-sectional study	One month after the epidemic, the results showed that 7% of the study population had severe symptoms of post-epidemic stress. There were accidents (hyperexcitability, frequent reminders, and negative changes in mood and cognition). People with better sleep quality and early awakening had the fewest symptoms of post-traumatic stress.

Author/year	Aim	Instrument	Population/ sample size	Study design	Conclusion
Sun & et al. 2020 [26]	prevalence of and risk factors for acute posttraumatic stress disorder (PTSD) in Chinese people shortly after the COVID-19 outbreak.	PTSD Checklist for DSM-5 (PCL-5), Sleep Quality Index (PSQI) (PCL-5)	Chinese people/2091	Cross-sectional study	One month after the epidemic, the results showed that 1.4% of the study population developed post-traumatic stress symptoms. Predictors of post-traumatic stress included the female population, people with a history of recent exposure in Wuhan, people at risk of infection, and poor sleep quality.
Hu & et al. 2020 [27]	to validate this observation and find potential risk factors, if applicable	International Classification of Diseases 10th Edition (ICD-10)	Chines Adult population/13783	Cross-sectional study	After eliminating seasonal factors such as spring festivities, a positive relationship was found between the prevalence of schizophrenia and the Covid-19 epidemic for the first time. Also in the middle age group (39-50), a large increase in the incidence of schizophrenia was observed for the first time.
Qi & et al. 2020 [28]	to evaluate sleep disturbances of fMW and made a comparison with non-fMW.	Pittsburgh Sleep Quality Index (PSQI), Athens Insomnia Scale (AIS) and Visual Analogue Scale (VAS)	medical workers from multiple hospitals in Hubei Province, China/1306	Cross-sectional study	Frontline staff had lower scores on sleep quality, insomnia, and depressive symptoms, and they were more anxious than other health care workers. Women showed lower sleep quality and more sleep disturbance than men compared to the subgroup.
Xiao 2020 [6]	Social capital and sleep quality in isolated individuals during the Covid-19 epidemic	Personal Social Capital Scale 16 (PSCI-16), Self-Rating Anxiety Scale (SRAS), the Stanford Acute Stress Reaction (SASR), Pittsburgh Sleep Quality Index (PSQI)	Isolated people For 14 days/170	Cross-sectional study	Low levels of social capital were associated with increased levels of anxiety and stress. But with increasing levels Social capital had a positive relationship with increasing the quality of sleep. Anxiety was associated with stress and decreased sleep quality, and the combination of anxiety and stress reduced the positive effects of social capital on sleep quality.

Author/year	Aim	Instrument	Population/ sample size	Study design	Conclusion
Li 2020 [29]	The effect of declaring the Covid-19 epidemic on psychological consequences	Online Ecological Recognition (OER)	Socially prosperous class/17865	Cross-sectional study	After the announcement of the Covid epidemic - 19 negative emotions (anxiety, depression, and violence) increased and vice versa positive emotions (life satisfaction and happiness) decreased. The subjects were most concerned about their own health and that of their families.
Li, & et al. 2020 [30]	Adjacent psychiatric traumatization at the community level and medical and non-medical teams helping to control Covid-19	A mobile app-based	community members and nurses/730	cross-sectional study	Proximity psychological trauma was assessed with psychological and physiological scores among Frontline nurses were lower in treatment than nonlinear frontline nurses. The scores of proximity psychological trauma to the general public were higher than front-line nurses, but did not differ from non-front-line nurses.
Moghani & et al. 2020 [31]	Assessing the level of anxiety of the Iranian community in Covid-19	Online questionnaire	General population/10754	Descriptive	Anxiety levels in women, Young people 21-40 years old, and People who had at least one sick family member or friend, It was higher.
Taghizadeh & et al. 2020 [32]	Anxiety and depression in medical staff and the community	Hospital Anxiety and Depression Scale (HADS)	General population/2045	Descriptive-cross-sectional	65.6% and 423% of the samples had moderate to severe anxiety and depression, respectively. The prevalence of anxiety was higher in the age range of 30-39 years. Anxiety and depression in doctors, nurses, and people suspected of having Covid-19 were higher than in other occupations and the general public.
Jahanbakhshi & et al. 2020 [33]	Anxiety of Iranian adults during Quaid; Predicting more distress than Chinese	Covid-19 Peritraumatic Distress Index (CPDI)	Adult General population/1058	Descriptive-cross –sectional	The level of psychological distress in Iranians was 33.54 on average, which was higher than the average level of stress in the Chinese at 23.65.

Author/year	Aim	Instrument	Population/ sample size	Study design	Conclusion
Kaveh & et al. 2020 [34]	Anxiety level in the treatment staff during Covid-19	Beck Anxiety Inventory (BDI)	Hospital medical staff/1038	Descriptive-cross –sectional	39.6% of participants had moderate to severe anxiety. The level of anxiety of women and nurses was higher than in other samples.
Ansari & et al. 2020 [35]	Factors related to the psychological state of individuals in Covid-19	Hospital Anxiety and Depression Scale (HADS)	Adult General population/788	Descriptive-cross –sectional	Mean anxiety and depression scores of the samples, respectively; were 7/08 ± 3.68 and 6.27 ± 71.3. Anxiety and depression scores were higher in widows, women, and those with cardiovascular disease.
Eisazadeh & et al. 2020 [36]	Psychological consequences of Covid-19 patients	Semi- Structure Interview	Adult General population/9	Qualitative Content Analysis	Fear of death, anxiety, depression and decreased social activity and feelings of exclusion from society and reduced contact with family and community and the experience of the social stigma of having Covid-19 disease in the individual or family members were expressed.
Othman & et al. 2020 [37]	Depression, Anxiety, and Stress in the Time of COVID-19 Pandemic in Kurdistan Region, Iraq. Kurdistan Journal of Applied Research	Depression, Anxiety and Stress Scale (DASS-21)	Adult General population/548	Descriptive-cross-sectional	45% had depression, 47% anxiety, and 18% stress. In regression analysis, the female gender was the most important factor for the high level of depression, anxiety, and stress. Depression, anxiety, and stress were higher in people with higher education.
Suryadevara & et al. 2020 [38]	Mental Health Status among the South Indian Pharmacy Students during Covid-19 Pandemic Quarantine Period: A Cross-Sectional Study.	Depression, Anxiety and Stress Scale (DASS-21)	Pharmacy students/500	Descriptive-cross sectional	31.5%, 26%, and 19% of students had severe to very severe anxiety, depression, and stress, respectively.

Author/year	Aim	Instrument	Population/ sample size	Study design	Conclusion
Garcia-Priego 2020 [39]	Anxiety, depression, attitudes, and internet addiction during the initial phase of 2019 coronavirus disease (COVID-19) epidemic	Hospital Anxiety and Depression Scale (HADS), Internet Addiction Test (IAT)	Adult General population/561	Descriptive-cross –sectional	Fifty percent had anxiety, 27.6 percent had depression, and 62.7 percent had Internet addiction in the first few weeks of quarantine. Anxiety, depression in young people, and people addicted to the Internet with sleep problems were more.
Pieh & et al. 2020 [40]	Mental health during COVID-19 lockdown: A comparison of Austria and the UK. Available	Depression (PHQ-9), anxiety (GAD-7), stress (PSS-10), and sleep quality (ISI)	Adult General population/2015	Descriptive-cross –sectional	8.4% and 24.6% had severe depression in Astaria and England, 6% and 18.9% had severe anxiety in Austria and the UK, respectively, and 15.8% and 28.2% in the UK had sleep problems following COVID-19. The average perceived stress score in Staria and England was 16 ± 7.5 and 17.7 ± 7/9 respectively.

Table 1.
Summary of studies.

in the community [4, 18, 22, 25–27, 31, 33, 35–37, 39, 40]. A study has been done on the patients 'families [20]. A study has been done exclusively in the patients' community [15]. Studies have also been done on isolated people in the community [6, 17]. Also, studies have been done on the medical staff [19, 21, 23, 24, 28, 30, 32, 34, 38]. Studies have been conducted jointly between patients, the community, staff, and students [21, 22]. A study also shows a psychological comparison between the general public and nurses [30]. Schizophrenia, mental distress, insomnia and sleep disturbances, and Internet addiction were among the various studies. Anxiety levels of community members, patients, and treatment staff were reported to be moderate to severe in different studies of [6–65.6%] percent [4, 6, 15–18, 21–23, 28, 29, 40]. Symptoms of depression were moderate to severe [8.4–50.4%] in isolated individuals, patients, medical staff, families of medical staff, and the affluent class of society [4, 15–17, 19, 20, 29].

Generalized anxiety disorder also occurs in medical and non-medical staff and the families of medical staff [34%] were reported [19, 20]. Stress levels in isolated individuals, affluent class, and the general public were expressed from [8.1% to 73.4%] [6, 25]. A study was shown on adults in the community aged 39–50 years [27]. Psychological disturbance and distress were reported in quarantined and isolated individuals, the general adult population, and the medical staff on average to severe [39.1–71.5%] [16–18, 24, 33]. Internet addiction was also reported [62.7%] [39]. Sleep disorders were shown as low quality of sleep and insomnia in the community, medical and non-medical staff about [18.1–36.1%] [6, 19, 21, 25–28, 39]. Vicarious traumatization was also, reported in a study in community, frontline, and non-front line nurses [30], so in community and non-frontier nurses who suffered from psychological damage in the form of symptoms of loss of appetite, fatigue, irritability, fear, inattention, numbness, despair, and insomnia were expressed. Behavioral disorders such as violence and aggression were reported in the affluent class of society [29, 32]. Psychosocial consequences following having Covid-19 disease in an individual or family member were reported in a study in Iran [36]. In some community studies, women were more vulnerable to psychological and sleep disorders [17, 23, 28, 31, 34, 35, 37]. Unemployed people [25%] also suffered from anxiety and psychological distress [18]. The level of psychological distress in Iranians with an average of [34.54] and a standard deviation was [14.92] which was higher than the average level of stress in Chinese with a value of 23.65 with a standard deviation of [5.45] [33]. Also, in front-line staff studies, about [41.5] were more likely to suffer from depression, anxiety, insomnia, and mental distress [16, 23, 28]. In some studies, younger people were more prone to generalized anxiety disorder and psychological distress [17, 19, 31, 39]. This study aimed to investigate the prevalence of various psychological disorders in the face of the coronavirus Covid-19 pandemic. Based on the results, the prevalence of various mental disorders was studied in 28 studies. In these studies, different groups including patients, patients' families, healthy people in the community, and medical staff were examined. Most of the 28 studies on the prevalence of mental disorders and related factors were related to the general public [13 studies] and medical staff [9 studies].

The most common mental disorders in the studied studies were depression and anxiety disorders so the level of anxiety in the community, patients, and medical staff were reported in different studies from moderate to severe [6–65.6%] [4, 6, 15–17, 21–23, 28, 29, 40]. Generalized anxiety disorder was also reported in medical and non-medical staff and the families of medical staff [about 34%] [19, 20]. The use of measures such as accurate updating of health information, especially about the number of people who have improved, has been associated with low- stress levels in the Covid-19 epidemic in Chinese society. Additional information about medications or vaccines, transmission routes, and updates on the number of infected cases and locations [e.g., real-time, online tracking map] were also associated with lower levels of anxiety [20], which can be of interest to the health authorities of other communities in the Covid-19 epidemic. In this study, the prevalence of moderate to severe anxiety was in the community, patients, and medical staff and the anxiety of medical staff was higher than normal in the community. Psychological problems such as anxiety, fear, and stress are more common in patients with Covid-19 or people who suspect it and the families of these patients or those with whom they are in contact. Epidemiologists, doctors, and all health professionals can also be affected by these disorders [22]. Also, the results of the above studies showed that nurses are more vulnerable to serious psychological damage in their work environment than physicians and other treatment staff [28]. Consistent with the findings of the present study, the results of a study during the SARS epidemic in Taiwan showed that nurses suffered from severe psychological problems such as anxiety and depression and militancy, and mental distress [3, 41]. Also during the MERS-CoV epidemic in Saudi Arabia, nurses became frightened and nervous after experiencing stressful patient care experiences [42]. However, in this study, compared to previous studies, the percentage of mental disorders is higher.

5. Discussion

The aim of this study was to investigate the prevalence of various psychological disorders in face of the coronavirus Covid-19 epidemic. Based on the results, the prevalence of various mental disorders was evaluated in 28 studies. In these studies, different groups including patients, patients' families, healthy people in the community, and medical staff were examined. Most of the 28 studies on the prevalence of mental disorders and related factors were related to the general public (13 studies) and medical staff (9 studies). The most common mental disorders in the studied studies were Depression and Anxiety Disorder, so the level of anxiety in the community, patients, and staff were reported in various studies from moderate to severe (6–65.6%) [6, 21–23, 28, 29, 40, 15–19]. Disseminated anxiety disorder was also reported in medical and non-medical staff and about 34% of the staff of medical staff [19, 20]. Particularly in terms of the number of people who recovered, the low level of stress in the Covid-19 epidemic was associated with 19 Chinese communities. Additional information about drugs or vaccines, routes of transmission, and updates on the number of infected cases and location (e.g., real-time, map Online tracking) was also associated with lower levels of anxiety [20], which could be of concern to health officials in other communities in the Covid-19 epidemic.

In this study, the prevalence of moderate to severe anxiety was in the community, patients, and medical staff and the anxiety of medical staff were higher than normal in the community. Psychological problems such as anxiety, fear, and stress are often present in patients with Covid-19 or people who suspect it and the families of these patients or those with whom they are in contact. Also, epidemiologists, physicians, and all health professionals can be affected [22]. The results of the above studies also showed that nurses are more psychologically exposed to serious psychological damage in their work environment than physicians and other medical staff [28]. Results of the present study The results of a study during the SARS epidemic in Taiwan showed that nurses suffered from severe psychological problems such as anxiety, depression, militancy, and mental distress [3, 41]. Patients were taken care of, but in this study, compared to previous studies, the percentage of mental disorders is higher.

Another finding of the study was the higher prevalence of anxiety, depression, and stress in quarantined people, patients, treatment staff, and families of treatment staff as well as the affluent segment of society (8.1–73.4%) [4, 6, 17]. Similar to this finding, other studies have found long-term quarantine to cause psychological problems, including anxiety and depressive disorder [11]. People who are quarantined at home avoid stress and feel lonely due to lack of space for physical activity, stress due to limited social interactions, and anxiety due to fear of transmitting the infection to family members, so their mental health needs more attention [43]. Other studies have also found that social support and social activity in the community are effective in reducing the level of depression and anxiety and better mental health [6, 44]. Post-traumatic stress disorder was also reported at approximately (4.6–7%) among adults living in cities affected by the Covid-19 epidemic crisis. Other studies have noted this point that many quarantined people have experienced psychological distress, including post-traumatic stress disorder (PTSD) and depression, and the longer they are quarantined, the more likely they are to experience PTSD symptoms [6]. In most of the studies, a high percentage of the general public (97%) were concerned about the prevalence of Covid-19 and 98% had a slight disturbance in their daily work and life, as well as an anxiety score. On the contrary, the results of this study were conducted during a study of the H1N1 flu outbreak. The results showed that about 10–30% of the general public were concerned about being infected with the virus and the disease [12]. Decreased contact with family and community and experience of the social stigma of having Covid-19 disease in the individual or family members were also reported in a qualitative study in Iran [36].

In a study of the Ebola outbreak, a wide range of psychosocial effects was reported on individuals during an outbreak of infection, including fear of illness or death, feelings of weakness, disability, and social stigma [11]. In most of the studies, women were more vulnerable to psychological disorders and sleep disorders [18, 23, 28, 31, 34, 35, 37]. Although the prevalence of the disease in Iran was higher in men in than women [45], the results of the present study with most studies in Iran and The world, including the study of Ahmadvand, Khosravi, and Meyer, is consistent [46–48]. Evidence suggests that the higher prevalence of mental disorders in women than men may be more related to women 's limitations in social participation, biological factors, and environmental stress [49]. A history of positive contact with people with symptoms and people with higher education were more aware of the risk of SARS and had moderate anxiety levels and took more precautions [14]. They performed against the infection, which is somewhat different from the results of this epidemic. In some studies, young people were more prone to generalized anxiety disorder and mental distress [18, 19, 31, 39]. That people experience more, also during the outbreak of SARS, significant psychological effects have been reported, especially in young people compared to older people [13, 50], which is similar to the results of our study. The findings of the study emphasize the need to pay attention to the health of people who have not been affected by the virus, especially those who quit when the disease broke out or people who are active in sports, who have been forced to stop physical activity due to the outbreak of the disease. Also, people who are healthy themselves but have been in contact with infected people through family or work relationships because they had lower health, more anxiety, and less life satisfaction [18], as well as support for patients, family members, and providers. Health services during the epidemic were among the items mentioned in the studies. Things like paying more attention to vulnerable groups such as youth, the elderly, women, and migrant workers, accessing and strengthening medical resources, and the public health service system, especially after the initial midwifery examination and management of the Covid-19 epidemic. Nationwide strategy and coordination for psychological first aid during major disasters, which potentially.

Presented through medicine Telemedicine is one of the interventions that should be established, and finally, a comprehensive program to reduce stress should be designed through prevention and intervention including epidemiological monitoring, screening, referral, and targeted intervention to prevent further mental health problems [23]. Research timing can explain the difference in results. For the reasons mentioned above, what seems to increase the prevalence of mental disorders in the treatment of coronary heart disease is the application of traffic regulations, followed by the closure of recreational and sports facilities, unemployment, and the resulting economic pressures. He noted the low income of some citizens. According to the results of studies and the impact of COVID-19 disease in different segments of society, including patients, the general public, medical staff, and their families, it is necessary to do timely and effective psychological interventions. In addition to medical care for patients, especially pneumonia patients who need serious quarantine, the detection of psychological problems in the disease process online, is emphasized [21]. During the Corona epidemic in some countries, including China, psychological counseling services, including the telephone and, the Internet for counseling or intervention programs, became widespread, and the China Provincial Council announced that it was launching online institutions in response to the outbreak [49].

One of the limitations of the present study is that all research has been done in a short period of time, and due to the fact that new studies on the psychological consequences of this disease are updated every day, we were able to publish the studies until the end. May 2019 and evaluate in this study. However, due to a large number of participants and the study population, which has been done among all classes, including patients, medical and non-medical staff, patients' families, quarantined people, and adults in general, this limitation is largely overshadowed.

6. Conclusion

According to the findings of the present study, Covid-19 causes a high prevalence and a wide range of psychological disorders such as (stress, anxiety, depression, post-traumatic stress disorder, schizophrenia, psychological distress, insomnia and sleep disturbance, and Internet addiction) in different individuals and groups. And especially the treatment and care staff. Because treatment and care staff are at the forefront of this incident, hospitals should strive to provide psychological support to nurses and provide timely psychological assistance and training to deal with the problem by empowering nurses to manage emotions and effective coping strategies. Other people in the community and patients also need training and support to deal with the psychological effects of the disease.

Acknowledgements

The Clinical Research Development Unit of Baqiyatallah Hospital, Behavioral Sciences Research Center, and the Vice Chancellor for Research, School of Nursing, Baqiyatallah University of Medical Sciences are hereby thanked and appreciated.

Conflict of interest

The authors declare no conflict of interest.

Author details

Robabe Khalili* and Leila Karimi
Nursing Faculty, Behavioral Sciences Research Center, Life Style Institute, Baqiyattallah University of Medical Sciences, Tehran, Iran

*Address all correspondence to: khalili1120@gmail.com

References

[1] Xiao C. A novel approach of consultation on 2019 novel coronavirus (COVID-19)-related psychological and mental problems: Structured letter therapy. Psychiatry Investigation. 2020;**17**(2):1756. DOI: 10.30773/pi.2020.0047

[2] World meters. 2020

[3] Xiao H, Zhang Y, Kong D, Li S, Yang N. Social capital and sleep quality in individuals who selfisolated for 14 days during the coronavirus disease 2019 (COVID-19) outbreak in January 2020 in China. Medical Science Monitor. 2020:26. DOI: 10.12659/MSM.923921

[4] Sirati Nir M, Karimi L, Khalili R. Research paper the perceived stress level of health care and non-health care in exposed to covid-19 pandemic. Iranian Journal of Psychiatry and Clinical Psychology. 2020;**26**(3 Spec):294-305. DOI: 10.32598/ijpcp.26.3405.1

[5] WHO organization of mental health services in developing. Countries sixteen report of WHO. Available from: http://www.healthnettpo.org/mentalhealth

[6] Cumbie SA, Conley VM, Burman ME. Advanced practice nursing model for comprehensive care with chronic illness: Model for promoting process engagement. Advances in Nursing Science. 2004;**27**(1):70-80. DOI:10.1097/00012272-200401000-00008

[7] Kaplan H SBAocpTbPN. Abstract of Clinical Psychiatry. 1st ed. Tehran: Hayyan; 1996

[8] Melo-Oliveira ME, Sá-Caputo D, Bachur JA, Paineiras-Domingos LL, Sonza A, Lacerda AC, et al. Reported quality of life in countries with cases of COVID19: A systematic review. Expert Review of Respiratory Medicine. 2021;**15**(2):213-220. DOI: 10.1080/17476348.2021.1826315

[9] Chen R, Chou KR, Huang YJ, Wang TS, Liu SY, Ho LY. Effects of a SARS prevention programme in Taiwan on nursing staff's anxiety, depression and sleep quality: A longitudinal survey. International Journal of Nursing Studies. 2006;**43**(2):215-225. DOI: 10.1016/j.ijnurstu.2005.03.006

[10] Marjanovic Z, Greenglass ER, Coffey S. The relevance of psychosocial variables and working conditions in predicting nurses' coping strategies during the SARS crisis: An online questionnaire survey. International Journal of Nursing Studies. 2007;**44**(6):991-998. DOI: 10.1016/j.ijnurstu.2006.02.012

[11] Hall RC, Hall RC, Chapman MJ. The 1995 Kikwit Ebola outbreak: lessons hospitals and physicians can apply to future viral epidemics. General Hospital Psychiatry. 2008;**30**(5):446-452. DOI: 10.1016/j.genhosppsych.2008.05.003

[12] Rubin GJ, Potts H, Michie S. The impact of communications about swine flu (influenza A H1N1v) on public responses to the outbreak: Results from 36 national telephone surveys in the UK. Health Technology Assessment. 2010;**14**(34):183-266. DOI: 10.3310/hta14340-03

[13] Sim K, Chan YH, Chong PN, Chua HC, Soon SW. Psychosocial and coping responses within the community health care setting towards a national outbreak of an infectious disease. Journal of Psychosomatic Research.

2010;**68**(2):195-202. DOI: 10.1016/j.jpsychores.2009.04.004

[14] Leung G, Lam T, Ho L, Ho S, Chan B, Wong I, et al. The impact of community psychological responses on outbreak control for severe acute respiratory syndrome in Hong Kong. Journal of Epidemiology & Community Health. 2003;**57**(11):857-863. DOI: 10.1136/jech.57.11.857

[15] Yang L, Wu D, Hou Y, Wang X, Dai N, Wang G, et al. Analysis of psychological state and clinical psychological intervention model of patients with COVID-19. MedRxiv. 2020 Jan 1. DOI: 10.1101/2020.03.22.20040899

[16] Lai J, Ma S, Wang Y, Cai Z, Hu J, Wei N, et al. Factors associated with mental health outcomes among health care workers exposed to coronavirus disease 2019. JAMA Network Open. 2020;**3**(3):e203976. DOI: 10.1001/jamanetworkopen.2020.3976

[17] Qiu J, Shen B, Zhao M. A nationwide survey of psychological distress among Chinese people in the COVID-19 epidemic: Implications and policy recommendations. General Psychiatry. 2020;**33**(2):e100213. DOI: 10.1136/gpsych-2020-100213

[18] Zhang SX, Wang Y, Rauch A, Wei F. Health, distress and life satisfaction of people in China one month into the COVID-19 outbreak. Distress and Life Satisfaction of People in China One Month into the COVID-19 Outbreak (3/12/2020). 2020 Mar 12. DOI: 10.2139/ssrn.3555216

[19] Huang Y, Zhao N. Generalized anxiety disorder, depressive symptoms and sleep quality during COVID-19 epidemic in China: A web-based crosssectional survey. medRxiv. 2020. DOI: 10.21203/rs.3.rs-17172/v1

[20] Ying Y, Ruan L, Kong F, Zhu B, Ji Y, Lou Z. Mental health status among family members of health care workers in Ningbo, China, during the coronavirus disease 2019 (COVID-19) outbreak: a cross-sectional study. BMC psychiatry. Dec 2020;**20**(1):1-0. DOI: 10.1101/2020.03.13.20033290

[21] Liu S, Yang L, Zhang XY, Liu Z. Servicios de salud mental en línea en China durante el brote de COVID-19. The Lancet Psychiatry. 2020;**7**(4):E17-8. DOI: 10.1016/ S2215-0366(20)30077-8

[22] Kwok KO, Li KK, Chan HH, Yi YY, Tang A, Wei WI, et al. Community responses during early phase of COVID-19 epidemic, Hong Kong. Emerging infectious diseases. Jul 2020;**26**(7):1575. DOI: 10.1101/2020.02.26.20028217

[23] Jiang Y. Psychological Impact and Coping Strategies of Frontline Medical Staff in Hunan Between January and March 2020 During the Outbreak of Coronavirus Disease 2019 (COVID 19) in Hubei, China. Medical Science Monitor. 2020;**26**:e924171. DOI: 10.12659/ MSM.924171

[24] Dai Y, Hu G, Xiong H, Qiu H, Yuan X. Psychological impact of the coronavirus disease 2019 (COVID-19) outbreak on healthcare workers in China. medRxiv. 2020. DOI: 10.1101/2020.03.03.20030874

[25] Liu N, Zhang F, Wei C, Jia Y, Shang Z, Sun L, et al. Prevalence and predictors of PTSS during COVID-19 Outbreak in China Hardest-hit Areas: Gender differences matter. Psychiatry Research. May 2020;**287**:112921. DOI: 10.1016/j.psychres.2020.112921

[26] Sun L, Sun Z, Wu L, Zhu Z, Zhang F, Shang Z, et al. Prevalence and risk factors of acute posttraumatic stress symptoms during the COVID-19

outbreak in Wuhan, China. MedRxiv. 23 Apr 2020;**10**(2020.03):06-20032425. DOI: 10.1101/2020.03.06.20032425

[27] Hu W, Su L, Qiao J, Zhu J, Zhou Y. COVID-19 outbreak increased risk of schizophrenia in aged adults. 2020;**1**:2-4

[28] Qi J, Xu J, Li BZ, Huang JS, Yang Y, Zhang ZT, et al. The evaluation of sleep disturbances for Chinese frontline medical workers under the outbreak of COVID-19. Sleep medicine. 1 Aug 2020;**72**:1-4. DOI: 10.1101/2020.03.06.20031278

[29] Li S, Wang Y, Xue J, Zhao N, Zhu T. The impact of COVID-19 epidemic declaration psychological consequences. A Study on Active on Weibo Usres. 2020:**17**(6);2032. DOI: 10.3390/ ijerph17062032

[30] Li Z, Ge J, Yang M, Feng J, Qiao M, Jiang R, et al. Vicarious traumatization in the general public, members, and non-members of medical teams aiding in COVID-19 control. Brain, behavior, and immunity. 1 Aug 2020;**88**:916-919. DOI: 10.1101/2020.02.29.20029322

[31] Moghanibashi-Mansourieh A. Assessing the anxiety level of Iranian general population during COVID-19 outbreak. Asian Journal of Psychiatry . Jun 2020;**51**:102076. DOI: 10.1016/j. ajp.2020.102076

[32] Taghizadeh F, Hassannia L, Moosazadeh M, Zarghami M, Taghizadeh H, Dooki AF, et al. Anxiety and depression in health workers and general population during COVID19 Epidemic in IRAN: A web-based cross-sectional study. medRxiv. 2020 Jan 1. DOI: 10.1101/2020.05.05.20089292

[33] Jahanshahi AA, Dinani MM, Madavani AN, Li J, Zhang SX. The distress of Iranian adults during the Covid-19 pandemic–More distressed than the Chinese and with different predictors. Brain, behavior, and immunity. Jul 2020;**87**:124. DOI: 10.1016/j. bbi.2020.04.081

[34] Kaveh M, Davari-tanha F, Varaei S, Shirali E, Shokouhi N, Nazemi P, et al. Anxiety levels among Iranian health care workers during the COVID-19 surge: A cross-sectional study. MedRxiv. 2020 Jan 1. DOI: 10.1101/2020.05.02.20089045

[35] Ansari Ramandi MM, Yarmohammadi H, Beikmohammadi S, Hosseiny Fahimi BH, Amirabadizadeh A. Factors affecting the psychological status of an Iranian population during Coronavirus pandemic. Caspian Journal of Internal Medicine. 2020;**11**(1):2-0

[36] Eisazadeh F, Aliakbari Dehkordi M, Aghajanbigloo S. Psychological consequences of patients with coronavirus (COVID-19): A qualitative study. Biquarterly Iranian Journal of Health Psychology. 2020;**2**(2):9-20

[37] Othman N. Depression, anxiety, and stress in the time of COVID-19 pandemic in Kurdistan region, Iraq. Kurdistan Journal of Applied Research. 5 May 2020:37-44. DOI: 10.24017/covid.5

[38] Vidyadhara S, Chakravarthy A, Kumar AP, Harsha CS, Rahul R. Mental health status among the South Indian Pharmacy students during Covid-19 pandemic's quarantine period: a cross-sectional study. MedRxiv. 2020 Jan 1. DOI: 10.1101/2020.05.08.20093708

[39] Priego-Parra BA, Triana-Romero A, Pinto-Gálvez SM, Ramos CD, Salas-Nolasco O, Reyes MM, et al. Anxiety, depression, attitudes, and internet addiction during the initial phase of the 2019 coronavirus disease (COVID-19)

epidemic: A cross-sectional study in México. MedRxiv. 2020 Jan 1. DOI: 10.1101/2020.05.10.20095844

[40] Pieh C, Budimir S, Probst T. Mental health during COVID-19 lockdown: A comparison of Austria and the UK. SSRN Electronic Journal. May 2020;**10**. DOI: 10.2139/ssrn.3592372

[41] Chen WK, Cheng YC, Chung YT, Lin CC. The impact of the SARS outbreak on an urban emergency department in Taiwan. Medical care. 1 Feb 2005:168-172. DOI: 10.1097/00005650-200502000-00010

[42] Khalid I, Khalid TJ, Qabajah MR, Barnard AG, Qushmaq IA. Healthcare workers emotions, perceived stressors and coping strategies during a MERS-CoV outbreak. Clinical Medicine & Research. 2016;**14**(1):7-14. DOI: 10.3121/cmr.2016.1303

[43] Valencia-Garcia D, Simoni JM, Alegría M, Takeuchi DT. Social capital, acculturation, mental health, and perceived access to services among Mexican American women. Journal of Latina/o Psychology. 2012;**1**(S):78-89. DOI: 10.1037/2168-1678.1.S.78

[44] Li C, Jiang S, Fang X. Effects of multidimensional social capital on mental health of children in poverty: An empirical study in Mainland China. Journal of Health Psychology. 2020;**25**(6):853-867. DOI: 10.1177/1359105317737608

[45] Farnoosh G, Ghanei M, Khorramdelazad H, Alishiri G, Farahani AJ, Shahriary A, et al. Are Iranian sulfur mustard gas-exposed survivors more vulnerable to SARS-CoV-2? Some similarity in their pathogenesis. Disaster medicine and public health preparedness. Dec 2020;**14**(6):826-832. DOI: 10.1017/dmp.2020.156

[46] Meyer C, Rumpf H, Hapke U, Dilling H, John U. Lifetime prevalence of mental disorders in general adult population. Results of TACOS study. Der Nervenarzt. 2000;**71**(7):535-542. DOI: 10.1007/s001150050623

[47] Ahmadvand A, Sepehrmanesh Z, Ghoreyshi F, Assarian F, Moosavi GA, Saee R, et al. Prevalence of mental disorders in general population of Kashan City. Iranian Journal of Epidemiology. 2010;**6**(2):16-24

[48] Khosravi S. Epidemiology of mental disorders among over 15 years old population in rural and urban area of Borujen, 1994. Journal of Shahrekord University of Medical Sciences. 2003;**4**(4):31-39

[49] The State Council of China. A notification to set up nationwide psychological assistance hotlines against the 2019-nCoV outbreak. Published February 2, 2020. Accessed March 3, 2020. Available from: http://www.gov.cn/xinwen/2020-02/02/content_5473937.htm

[50] Van Bortel T, Basnayake A, Wurie F, Jambai M, Koroma AS, Muana AT, et al. Psychosocial effects of an Ebola outbreak at individual, community and international levels. Bulletin of the World Health Organization. 2016;**94**(3):210-214. DOI: 10.2471/BLT.15.158543

Chapter 12

Overarching Goal and Intervention for Healthy Aging in Older People during and after the COVID-19 Pandemic: Impact of Rehabilitation

Koki Kawamura, Shinichiro Maeshima, Aiko Osawa and Hidenori Arai

Abstract

The coronavirus disease 2019 (COVID-19) pandemic has had a major impact on society and our lives. Many older people and those with underlying medical conditions have refrained from social activities and become housebound, increasing the risk of frailty. Therefore, we developed the Home Exercise Program for Older People, a multidisciplinary program that makes it easier for older people to exercise at home. We also provide outpatient rehabilitation for not only those affected by COVID-19, but also older people with frailty who have become confined under the COVID-19 pandemic. In this chapter, we overview the situations and lives of older people in Japan under the COVID-19 pandemic and discuss preventive strategies.

Keywords: COVID-19, SARS-CoV-2, rehabilitation, frailty, NCGG-HEPOP®

1. Introduction

1.1 Worldwide spread of COVID-19 and refraining from leaving the home among the aged

The spread of the coronavirus infection caused by the novel severe acute respiratory syndrome coronavirus 2 has had a major impact on people's lives [1, 2]. Within approximately 1 month after the global outbreak of coronavirus disease 2019 (COVID-19), when it was declared a pandemic by the World Health Organization, the average number of steps taken by 455,404 people in 187 countries was reported to have decreased by 27.3% [3]. In Japan, a state of emergency was declared, and many people were forced to refrain from going out and to restrict their social activities. They were also encouraged to stay indoors to avoid the "Three Cs" (closed spaces, crowded places, and close-contact settings). Because higher mortality rates were reported among older patients and those with underlying medical conditions [4], older individuals more strictly refrained from activities. In fact, in a survey of 1600 older persons aged 65 years and older, physical activity levels were approximately 30% lower than before the spread of COVID-19 [5, 6].

Although a trend toward less restraint with respect to engagement in activities has recently been seen, many older people remain at increased risk of frailty or deteriorating to a level requiring nursing care as the COVID-19 pandemic continues unabated. The risk of frailty or deterioration to the state of requiring long-term care is therefore increasing.

1.2 Definition of frailty

Frailty, a condition in which older people lose the ability to perform activities, is defined as "a state of multiple declines in physical functions with reserve capacity approaching or exceeding a clinically disabling threshold, assuming there is a threshold for clinical impairment" and falls between normal health and the need for nursing care [7, 8]. Frailty progresses because of not only the age-related deterioration of physical functions such as muscle strength, balance, and walking ability, but also psychological problems such as cognitive impairment and depression, and social problems such as living alone and economic deprivation, which can lead to outcomes such as functional disability, the need for nursing care, and even death [7, 9–11]. Both the prevention and remediation of frailty are important because decreased activity levels in older people increase the risk of developing frailty and, with respect to older people with underlying medical conditions, the risk of requiring long-term care [12, 13]. Frailty is characterized by vulnerability to functional decline even under mild stress and is notably reversible, allowing a return to a robust state, if appropriate measures are taken. Frailty encompasses not only physical, but also mental, cognitive, social, and other aspects (**Figure 1**). The physical aspect of frailty is based on the concept of the phenotype model proposed by Fried et al. [7]. Rockwood et al. have also proposed the deficit accumulation model [14]. The deficit accumulation model is useful for comprehensive assessment of functional impairment in the selection of clinical interventions and prediction of life expectancy and risk of institutionalization, including for those with disabilities or at end-of-life stages. Of the two models, the accumulation model is more complex to use in clinical practice, so the phenotypic

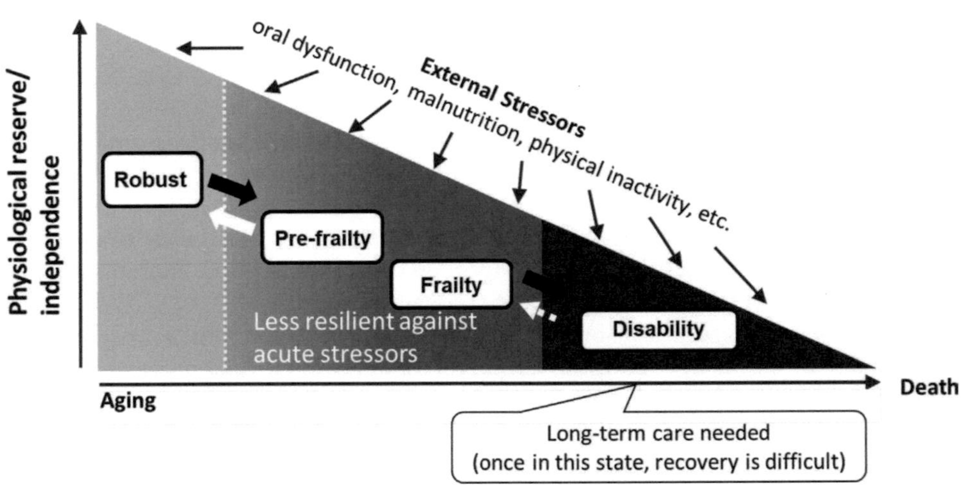

Figure 1.
Conceptual diagram of frailty for older people, there is concern about the progression of frailty, in which a small amount of stress can lead to major deteriorations in health. Prepared by the author with reference to Kuzuya M (2009) [13].

model definition is often used in studies of community-dwelling elderly, and the phenotypic model focusing on physical aspects will be used in this paper.

1.3 Assessment of frailty

The Cardiovascular Health Study (CHS) criteria proposed by Fried [7] are often used to consider disability prevention for older individuals living in the community. These criteria assess five items—fatigue, weight loss, decreased physical activity, decreased walking speed, and decreased muscle strength—with those meeting the criteria for three or more items being considered to be frail, and one or two items pre-frail. The revised Japanese version of the CHS criteria (J-CHS) [15] and the Frailty Screening Index [16] are commonly used in Japan. The former includes measures of walking speed and grip strength and focuses on the physical aspects of frailty, whereas the latter is a more general assessment, as all questions are binary choice and some focus on memory. The Kihon Checklist, which has been used to identify people eligible for secondary prevention projects and lifestyle support services, is also used. A total score of eight points or more is considered to indicate frailty, and a score of 4–7 points pre-frailty, suggesting an increased risk of requiring nursing care and even death [17].

1.4 Evidence of interventions for frailty

Intervention studies on older individuals with reduced mobility have reported the effectiveness of muscle strengthening exercises, stretching, aerobic exercises, and balance exercises on lower limb muscle strength, and many of these studies have reported that exercises combining two or more of these exercises are more effective [18]. However, evidence for interventions in older adults with frailty remains weak because the definition of "frailty" differs from country to country and study to study, and the target population is not sufficiently uniform. It is therefore desirable to establish the same definition of frailty, clarify the inclusion criteria, and accumulate larger samples.

2. Survey of the effects of COVID-19 on older people with underlying medical conditions

2.1 Survey on the influence of the spread of COVID-19 on living at home

The Asian Working Group on Sarcopenia (AWGS) recommends establishing a balance between the prevention of COVID-19 and maintenance of function [19], as well as providing continued physical activity and daily living instructions to sustain activity levels and exercise opportunities while working to prevent infection and avoid functional decline. A systematic review of the impact of the spread of infection on rehabilitation found that all patients with COVID-19, regardless of infection status, had limited rehabilitation services [20], and a follow-up study found that community-dwelling older adults who lived alone or were less socially active tended to remain less active [21]. Older individuals with frailty or underlying conditions who live alone and have little social interaction may be at a particularly increased risk of developing frailty and disability.

Our hospital provides rehabilitation services to older patients not only during inpatient care, but also on an outpatient and home-visit basis. Under this situation, with the aim of discussing future interventions to maintain activity levels and function in older patients with underlying diseases, we conducted a survey on the impact of the spread of COVID-19 in older patients undergoing rehabilitation at our hospital [22].

2.2 Impact of the pandemic in the patients who received rehabilitation

We surveyed 175 patients aged 65 years or older receiving outpatient or in-home rehabilitation at our center regarding their activities before and during the spread of COVID-19. The results indicated that the frequency of going out for errands tended to decrease during the period of infection spread. On the other hand, the frequency of going out for health reasons tended to be divided into two groups: those who consciously went out and those who refrained from and reduced the frequency of going out. Regarding exercise, approximately half of the respondents reported engaging in some form of exercise during the COVID-19 pandemic, with the most common reference material being "nothing in particular" (**Figure 2**). The frailty group was classified into three groups based on scores on the Kihon Checklist and whether they required nursing care [17, 23]. Both the frailty and nursing care groups were significantly less likely to go out after the start of the infection spread (**Figure 3**).

2.3 Outcomes of older patients hospitalized with COVID-19

The number of infected patients in Japan increased dramatically around January 2022 as the Omicron variant, which is associated with a lower mortality rate but greater infectiousness compared with the Delta variant, became the dominant strain [24]. Older individuals with pre-hospitalization frailty were found to be more likely to experience disability during acute treatment and a reduced ability to perform activities of daily living, even in relatively mild cases of COVID-19, and to sometimes require continued rehabilitation even after treatment is completed [25, 26]. We conducted a study using the Clinical Frailty Scale (CFS) to determine whether patients admitted to our hospital with a positive COVID-19 test result could be discharged directly home from the COVID-19 ward after the completion of acute care, depending on the severity of their frailty. The cutoff value on the CFS for not being discharged home [14] was six points (moderate frailty) or higher, with a sensitivity of 77.8% and specificity of 81.8% [27].

3. Home exercise program for older people (NCGG-HEPOP®)

3.1 Development and Purpose of HEPOP®

To maintain the physical and mental functions of older individuals whose social activities were limited because of the prolonged spread of COVID-19 and other factors and to create materials that would allow nonprofessionals to provide appropriate advice regarding exercise and activity, the National Center for Geriatrics and Gerontology published a "Home Exercise Program for Older People" (NCGG-HEPOP®). This program was drafted mainly by therapists and completed by considering advice and opinions from specialist physicians from each department and multiple other professionals.

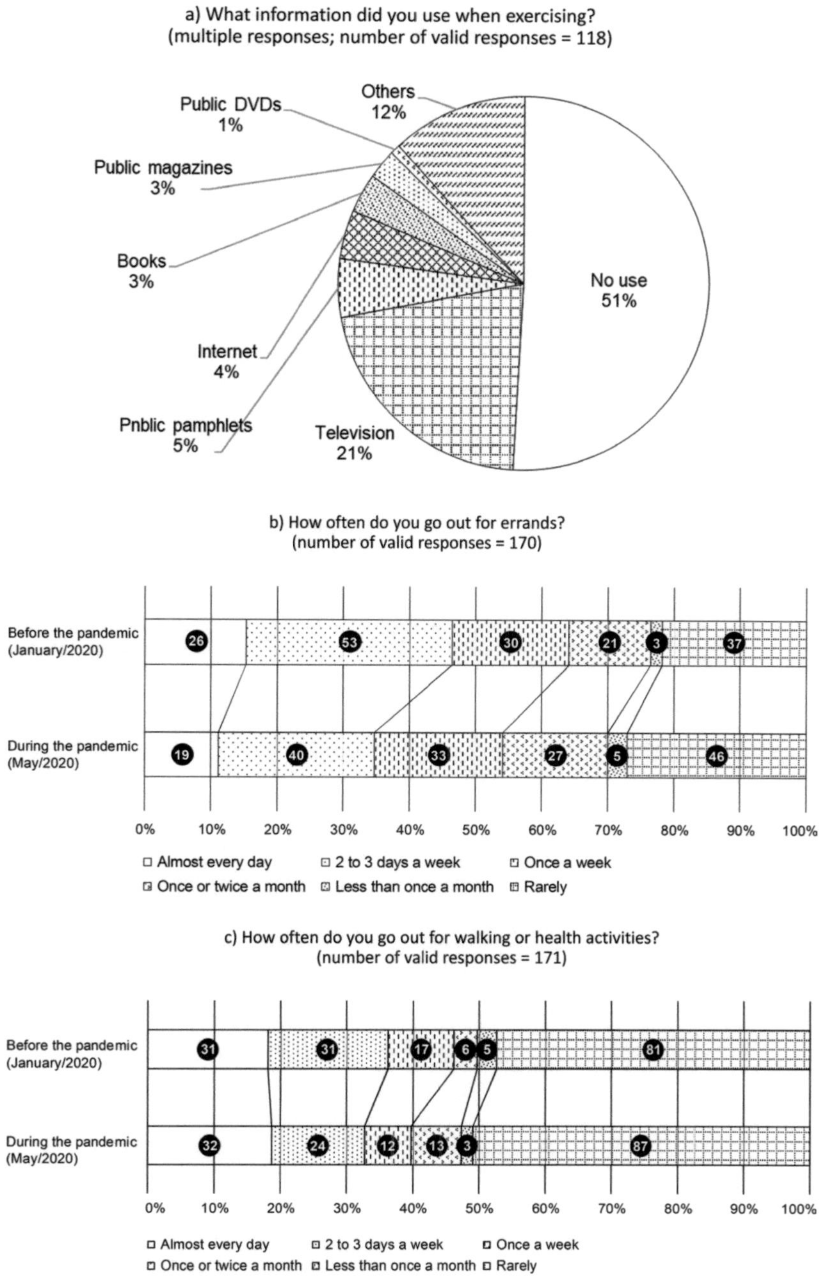

Figure 2.
Status of exercise and going out.

3.2 Contents of HEPOP®

In HEPOP®, a flowchart was created to enable the selection of an appropriate individual exercise and activity package and exercise and lifestyle guidance program (**Figures 4** and **5**) based on several questions [28]. For example, responses of "Yes"

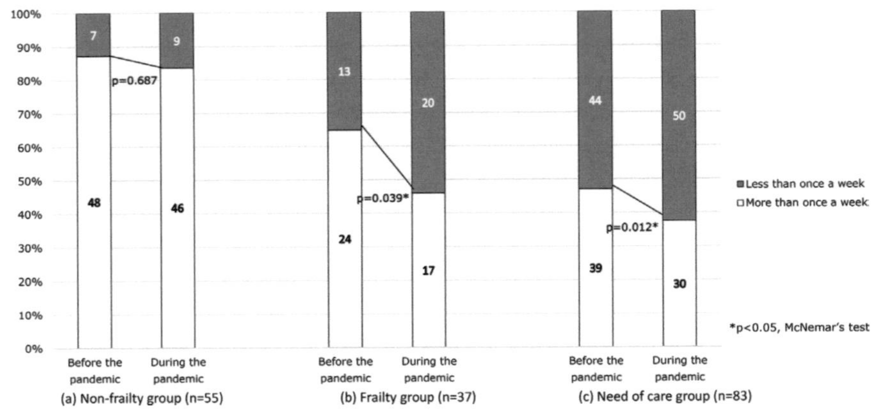

Figure 3.
Change in frequency of going out before and after the spread of infection. Before the pandemic = November/2019–January/2020. During the pandemic = March/2020–May/2020. (a) Kihon Checklist (KCL) score < 8, (b) KCL score ≥ 8, (c) Person in need of nursing care.

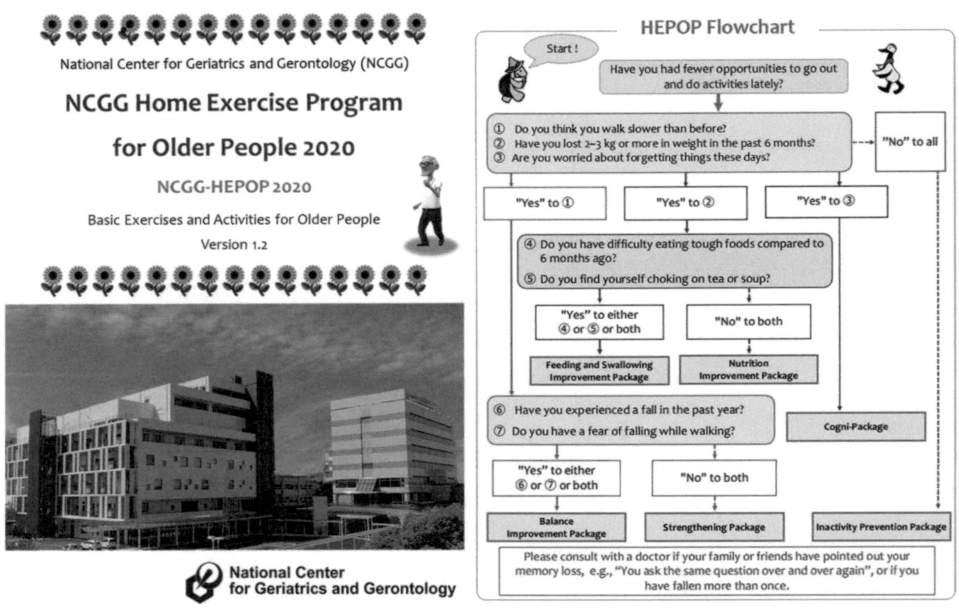

Figure 4.
Home exercise program for older people (HEPOP®).

to the items "Do you think you walk slower than before?" and "Have you experienced a fall in the past year?" recommends of balance improvement package. Five other packages were also created: Strengthening package, Inactivity prevention package, Cogni-package, Feeding and swallowing improvement package, and Nutrition improvement package [29, 30]. Each package includes more than 10 different programs and is classified into three levels according to the exercise difficulty and load, thereby allowing participants to select and combine exercises according to their abilities and condition on that particular day. Since the appropriate package may change depending on one's physical and mental condition, it was recommended to answer the flowchart questions once a month or after changes in one's physical or

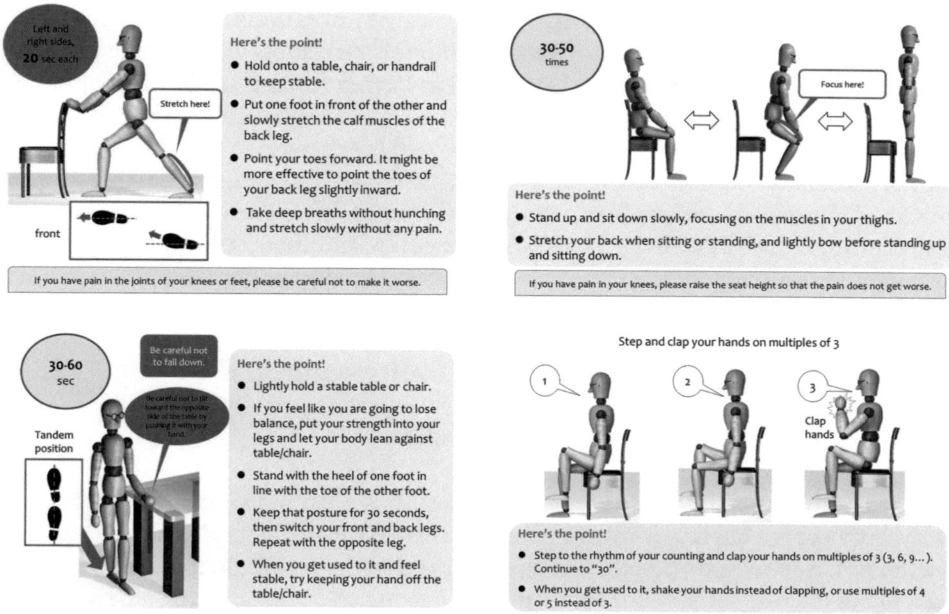

Figure 5.
HEPOP® exercises.

mental condition and to choose exercises and activities more appropriate for one's condition at that time.

3.3 Preparing and publishing shortened, video, and multi-language versions of HEPOP®

To disseminate HEPOP® widely around the world, we made it available for anyone to view and download free of charge from our website and also printed and distributed booklets. In addition, we produced a DVD that included some of the exercises with explanations [31] and distributed it to those who wanted to learn more, in addition to uploading the contents to YouTube. We also had the videos translated into English, Chinese, Thai, Russian, and other languages, with the aim of creating content that could be used by anyone around the world.

3.4 Application of HEPOP® and problems experienced during the COVID-19 pandemic

Study participants with various diseases, as described in the previous section (2.1), were given exercise instructions using HEPOP® and encouraged to exercise independently at home. Several weeks later, those who were non-frail, frail, or in need of care at the time of the intervention were surveyed to determine whether they had implemented the exercises [22]. Approximately 50% of those in the non-frail group and those in need of care were able to implement exercises at least once a week, whereas the frail group had a lower frequency, in the 30% range. The non-frail group was more likely to exercise because they already had a higher rate of exercise, whereas those in need of nursing care used some kind of nursing care service and required more involvement from a third party. On the other hand, the individuals with frailty were less likely to participate in social activities because of limitations in their communities, such as a lack of social gatherings and senior citizen clubs, which are the main hubs for social participation activities, as well as having fewer friends and neighbors, which may have resulted in less social participation and consequently fewer exercise opportunities [32, 33]. As the spread of COVID-19 is expected to be prolonged, and the associated limitations on social participation are presumed to further increase the risk of functional decline [34], we would like to build on these results and expand the use of tools such as HEPOP® for frail older adults and their family and medical caregivers to complement the opportunities for and quality of exercise.

4. Outpatient clinic for locomotive and frailty syndrome

4.1 What is a locomotive-frailty outpatient clinic?

To properly assess and improve the holistic health of older individuals with or at risk of frailty, our hospital has been providing a comprehensive medical service since 2016, when we established the world's first locomotive-frailty outpatient clinic. In this clinic, a multidisciplinary team of geriatricians, orthopedic surgeons, and rehabilitation physicians, as well as physical therapists, dietitians, pharmacists, and social workers, conduct evaluations to determine an appropriate treatment plan for patients and propose and implement intervention methods. For example, dietitians provide dietary and nutritional guidance to patients with malnutrition and obesity problems, and physical therapists provide exercise guidance to patients with decreased muscle strength and balance. The prevalence of frailty among the patients seen in our clinic was found to be 30.9%, which is higher than the 6.1% and 11.3% [8] reported in a survey of older adults living in the community.

4.2 Early detection of high-risk patients in need of care

One of the main roles of our locomotive-frailty outpatient clinic is the easy and early detection of patients at particularly high risk of worsening to the need for care and the provision of appropriate preventive caregiving measures. In our previous study of risk factors for worsening to the need for long-term care in 233 patients (mean age 78 ± 6 years) who had visited our locomotive-frailty outpatient clinic [35], we found an association between scores on the Short Physical Performance Battery (SPPB), which is used in AWGS 2019 [36], and whether a person was certified as requiring long-term care 1 year later. Specifically, an SPPB cutoff score of nine points or less was associated with an increased risk of new or worsened long-term care need certification after 1 year (area under the receiver operating characteristic curve 0.74, sensitivity 65%, specificity 75%) (**Table 1**).

5. Rehabilitation for older patients with frailty

5.1 Voluntary exercise efforts and behavior modification

Behavior modification is one of the most important perspectives in implementing rehabilitation for patients with frailty and those at risk of needing care. Even if high-quality exercise regimens are provided by professionals such as physical therapists or HEPOP®, simply providing it to the individual does not prevent caregiving.

	Usual walking speed (m/s)	SPPB (score)
Cutoff value	0.92	9
P	<0.001	<0.001
Sensitivity	62.2%	64.9%
Specificity	77.0%	75.0%
Maximum youden's index	0.392	0.399
AUC [95%CI]	0.740 [0.656–0.825]	0.737 [0.647–0.827]

SPPB, Short Physical Performance Battery; AUC, area under the curve; CI, confidence interval.

Table 1.
Cutoff values for usual walking speed and the SPPB.

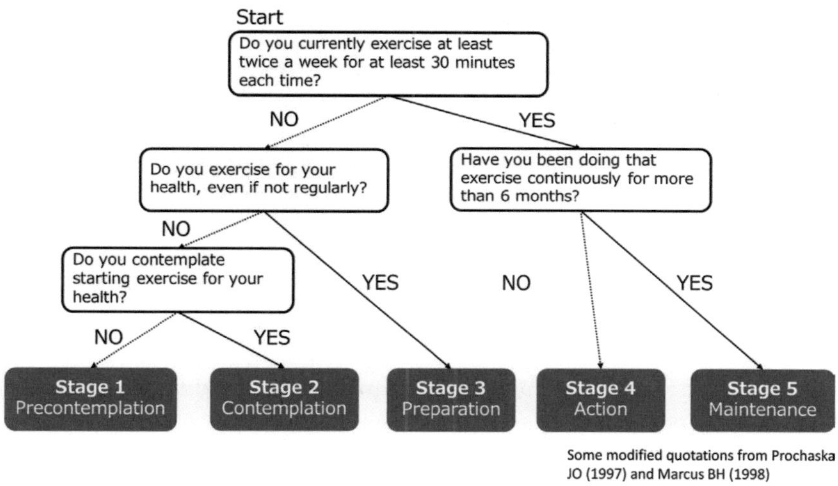

Figure 6.
Transtheoretical model flowchart some modified quotations from Prochaska JO (1997) and Marcus BH (1998) [37, 38].

In our clinic, we use the transtheoretical model of health behavior change (TTM) [37, 38], a stage classification based on behavioral modification, preparation for exercise, and duration of practice, to assess exercise awareness and provide stage-appropriate interventions when conducting rehabilitation and exercise interventions for people with frailty (**Figure 6**). Some people have always been regular exercisers, whereas others have always wanted to exercise, but have not been able to do so regularly. The method of involvement varies depending on the stage, and one of the goals is to get patients to progress to further stages. A meta-analysis of practice reports for people with diabetes found that introducing practices, setting up step-by-step exercise, working toward habituation, and providing feedback on assessment results significantly improved HbA1c levels in people with diabetes after the intervention [39].

Further study is needed to determine the effectiveness of this model for older patients with frailty. However, those in stages 2 and 3 may share a schedule and specific targets to make it easier for them to continue exercising. In stages 4 and 5, we instruct patients on the appropriate amount of exercise, the selection of an exercise program, and the correct posture so that they do not exercise incorrectly or overuse the exercise program. In stage 1, which involves the initial explanation of the benefits of exercise, followed by family participation, an immediate effect may be seen.

5.2 Changes in motor function and behavior modification stage after exercise

This section presents the findings of our clinical study on outpatient rehabilitation for older individuals who were referred from the locomotive-frailty outpatient clinic at our hospital because of declines in muscle strength and balance. Rehabilitation consisted mainly of exercise instruction at home by a physical therapist using HEPOP®. The following points were tried and tested: (1) regular evaluations were conducted to provide feedback to the patients, (2) the amount and frequency of exercise were gradually increased based on the evaluation results, (3) the importance of voluntary exercise at home was explained and the patients were asked to record their daily exercise status, (4) low-intensity, high-frequency strength exercises were performed at home, whereas high-intensity, high-difficulty balance exercises were performed at the hospital under the supervision of a physical therapist, and (5) the frequency of visits to the hospital was reduced from once a week to once a week or longer as the exercise habits became more firmly established. After 3 months of outpatient rehabilitation among 36 older individuals aged 65 years and over, we found significant improvements in walking time, on the Timed Up and Go test (TUG), and on the five times sit-to-stand test (paired *t* test, $p < 0.05$). In addition, 75% of the participants improved their TTM stage by one stage or more (McNemar's test, $p < 0.05$). Based on these findings, we believe that home exercise instruction using HEPOP® may be effective for improving physical function and promoting behavioral modification in older individuals.

5.3 A Case in which frailty improved with appropriate exercise guidance despite the COVID-19 pandemic

We present a case in which physical function was improved by exercise instruction in a homebound older adult who had originally established an exercise habit, but whose activity was restricted during the COVID-19 pandemic. An older man in his 70s with a history of a classic lumbar vertebral compression fracture had subjective symptoms of stumbling when walking after refraining from activity due to the ongoing pandemic. Prior to visiting our institution, he was attending a gym for training five to six times a week. He mainly performed aerobic exercises using an ergometer and treadmill, and his behavioral modification stage was 5. However, he was not performing muscle strengthening exercises or balance training. When COVID-19 began to spread, it limited his access to the training gym and thus reduced his activity levels. Therefore, exercise instruction from a physical therapist was started once a week at an outpatient rehabilitation center. At the time of his initial examination, he had a J-CHS score of 1 (Pre-frailty), a walking speed of 1.1 m/s, a TUG time of 7.7 s, knee extension muscle strength of 42.3 kgf on the right and 36.9 kgf on the left, and a one-leg standing time of 8.7 s. Outpatient rehabilitation included exercise instruction using HEPOP®, routine home exercise checks using a notebook, standing balance exercises, and resistance training instruction for 3 months (**Figure 7**). After the intervention, he started to perform machine training in addition to aerobic exercise at the gym, which he resumed, and was also able to perform HEPOP exercises daily at home. As a result, 3 months after the intervention, his complaint of stumbling when walking disappeared and his physical functions improved (walking speed 1.3 m/s, TUG time 6.2 s, and one-leg standing time 17.1 s). His knee extension muscle strength improved to 43.3 kgf on the right and 40.8 kgf on the left. Although this patient was in behavioral modification

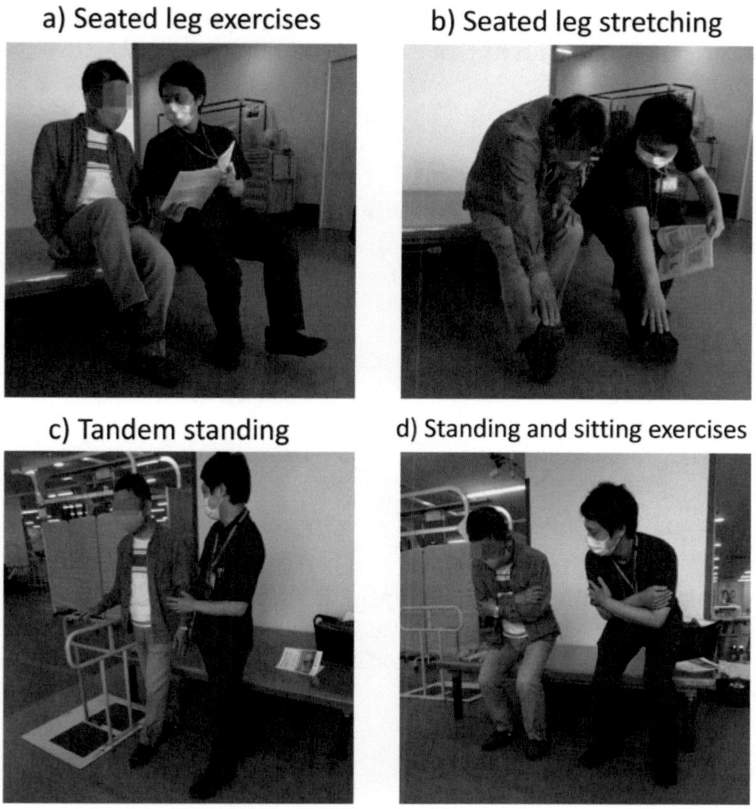

Figure 7.
Actual exercise instruction for older people using HEPOP®.

stage 5, we found that his exercise content was skewed, his balance ability had declined, and he had no exercise routine other than those performed at the gym. Therefore, even in patients with apparently good exercise habits and motivation, a specialized evaluation may reveal decreased or declining function, and a review of exercise content and improvement of function may be achieved by taking a more targeted approach. It is assumed that many older people are at risk for such functional decline as a result of the COVID-19 pandemic, so assessment and intervention in outpatient frailty clinics may play an important social role during this prolonged situation.

6. Conclusion

This chapter introduced the risk of frailty due to COVID-19 and key points regarding exercise guidance in the community and medical institutions. There is some concern that the prolonged COVID-19 pandemic has reduced the frequency of outings and opportunities for exercise and activity among many older adults, thereby increasing their risk of deteriorated physical and mental functions. In addition, in this situation, rehabilitation and other medical services are difficult to provide, and older adults with frailty are at a higher risk of decreased physical function and the need for increased caregiving. We hope that the use of guides for activities that can be performed at home according to each individual function, the provision of comprehensive support mainly through community collaboration, and ongoing assessments and support by medical professionals can help older adults living at home continue to live healthy lives.

Acknowledgements

The present studies were performed with the support of the NCGG, Japan, through grants for longevity medical research and development expenses (20–12, 20–27, 21–37, 22–22, 22–24).

Conflict of interest

The authors declare no conflict of interest.

Ethical considerations

All study protocols complied with the principles laid out in the Declaration of Helsinki, and written informed consent was obtained from each participant. The ethics review board of the National Center for Geriatric and Gerontology approved this study [Approval No. 881-9, 1413-2, 1582].

Author details

Koki Kawamura, Shinichiro Maeshima*, Aiko Osawa and Hidenori Arai
National Center for Geriatrics and Gerontology, Obu, Japan

*Address all correspondence to: shinichiromaeshima@gmail.com

References

[1] World Health Organization. WHO Coronavirus (COVID-19) Dashboard. 2022. Available from: https://covid19.who.int/ [Accessed: June 5, 2022]

[2] Ministry of Health LaW. About COVID-19. 2022. Available from: https://www.mhlw.go.jp/stf/seisakunitsuite/bunya/0000164708_00079.html [Accessed: June 5, 2022]

[3] Tison GH, Avram R, Kuhar P, et al. Worldwide effect of COVID-19 on physical activity: A descriptive study. Annals of Internal Medicine. 2020;**173**:767-770. DOI: 10.7326/M20-2665

[4] Ruan S. Likelihood of survival of coronavirus disease 2019. The Lancet Infectious Diseases. 2020;**20**(6):630-631. DOI: 10.1016/S1473-3099(20)30257-7

[5] Onder G, Rezza G, Brusaferro S. Case-fatality rate and characteristics of patients dying in relation to COVID-19 in Italy. The Journal of the American Medical Association. 2020;**323**(18):1775-1776. DOI: 10.1001/jama.2020.4683

[6] Yamada M, Kimura Y, Ishiyama D, et al. Effect of the COVID-19 epidemic on physical activity in community-dwelling older adults in Japan: A cross-sectional online survey. The Journal of Nutrition, Health & Aging. 2020;**24**:948-950. DOI: 10.1007/s12603-020-1424-2

[7] Fried LP, Tangen CM, Walston J, et al. Frailty in older adults: Evidence for a phenotype. The Journals of Gerontology. Series A, Biological Sciences and Medical Sciences. 2001;**56**:M146-M157. DOI: 10.1093/gerona/56.3.m146

[8] Gobbens RJ, Luijkx KG, Wijnen-Sponselee MT, Schols JM. In search of an integral conceptual definition of frailty: Opinions of experts. Journal of the American Medical Directors Association. 2010;**11**(5):338-343. DOI: 10.1016/j.jamda.2009.09.015

[9] Makizako H, Shimada H, Doi T, et al. Impact of physical frailty on disability in community-dwelling older adults: A prospective cohort study. BMJ Open. 2015;**5**(9):e008462. DOI: 10.1136/bmjopen-2015-008462

[10] Vermeiren S, Vella-Azzopardi R, Beckwee D, et al. Frailty and the prediction of negative health outcomes: A meta-analysis. Journal of the American Medical Directors Association. 2016;**17**(12):1163.e1-1163.e17. DOI: 10.1016/j.jamda.2016.09.010

[11] Negrini F, Sire AD, Andrenelli E, et al. Rehabilitation and COVID-19: A rapid living systematic review 2020 by Cochrane Rehabilitation Field. Update as of October 31st, 2020. European Journal of Physical and Rehabilitation Medicine. 2021;**57**(1):166-170. DOI: 10.23736/S1973-9087.20.06723-4

[12] Sugishita M, Koshizuka Y, Sudou S, et al. The validity and reliability of the Japanese version of the mini-mental state examination MMSE-J with the original procedure of the attention and calculation task (2001). Japanese Journal of Cognitive Neuroscience. 2018;**20**(2):91-110. DOI: 10.11253/ninchishinkeikagaku.20.91

[13] Kuzuya M. Impact of sarcopenia and frailty on elderly health. Japanese Journal of Geriatrics. 2009;**46**(4):279-285 (in Japanese)

[14] Rockwood K, Song X, MacKnight C, et al. A global clinical measure of fitness

and frailty in elderly people. CMAJ. 2005;**173**(5):489-495. DOI: 10.1503/cmaj.050051

[15] Satake S, Arai H. The revised Japanese version of the Cardiovascular Health Study criteria (revised J-CHS criteria). Geriatrics & Gerontology International. 2020;**20**(10):992-993. DOI: 10.1111/ggi.14005

[16] Yamada M, Arai H. Predictive value of frailty scores for healthy life expectancy in community-dwelling older Japanese adults. Journal of the American Medical Directors Association. 2015;**16**(11):1002.e7-1002.11. DOI: 10.1016/j.jamda.2015.08.001

[17] Satake S, Shimokata H, Senda K, et al. Validity of total Kihon checklist score for predicting the incidence of 3-year dependency and mortality in a community-dwelling older population. Journal of the American Medical Directors Association. 2017;**18**(6):552.e1-552.e6. DOI: 10.1016/j.jamda.2017.03.013

[18] Sherrington C, Michaleff ZA, Fairhall N, et al. Exercise to prevent falls in older adults: An updated systematic review and meta-analysis. British Journal of Sports Medicine. 2017;**51**(24):1750-1758. DOI: 10.1136/bjsports-2016-096547

[19] Lim WS, Liang CK, Assantachai P, et al. COVID-19 and older people in Asia: Asian working group for Sarcopenia calls to actions. Geriatrics & Gerontology International. 2020;**20**(6):547-558. DOI: 10.1111/ggi.13939

[20] Andrenelli E, Negrini F, Sire AD, et al. Systematic rapid living review on rehabilitation needs due to Covid-19: update to May 31st, 2020. European Journal of Physical and Rehabilitation Medicine. 2020;**56**(4):508-514. DOI: 10.23736/S1973-9087.20.06435-7

[21] Yamada M, Kimura Y, Ishiyama D, et al. Recovery of physical activity among older Japanese adults since the first wave of the COVID-19 pandemic. The Journal of Nutrition, Health & Aging. 2020;**24**(9):1036-1037. DOI: 10.1007/s12603-020-1516-z

[22] Kawamura K, Kamiya M, Suzumura S, et al. Impact of the coronavirus disease 2019 outbreak on activity and exercise levels among older patients. The Journal of Nutrition, Health & Aging. 2021;**25**(7):921-925. DOI: 10.1007/s12603-021-1648-9

[23] Satake S, Senda K, Hong YJ, et al. Validity of the Kihon Checklist for assessing frailty status. Geriatrics & Gerontology International. 2016;**16**(6):709-715. DOI: 10.1111/ggi.12543

[24] Bouzid D, Visseaux B, Kassasseya C, et al. Comparison of patients infected with delta versus Omicron COVID-19 variants presenting to paris emergency departments: A retrospective cohort study. Annals of Internal Medicine. 2022;**175**(6):831-837. DOI: 10.7326/M22-0308

[25] Evans SJ, Sayers M, Mitnitski A, Rockwood K. The risk of adverse outcomes in hospitalized older patients in relation to a frailty index based on a comprehensive geriatric assessment. Age Aging. 2014;**43**(1):127-132. DOI: 10.1093/ageing/aft156

[26] Pranata R, Henrina J, Lim MA, et al. Clinical frailty scale and mortality in COVID-19: A systematic review and dose-response meta-analysis. Archives of Gerontology and Geriatrics. 2021;**93**:104324. DOI: 10.1016/j.archger.2020.104324

[27] Kawamura K, Osawa A, Tanimoto M, et al. Prediction of the possibility of return to home based

on frailty assessment at the time of admission to the COVID-19 Treatment Unit. Geriatrics & Gerontology International. 2022 (in press)

[28] NCGG-HEPOP Committee of NCGG-HEPOP 2020: National Center for Geriatrics and Gerontology – Home Exercise Program for Older People 2020; Basic Exercise and Activities for Older People (English). 2020. Available from: https://www.ncgg.go.jp/hospital/english/hepop/ [Accessed: June 6 2022]

[29] Osawa A, Maeshima S, Kondo I, Arai H. Balancing infection control and frailty prevention during and after the COVID-19 pandemic: Introduction of the NCGG Home Exercise Program for Older People 2020. Geriatrics & Gerontology International. 2020;**20**(9):846-848. DOI: 10.1111/ggi.13991

[30] Bando H, Murakami M, Moriyasu A. Introduction of home exercise program for current circumstance worldwide. International Journal of Complementary & Alternative Medicine. 2021;**14**(4):196-198

[31] Kamiya A, Noguchi M, Kibayashi T, et al. Video demonstrating NCGG-HEPOP 2020 exercises for older adults Affiliations expand. Geriatrics & Gerontology International. 2021;**21**(9):871-872. DOI: 10.1111/ggi.14241

[32] Imuta H, Yasumura S, Abe H, Fukao A. The prevalence and psychosocial characteristics of the frail elderly in Japan: A community-based study. Aging (Milano). 2001;**13**(6): 443-453 PMID: 11845972

[33] Shimada H, Makizako H, Doi T, et al. Combined prevalence of frailty and mild cognitive impairment in a population of elderly Japanese people. Journal of the American Medical Directors Association. 2013;**14**(7):518-524. DOI: 10.1016/j.jamda.2013.03.010

[34] Woods NF, LaCroix AZ, Gray SL, et al. Frailty: Emergence and consequences in women aged 65 and older in the Women's Health Initiative Observational Study. Journal of the American Geriatrics Society. 2005;**53**(8):1321-1330. DOI: 10.1111/j.1532-5415.2005.53405.x

[35] Kawamura K, Kondo I, Osawa A, et al. Walking speed and Short Physical Performance Battery are associated with conversion to long-term care need: A study in outpatients of a locomotive syndrome-frailty clinic. Geriatrics & Gerontology International. 2021;**21**(10):919-925. DOI: 10.1111/ggi.14258

[36] Chen LK, Woo J, Assantachai P, et al. Asian Working Group for Sarcopenia: 2019 consensus update on sarcopenia diagnosis and treatment. Journal of the American Medical Directors Association. 2020;**21**(3):300-307.e2. DOI: 10.1016/j.jamda.2019.12.012

[37] Prochaska JO, Velicer WF. The transtheoretical model of health behavior change. American Journal of Health Promotion. 1997;**12**(1):38-48. DOI: 10.4278/0890-1171-12.1.38

[38] Marcus BH, Emmons KM, Simkin LR, et al. Evaluation of motivationally tailored vs. standard self-help physical activity interventions at the workplace. American Journal of Health Promotion. 1998;**12**(4):246-253. DOI: 10.4278/0890-1171-12.4.246

[39] Kevin A, Gearoid O, Francis MF, et al. Behaviour change techniques targeting both diet and physical activity in type 2 diabetes A systematic review and meta-analysis. International Journal of Behavioral Nutrition and Physical Activity. 2017;**14**(1):18. DOI: 10.1186/s12966-016-0436-0

Chapter 13

The Advantages of an Integrative Approach in the Primary Healthcare of Post-COVID-19 and ME/CFS Patients

Diana Araja, Angelika Krumina, Uldis Berkis, Zaiga Nora-Krukle and Modra Murovska

Abstract

The coronavirus disease caused by the SARS-CoV-2 virus (COVID-19) pandemic has changed not only global epidemiological and economic developments but also the lives of every individual, with particular severity for patients. The number of acute illness cases grew rapidly, significantly increasing the workload of hospitals, and simultaneously, new chronic diseases emerged, such as persistent post-COVID-19 syndrome (PPCS), with unclear etiology, symptoms, and complexity—similar to myalgic encephalomyelitis/chronic fatigue syndrome (ME/CFS). Accordingly, the burden of chronic diseases poses new long-term challenges for primary healthcare and requires new approaches to patient care. This chapter provides insight into the integrative approach to healthcare and focuses on potentially new solutions by implementing an integrative attitude to the treatment of post-COVID-19 and ME/CFS patients in primary healthcare. Integrative health coaching contributes the holistic approach to patients' overall health and resilience through cognitive practice and patient active engagement. The findings of this chapter can enrich the person-centered approach and healthcare system strengthening through holistic measures and systems thinking.

Keywords: persistent post-COVID-19 syndrome (PPCS), myalgic encephalomyelitis/chronic fatigue syndrome (ME/CFS), integrative approach, coaching, patient-reported outcomes (PROs)

1. Introduction

The coronavirus disease caused by the SARS-CoV-2 virus (COVID-19) pandemic induced overload in acute healthcare and significantly increased the burden of chronic diseases. One of the new manifestations of chronic diseases is the post-COVID-19 disorder, for which a common definition has not yet been established, but which creates the preconditions for expanding the prevalence of related diseases. The results of an online survey of 3762 participants with confirmed (diagnostic/antibody positive; 1020) or suspected (diagnostic/antibody negative or untested; 2742) COVID-19, performed in 56 countries, from September 6, 2020 to November 25, 2020, demonstrated that 1700 respondents (45.2%) required a reduced work schedule compared to pre-illness, and an additional 839 (22.3%) were not working at the time of survey due to illness. After 6 months of the post-COVID conditions, the most frequent symptoms were fatigue, post-exertional malaise, and cognitive dysfunction. Cognitive dysfunction or memory issues were common across all age groups (~88%) [1]. Already in July 2020, Dr. Anthony Fauci, the Director of the National Institute for Allergy and Infectious Diseases (US Department of Health and Human Services), assumed that patients post-COVID-19 can develop “a post-viral syndrome that's very strikingly similar to myalgic encephalomyelitis/chronic fatigue syndrome” [2].

The authors, in one of the previous studies on the COVID-19 pandemic consistencies in healthcare [3], revealed that since October 2020, several articles have reported myalgic encephalomyelitis/chronic fatigue syndrome (ME/CFS) as a potentially post-COVID-19-associated disease [4–11]. The literature reviews on the potential causal interaction between post-COVID-19 and ME/CFS also appeared in the following period [12–19]. The reviews' results highlighted problems associated with the definitions and diagnostic criteria for ME/CFS and post-COVID-19 disorder. There were various manifestations of the interaction between post-COVID-19 and ME/CFS, from the similarity of the symptoms to the assumption that it is the same disease [3]. Over time, the COVID-19 long-haulers reported an overall reduction of most symptoms including unrefreshing sleep and post-exertional malaise, but an intensification of neurocognitive symptoms. When compared to ME/CFS, the COVID-19 sample was initially more symptomatic for the immune and orthostatic domains but over time, the long-haulers evidenced significantly less severe symptoms than those with ME/CFS, except in the orthostatic domain [20]. However, almost all publications indicated the need for further research into the similarities and differences between post-COVID-19 and ME/CFS to determine the nature of these conditions and define risk factors, prevalence, and possible interventions [3].

Concerning the definitions, ME/CFS commonly is defined as a poorly understood, serious, complex, multisystem disorder, characterized by symptoms lasting at least 6 months, with severe incapacitating fatigue not alleviated by rest, and other symptoms—many autonomic or cognitive in nature—including profound fatigue, cognitive dysfunction, sleep disturbances, muscle pain, and post-exertional malaise, which lead to substantial reductions in the functional activity and quality of life [21]. The common definition of post-COVID-19 disorder has not yet been established, but the results of some studies suggest, for instance, that it is composed of heterogeneous sequelae that often affect multiple organ systems, with significant impacts on morbidity, mortality, and quality of life [1]. Regarding the defining post-COVID-19 symptoms, based on the relapsing/remitting nature of post-COVID-19 symptoms, the following integrative classification was proposed by researchers: potentially infection-related symptoms (up to 4–5 weeks), acute post-COVID-19 symptoms (from week 5 to week 12), long post-COVID-19 symptoms (from week 12 to week 24), and persistent post-COVID-19 symptoms (lasting more than 24 weeks) [22]. Therefore, in the context of the time reference, ME/CFS is most closely associated with persistent post-COVID symptoms.

Persistent post-COVID symptoms were considered in light of a new “syndrome,” as the British Medical Association defines a syndrome “as a set of medical signs and symptoms which are correlated with each other and associated with a particular disease” [22]. Accordingly, the term “Persistent Post-COVID-19 Syndrome (PPCS)” was introduced in practice, as a pathologic entity, which involves persistent physical, medical, and cognitive sequelae following COVID-19, including persistent immunosuppression as well as pulmonary, cardiac, and vascular fibrosis [23]. Consequently, some authors note that the preliminary findings raise concern regarding a possible future ME/CFS-like pandemic in SARS-CoV-2 survivors [24].

The prevalence of ME/CFS in population varies from 0.19% to 7,6% [21]. Based on the earlier studies on other infections, researchers suggested that 10% of COVID-19 survivors could develop ME/CFS [2]. Accordingly, it is estimated that the US ME/CFS prevalence of 1.5 million prior to the COVID-19 pandemic (and an annual economic impact of $36–51 billion) could rise to between five and nine million people. This would incur an annual US economic impact of $149 to $362 billion in medical expenses and lost income, exclusive of other costs, such as disability benefits, social services, and lost wages of caretakers [25].

Considering the health-related quality of life (HRQoL) ME/CFS demonstrates a significant negative impact on general health, physical functioning, emotional health, vitality, cognitive health, and well-being, in different populations [12, 26–32]. Various tools are used to elaborate the HRQoL, such as EuroQoL-5 Dimensions (EQ-5D-3L) [26, 31] and (EQ-5D-5L) [12], 36-Item Health Survey (SF-36) [29, 31], Pediatric Quality of Life Inventory (PedsQL) [28], overall health status reported on a Visual Analogue Scale (VAS) [12, 27, 30], Abbreviated World Health Organization Quality of Life questionnaire (WHOQOL-BREF) [32], completed by people with ME/CFS, and Family Reported Outcome Measure (FROM-16) questionnaire [30, 32], completed by family members. Simultaneously, HRQol widely affected by all post-COVID-19 domains [24] mostly is assessed by EuroQoL-5 Dimension EQ-5D-5L and VAS [33–35].

The predominant score of ME/CFS and PPCS patients' healthcare is related to primary healthcare, given that patients of these syndromes are mostly treated on an outpatient basis [36–39]. The unifying issues for these diseases are also complex and multisystem nature, which requires coordinated integrative multidisciplinary teamwork to achieve treatment goals [34, 39]. Previous research demonstrated significant results of the interdisciplinary approach, such as the "Recovering from COVID" course, which took a whole system, biopsychosocial approach to understanding COVID-19 and post-viral fatigue and was led by an interdisciplinary team consisting of a clinical psychologist, physiotherapist, occupational therapist, dietitian, speech and language therapist, and a personal support navigator [34].

Moreover, COVID-19 is associated with high rates of psychiatric symptoms, including anxiety, depression, fatigue, sleep disruption, and posttraumatic stress, and consistent risk factors for psychiatric symptoms include the history of a psychiatric disorder and female gender [40]. Researchers notified that while the exact etiology remains unknown, and future research is needed, it is now recognized that overlapping symptomology between post-COVID-19 syndrome and ME/CFS provides a promising avenue for the development of post-COVID-19 rehabilitation [34].

Prior to the COVID-19 pandemic, it was assumed that primary care transformation will usher in a new era of advanced team-based care with extensive roles beyond the physician to build authentic healing relationships with patients [41]. The pandemic hampered the development of primary healthcare, with an emphasis on the hospital sector, but some achievements remain topical. In the context of integrity, the integrative and patient-centric view argues strongly that populations with physical, developmental, or cognitive disabilities—often with related chronic conditions or complex illnesses—endow the concept of healthcare integration with unique logic and meaning. Vulnerable individuals have complicated and ongoing needs (which frequently are part-medical, part-physical, part-psychological, and part-social), experience difficulties in everyday living, require a mix of services delivered sequentially or simultaneously by multiple providers, and receive both cure and care in the home, community, and institutional settings [42]. These statements mostly are applicable also for ME/CFS and post-COVID-19 conditions.

In order to organize person-centered health services for a growing number of people with multiple complex health and social care needs, a shift from fragmented to integrated health services delivery has to take place. For the organization of governance in integrated health services, it is important to better understand the underlying factors that drive collaboration, decision-making, and behavior between individuals and organizations [43]. There are multiple levels of integrated care, and four levels of health services delivery are investigated more often: the personal, the professional, the management, and the system level [43, 44]. In addition to the different levels, researchers present two crucial dimensions of integration: systemic integration, which includes the coherence of rules and policies in the health system, and normative integration, which comprises the role of shared values in coordination and collaboration [43–45].

In the scope of this research, the authors focus on two central levels of the integrative model—the personal level, assuming the relation with the person-centered approach, and the professional level of collaboration (**Figure 1**).

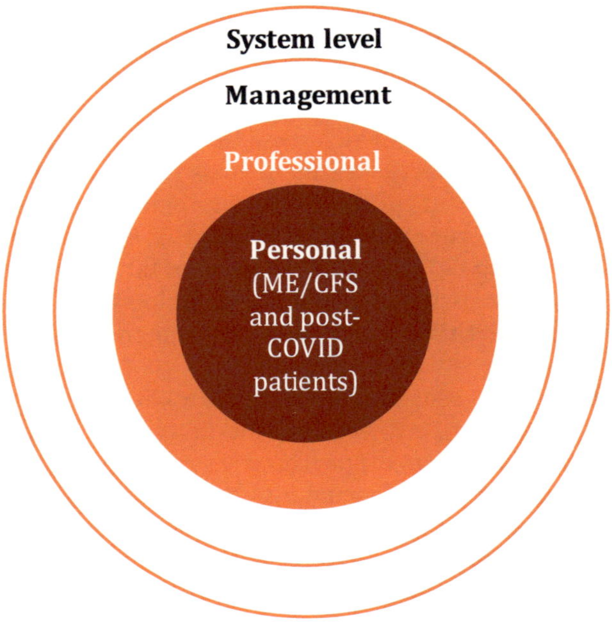

Figure 1.
The research focused on the personal and the professional level of integrated health services for myalgic encephalomyelitis/chronic fatigue syndrome (ME/CFS) and post-COVID-19 patients.

The following section provides an example of professional collaboration and patient outcomes in the integrative approach for ME/CFS and post-COVID-19 care.

2. Coaching as a supportive tool in integrative primary healthcare of post-COVID-19 and ME/CFS patients

Assuming that an integrative approach positively affects the treatment of chronic multimorbid conditions, this research aimed to identify opportunities to improve the health status of post-COVID-19 and ME/CFS patients by involving a professional coach in healthcare teamwork.

The theoretical foundation of coaching is based on psychological concepts [46]. Several types of models and theories form the basis of behavioral change in coaching. Those most frequently referred to in the literature include the Transtheoretical Model of Change (TTM), the Theory of Planned Behavior (TPB), Social Cognitive Theory (SCT), the Information-Motivation-Behavioral-Skills Model (IMB), Self-Determination Theory (SDT), Health Action Process Approach (HAPA), and Social Learning Theory (SLT) [47]. Each theory is distinct; however, coaching recognizes that individuals intrinsically learn in different ways, and thus the process could involve one or a combination of models or theories which may complement one another [46]. Practical coaching intends to facilitate, support, challenge, and guide a change to achieve a goal [48].

Regarding the coaching experience in healthcare during the COVID-19 pandemic, literature resources identified that COVID-19-specific tele-coaching effectively supported the risk-reduction behavior of patients with heart failure [49] and improved diabetes patients' health behavior [50], as well as coaching promoted medical staff well-being during COVID-19 [51] and demonstrated a positive effect on medical students' well-being [52]. On the whole, there are insufficient studies on the use of coaching in ME/CFS and post-COVID-19 patients.

To evaluate the complementary opportunities provided by coaching in post-COVID-19 in ME/CFS patients' healthcare, the longitude case study was performed in a primary care institution, in Latvia. The professional team consisted of a general practitioner, infectiologist, and coach. The coaching sessions were led by a certified coach of the Erickson Coaching International. Patient-centeredness, patient-determined goals, use of a self-discovery process, accountability, and consistent coaching relationship represent the key elements of coaching. Erickson coaching expands the coaching over and above these elements by strict focus at the solution (i.e. client's determined goal) not only throughout the individual coaching conversation but also throughout the entire coaching relationship (solution-focused Erickson coaching) [53].

Four patients, two ME/CFS and two post-COVID-19 patients with symptoms persistent for more than 6 months prior to diagnosis "Long-COVID-19," were invited to participate in this study. "Portraits" of the patients prepared by the supervising physicians are available in **Figure 2**. Virtual coaching sessions were held for each patient once a week for 4 weeks, in March and April 2022 (two additional sessions were conducted for Patient 2, by her request).

The work steps were devoted to the assessment of patients' HRQoL before and after the coaching course. In order to obtain comparable data for evaluation of the potential impact of the coaching process, HRQoL was assessed using the EuroQol-5D-5L measure (certified translation: EQ-5D-5L Latvian) as the patient-reported outcomes (PROs). The EuroQol EQ-5D-5L assesses HRQoL across five dimensions: mobility, self-care, usual activities, pain/discomfort, and anxiety/depression [54], and it was mentioned in previous research [12, 33–35]. Prior to the coaching course, patients were asked to assess their health across five dimensions, before the illness and at the present time. Accordingly, after the last coaching session, the patients had reassessed their health status.

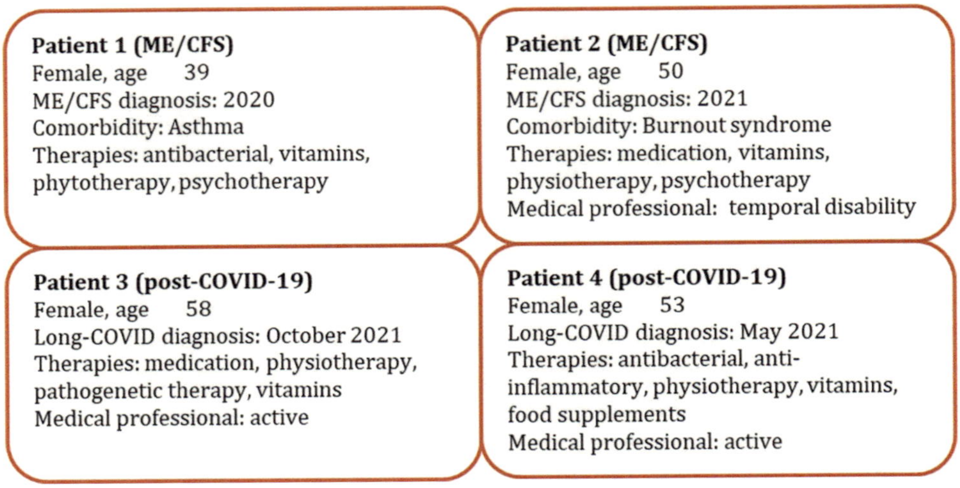

Figure 2.
"Portraits" of Myalgic encephalomyelitis/chronic fatigue syndrome (ME/CFS) and post-COVID-19 patients in the study.

The results of the PROs are shown in **Figure 3** (each dimension of health was scored from 1 (extreme problems) to 5 (no problems)). Descriptive and analytical statistical methods were utilized for the analysis of the obtained data.

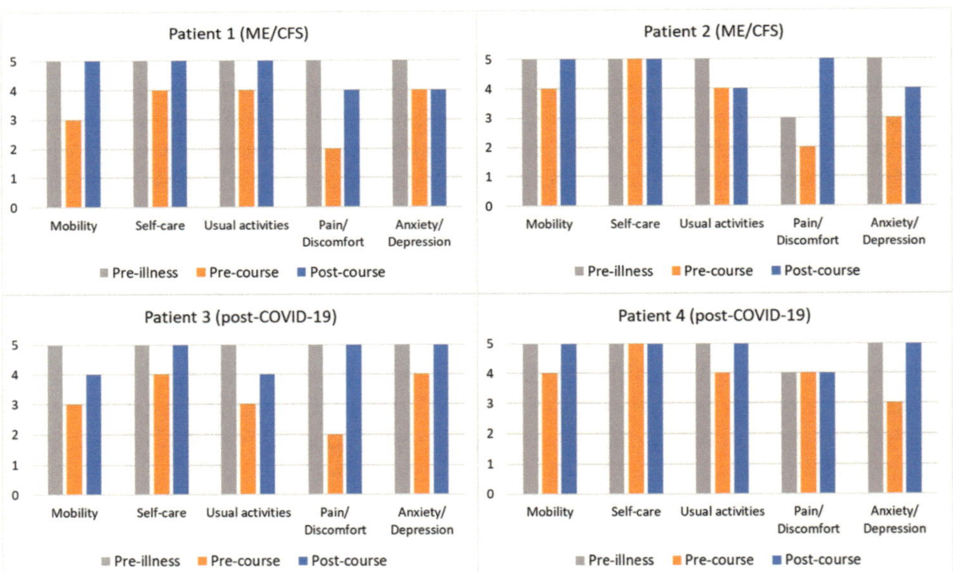

Figure 3.
Patient-reported health-related quality of life, as measured by the EuroQol-5D-5L framework (1—extreme problems, 2—severe problems, 3—moderate problems, 4—slight problems, and 5—no problems), in myalgic encephalomyelitis/chronic fatigue syndrome (ME/CFS) and post-COVID-19 patients: prior illness, prior coaching course, and after 4 weeks coaching course (Patient 2—after 6 weeks).

The results (**Figure 3**) show that Patient 1 (ME/CFS) and Patient 3 (post-COVID-19) demonstrated full-health HRQoL prior to illness, but Patient 2 (ME/CFS) and Patient 4 (post-COVID-19) had the pain and discomfort also before making the diagnosis. Self-care ability was less affected by the illness—by two points in sum for all patients; usual activities were more affected—by five points in sum for all patients; mobility was affected harder—by six points in sum for all patients; anxiety/depression was activated—by six points in sum for all patients; and pain/discomfort was most accelerated—by seven points in sum for all patients. After the coaching course, PROs demonstrate a stronger impact on pain/discomfort reduction—by eight points in sum for all patients, and on anxiety/depression—by four points in sum for all patients; while mobility was improved—by five points in sum for all patient, usual activities—by three points in sum for all patient, and self-care ability—by two points in sum for all patient (self-care ability was less affected by illness).

Additionally, the overall health self-assessment was performed by the VAS. Prior to the coaching, patients were asked to rate their health on a scale from 0 to 100 (where 0 means the worst health patient can imagine, and 100 means the best health patient can imagine), before the illness and at the present time. Accordingly, after the last coaching session, the patients had reassessed their health status. The results of the PROs by the VAS are shown in **Figure 4**.

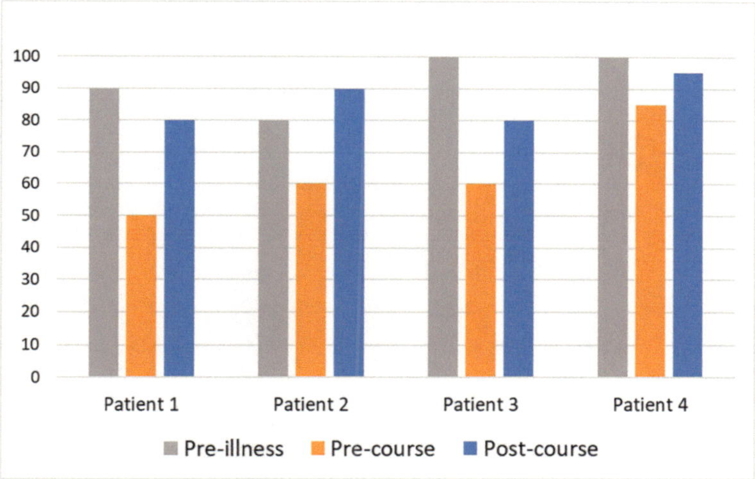

Figure 4.
Patient-reported health-related quality of life, as measured by the Visual Analogue Scale (0—the worst health patient can imagine, and 100—the best health patient can imagine), in myalgic encephalomyelitis/chronic fatigue syndrome (ME/CFS) and post-COVID-19 patients: prior illness, prior to the coaching course, and after 4 weeks coaching course (Patient 2—after 6 weeks).

PROs by the VAS (**Figure 4**) show that all patients reported a significant reduction in overall health status due to illness: Patient 1 (ME/CFS)—by 40%, Patient 2 (ME/CFS) and Patient 3 (post-COVID-19)—by 20%, and Patient 4 (post-COVID-19)—by 15%. After the coaching period, all patients demonstrated an improvement in overall health status by more than half: Patient 1 and Patient 2—by 30%, Patient 3—by 20%, and Patient 4—by 10%. Remarkably that ME/CFS patients reported greater improvement in overall health, and Patient 2 reported a higher score of overall health after the coaching course than it was before the diagnosis of illness.

In order to obtain more information on the health status of patients during the study, the physicians supervising these patients were also asked to assess patients' health state, prior to the coaching course and after the course. The assessment was performed by the VAS with a rating on a scale from 0 to 100 (where 0 means the worst health state of the patient, and 100 means the best health state of the patient). Three dimensions of health were defined for evaluation: overall health, emotional health, and cognitive health. The results of the assessment of the patients' health provided by the physicians are shown in **Figure 5**. Significant improvement was indicated in all dimensions of health in each patient. Remarkable that the physicians indicated a lower initial rate of the health states for ME/CFS patients in comparison with the health status of post-COVID-19 patients. Notably that the improvement also is greater in ME/CFS patients. Overall health state assessment after the coaching period is correlated with the results of PROs performed by VAS (**Figure 4**) (except for Patient 2 data in which patient's self-assessment is higher—probably by the fact that Patient 2 performed the last self-assessment after two additional weeks of coaching). The stabilization between all dimensions of health was a common tendency for all patients (**Figure 5**).

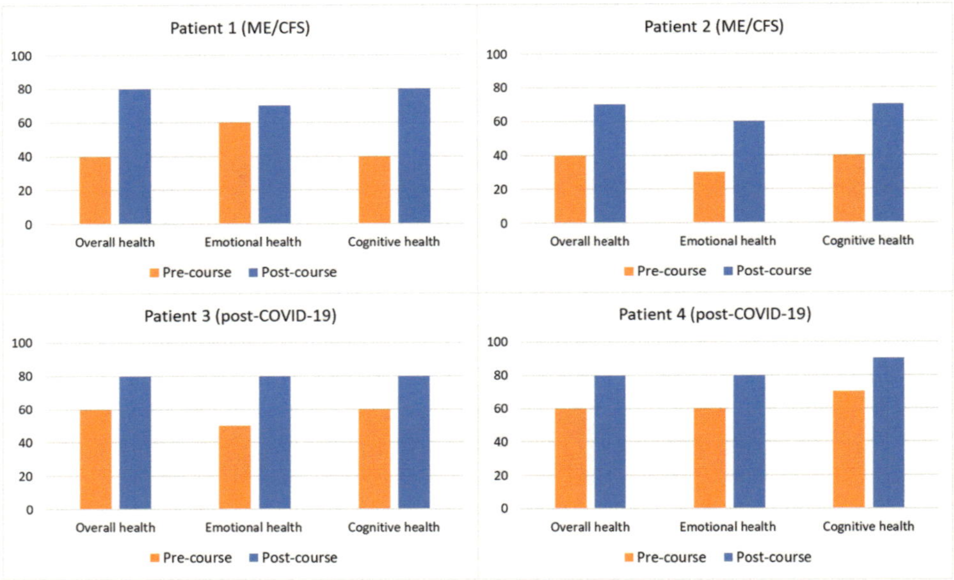

Figure 5.
Evaluation of the patient's overall health status, emotional health, and cognitive health, measured by the Visual Analogue Scale (0—the worst health state of the patient, and 100—the best possible health state of the patient), in myalgic encephalomyelitis/chronic fatigue syndrome (ME/CFS) and post-COVID-19 patients: prior to the coaching course, and after 4 weeks coaching course.

Overall results of the study demonstrate significant improvement in the health state of ME/CFS and post-COVID-19 patients, particularly, in overall health, emotional stability, and cognitive functionality. However, this case study has limitations, such as the following: data are not statistically significant for extrapolation to the whole population of patients; there are no sufficient data for comparison with data in other countries on coaching approach in healthcare of post-COVID-19 and ME/CFS patients; during the coaching period, patients continued to receive the standard treatment; therefore, coaching could be considered as a complementary tool in an integrative approach, but not as a monomethod. The strength of this research is focused on the great additional opportunity to resolve the problems arising in chronic diseases management, by affective collaboration and integrative approach, particularly, in primary healthcare.

This study can encourage the further investigation of coaching potential in healthcare, to receive more evidence on the effectiveness of this approach. Additionally, more sensitive evaluation instruments could be considered and would facilitate patients' self-assessment of such symptoms as anxiety, depression, fatigue, sleep disruption, and posttraumatic stress. At the same time, patients should be supported by teaching to work with the PROs tools in the process of health self-assessment. Eventually, in the scope of managerial and system level of integrative healthcare, it should be considered that the financing of the integrative approach can face the challenges in countries with strictly limited budget allocation for healthcare and social issues.

3. Conclusion

This chapter provided insight into the integrative approach to healthcare, with a particular focus on post-COVID-19 and ME/CFS disorders. Integrated healthcare consists of four main levels of health services delivery: the personal, the professional, the management, and the system level. In the framework of the practical research, the example of integration of coaching in the personal and professional level of primary healthcare of post-COVID-19 and ME/CFS patients demonstrated the potential for improvement in healthcare outcomes.

Acknowledgements

The study was supported by the Latvian Science Council's Fundamental and Applied Research project No. lzp-2019/1-0380 "Selection of biomarkers in ME/CFS for patient stratification and treatment surveillance/optimization," with the approval of the Research Ethics Committee of the Riga Stradins University (Decision No. 6-1/05/33–30 April 2020, Riga).

Conflict of interest

The authors declare no conflict of interest.

Author details

Diana Araja*, Angelika Krumina, Uldis Berkis, Zaiga Nora-Krukle and Modra Murovska
Institute of Microbiology and Virology, Riga Stradins University, Riga, Latvia

*Address all correspondence to: araja.diana@gmail.com

References

[1] Davis HE, Assaf GS, McCorkell L, et al. Characterizing long COVID in an international cohort: 7 months of symptoms and their impact. The Lancet. 2021;**38**:101019

[2] Komaroff AL, Bateman L. Will COVID-19 lead to myalgic encephalomyelitis / chronic fatigue syndrome? Frontiers in Medicine. 2021;**7**:606824

[3] Araja D, Berkis U, Murovska M. COVID-19 pandemic-revealed consistencies and inconsistencies in healthcare: A medical and organizational view. Health. 2022;**10**:1018. DOI: 10.3390/healthcare10061018

[4] Strayer DR, Youn D, Mitchell WM. Effect of disease duration in a randomized Phase III trial of rintatolimod, an immune modulator for Myalgic Encephalomyelitis/ Chronic Fatigue Syndrome. PLoS One. 2020;**15**(10):e0240403. DOI: 10.1371/ journal.pone.0240403

[5] Gaber T. Assessment and management of post-COVID fatigue. Progress in Neurology and Psychiatry. 2021;**25**(1): 36-39. DOI: 10.1002/pnp.698

[6] Friedman KJ, Murovska M, Pheby DFH, Zalewski P. Our evolving understanding of ME/CFS. Medicina. 2021;**57**(3):200. DOI: 10.3390/ medicina57030200

[7] Halpin SJ, McIvor C, Whyatt G, Adams A, Harvey O, McLean L, et al. Postdischarge symptoms and rehabilitation needs in survivors of COVID-19 infection: A cross-sectional evaluation. Journal of Medical Virology. 2021;**93**:1013-1022. DOI: 10.1002/ jmv.26368

[8] Simani L, Ramezani M, Darazam IA, Sagharichi M, Aalipour MA, Ghorbani F, et al. Prevalence and correlates of chronic fatigue syndrome and post-traumatic stress disorder after the outbreak of the COVID-19. Journal of Neuro Virology. 2021;**27**(1):154-159. DOI: 10.1007/ s13365-021-00949-1

[9] Townsend L, Moloney D, Finucane C, McCarthy K, Bergin C, Bannan C, et al. Fatigue following COVID-19 infection is not associated with autonomic dysfunction. PLoS One. 2021;**16**(2): e0247280. DOI: 10.1371/journal. pone.0247280

[10] Graham EL, Clark JR, Orban ZS, Lim PH, Szymanski AL, Taylor C, et al. Persistent neurologic symptoms and cognitive dysfunction in non-hospitalized Covid-19 'long haulers'. Annals of Clinical Translational Neurology. 2021;**8**(5):1073-1085. DOI: 10.1002/acn3.51350

[11] Toogood PL, Clauw DJ, Phadke S, Hoffman D. Myalgic encephalomyelitis/ chronic fatigue syndrome (ME/CFS): Where will the drugs come from? Pharmacological Research. 2021;**165**:105465. DOI: 10.1016/j. phrs.2021.105465

[12] Araja D, Berkis U, Lunga A, Murovska M. Shadow burden of undiagnosed myalgic encephalomyelitis/ chronic fatigue syndrome (ME/CFS) on Society: Retrospective and Prospective— in Light of COVID-19. Journal of Clinical Medicine. 2021;**10**:3017. DOI: 10.3390/ jcm10143017

[13] Wong TL, Weitzer DJ. Long COVID and Myalgic Encephalomyelitis/ Chronic Fatigue Syndrome (ME/ CFS)—A systemic review and

comparison of clinical presentation and symptomatology. Medicina. 2021;**57**:418. DOI: 10.3390/medicina57050418

[14] Poenaru S, Abdallah SJ, Corrales-Medina V. COVID-19 and post-infectious myalgic encephalomyelitis/chronic fatigue syndrome: A narrative review. Therapeutic Advances in Infectious Disease. 2021;**8**:1-16. DOI: 10.1177/20499361211009385

[15] Paul BD, Lemle MD, Komaroff AL, Snyder SH. Redox imbalance links COVID-19 and myalgic encephalomyelitis/chronic fatigue syndrome. PNAS. 2021;**118**(34):e2024358118. DOI: 10.1073/pnas.2024358118

[16] Komaroff AL, Lipkin WI. Review Insights from myalgic encephalomyelitis /chronic fatigue syndrome may help unravel the pathogenesis of postacute COVID-19 syndrome. Trends in Molecular Medicine. 2021;**27**(9):895-906. DOI: 10.1016/j.molmed.2021.06.002 89

[17] Deumer US, Varesi A, Floris V, Savioli G, López-Carrasco P, Rosati GM, et al. Myalgic encephalomyelitis/chronic fatigue syndrome (ME/CFS): An overview. Journal of Clinical Medicine. 2021;**10**:4786. DOI: 10.3390/jcm10204786

[18] Ceban F, Ling S, Lui LMW, Lee Y, Gill H, Teopiz KM, et al. Fatigue and cognitive impairment in Post-COVID-19 Syndrome: A systematic review and meta-analysis. Brain, Behavior, and Immunity. 2022;**101**:93-135. DOI: 10.1016/j.bbi.2021.12.020

[19] Rodríguez PS, Espinosa P, Aguilar AM, Muñoz MPR, Navarro MÁR. [Long COVID: Is it really myalgic encephalo-myelitis? Bibliographic review and considerations] [Article in Spanish]. Medicina de Familia Semergen. 2022;**48**(1):63-69. DOI: 10.1016/j.semerg.2021.03.006

[20] Jason LA, Islam MF, Conroy K, Cotler J, Torres C, Johnson M, et al. COVID-19 symptoms over time: Comparing long-haulers to ME/CFS. Fatigue: Biomedicine, Health & Behavior. 2021;**9**(2):59-68

[21] Pheby DFH, Araja D, Berkis U, Brenna E, Cullinan J, de Korwin JD, et al. The development of a consistent Europe-wide approach to investigating the economic impact of myalgic encephalomyelitis (ME/CFS): A report from the European Network on ME/CFS (EUROMENE). Health. 2020;**8**:88. DOI: 10.3390/healthcare8020088

[22] Fernández-de-las-Peñas C, Palacios-Ceña D, Gómez-Mayordomo V, Cuadrado ML, Florencio LL. Defining Post-COVID Symptoms (Post-Acute COVID, Long COVID, Persistent Post-COVID): An Integrative Classification. International Journal of Environmental Research and Public Health. 2021;**18**:2621. DOI: 10.3390/ijerph18052621

[23] Oronsky B, Larson C, Hammond TC, et al. A review of persistent post-COVID syndrome (PPCS). Clinical Reviews in Allergy and Immunology. 2021;**20**:1-9. DOI: 10.1007/s12016-021-08848-3

[24] Mantovani E, Mariotto S, Gabbiani D, Dorelli G, Bozzetti S, Federico A, et al. Chronic fatigue syndrome: An emerging sequela in COVID-19 survivors? Journal of Neurovirology. 2021;**27**(4):631-637. DOI: 10.1007/s13365-021-01002-x

[25] Mirin AA, Dimmock ME, Jason LA. Updated ME/CFS prevalence estimates reflecting post-COVID increases and associated economic costs and funding implications. Fatigue: Biomedicine, Health & Behavior. 2022;**10**(2):83-93. DOI: 10.1080/21641846.2022.2062169

[26] Hvidberg MF, Brinth LS, Olesen AV, Petersen KD, Ehlers L. The health-related quality of life for patients with myalgic encephalomyelitis/chronic fatigue syndrome (ME/CFS). PLoS One. 2015;**10**(7):e0132421. DOI: 10.1371/journal.pone.0132421

[27] Brenna E, Araja D, Pheby DFH. Comparative survey of people with ME/CFS in Italy, Latvia, and the UK: A Report on behalf of the Socioeconomics Working Group of the European ME/CFS Research Network (EUROMENE). Medicina. 2021;**57**:300. DOI: 10.3390/medicina57030300

[28] Roma M, Marden CL, Flaherty MAK, Jasion SE, Cranston EM, Rowe PC. Impaired health-related quality of life in adolescent myalgic encephalomyelitis/chronic fatigue syndrome: The impact of core symptoms. Frontiers in Pediatrics. 2019;**7**:26. DOI: 10.3389/fped.2019.00026

[29] Eaton-Fitch N, Johnston SC, Zalewski P, et al. Health-related quality of life in patients with myalgic encephalomyelitis/chronic fatigue syndrome: An Australian cross-sectional study. Quality of Life Research. 2020;**29**:1521-1531. DOI: 10.1007/s11136-019-02411-6

[30] Vyas J, Muirhead N, Singh R, et al. Impact of myalgic encephalomyelitis/chronic fatigue syndrome (ME/CFS) on the quality of life of people with ME/CFS and their partners and family members: An online cross-sectional survey. BMJ Open. 2022;**12**:e058128. DOI: 10.1136/bmjopen-2021-058128

[31] Krumina A, Vecvagare K, Svirskis S, Gravelsina S, Nora-Krukle Z, Gintere S, et al. Clinical profile and aspects of differential diagnosis in patients with ME/CFS from Latvia. Medicina. 2021;**57**:958. DOI: 10.3390/medicina57090958

[32] Brittain E, Muirhead N, Finlay AY, Vyas J. Myalgic encephalomyelitis/chronic fatigue syndrome (ME/CFS): Major impact on lives of both patients and family members. Medicina. 2021;**57**:43. DOI: 10.3390/medicina57010043

[33] Malik P, Patel K, Pinto C, Jaiswal R, Tirupathi R, Pillai S, et al. Post-acute COVID-19 syndrome (PCS) and health-related quality of life (HRQoL)—A systematic review and meta-analysis. Journal of Medical Virology. 2022;**94**(1):253-262. DOI: 10.1002/jmv.27309

[34] Harenwall S, Heywood-Everett S, Henderson R, et al. Post-Covid-19 Syndrome: Improvements in Health-Related Quality of Life Following Psychology-Led Interdisciplinary Virtual Rehabilitation. Journal of Primary Care and Community Health. 2021;**12**:1-12. DOI: 10.1177/21501319211067674

[35] Carenzo L, Protti A, Dalla Corte F, Aceto R, Iapichino G, Milani A, et al. Humanitas COVID-19 Task Force. Short-term health-related quality of life, physical function and psychological consequences of severe COVID-19. Annals of Intensive Care. 2021;**4**(11):91

[36] Bae J, Lin JMS. Healthcare utilization in myalgic encephalomyelitis/chronic fatigue syndrome (ME/CFS): Analysis of US Ambulatory Healthcare Data, 2000-2009. Frontiers in Pediatrics. 2019;**7**:185. DOI: 10.3389/fped.2019.00185

[37] Pavli A, Theodoridou M, Maltezou HC. Post-COVID syndrome: Incidence, clinical spectrum, and challenges for primary healthcare professionals. Archives of Medical Research. 2021;**52**(6):575-581. DOI: 10.1016/j.arcmed.2021.03.010

[38] Pinto M, Gimigliano F, De Simone S, Costa M, Bianchi AAM, Iolascon G.

Post-acute COVID-19 rehabilitation network proposal: From intensive to extensive and home-based IT supported services. International Journal of Environmental Research and Public Health. 2020;**17**(24):9335. DOI: 10.3390/ijerph17249335

[39] Parkin A, Davison J, Tarrant R, Ross D, Halpin S, Simms A, et al. Multidisciplinary NHS COVID-19 Service to Manage Post-COVID-19 Syndrome in the Community. Journal of Primary Care and Community Health. 2021;**12**:21501327211010994. DOI: 10.1177/21501327211010994

[40] Vanderlinda WM, Rabinovitza BB, Miaod IY, Oberlina LE, Bueno-Castellanoa C, Fridmana C, et al. A systematic review of neuropsychological and psychiatric sequalae of COVID-19: Implications for treatment. Current Opinion. 2021;**34**(4):420-433. DOI: 10.1097/YCO.0000000000000713

[41] Sawin G, O'Connor N. Primary care transformation. Primary Care. 2019;**46**(4):549-560. DOI: 10.1016/j.pop.2019.07.006

[42] Kodner DL, Spreeuwenberg C. Integrated care: Meaning, logic, applications, and implications – a discussion paper. International Journal of Integrated Care. 2002;**2**:e12. DOI: 10.5334/ijic.67

[43] Zonneveld N, Raab J, Minkman MMN. Towards a values framework for integrated health services: An international Delphi study. BMC Health Services Research. 2020;**20**:224. DOI: 10.1186/s12913-020-5008-y

[44] Valentijn PP, Schepman SM, Opheij W, Bruijnzeels MA. Understanding integrated care: A comprehensive conceptual framework based on the integrative functions of primary care. International Journal of Integrated Care. 2013;**13**:e010. DOI: 10.5334/ijic.886

[45] Valentijn PP. Rainbow of Chaos: A study into the theory and practice of integrated primary care. International Journal of Integrated Care. 2016;**16**(2):1-4

[46] Lonie JM, Austin Z, Nguyen R, Gill I, Tsingos-Lucas C. Pharmacist-based health coaching: A new model of pharmacist-patient care. RSAP. 2017;**13**:644-652. DOI: 10.1016/j.sapharm.2016.06.015

[47] Davis R, Campbell R, Hildon Z, Hobbs L, Michie S. Theories of behaviour and behaviour change across the social and behavioural sciences: A scoping review. Health Psychology Review. 2015;**9**:323-344. DOI: 10.1080/17437199.2014.941722

[48] Wolever RQ, Caldwell KL, Wakefield JP, et al. Integrative health coaching: An organizational case study. Explore Journal of Science Health. 2011;**7**:30-36. DOI: 10.1016/j.explore.2010.10.003

[49] Knoll K, Leiter SM, Rosner S, Trenkwalder T, Erben A, Kloss C, et al. Impact of tele-coaching during the COVID-19 pandemic on risk-reduction behavior of patients with heart failure. Telemedicine and e-Health. 2021;**28**(6):823-831. DOI: 10.1089/tmj.2021.0324

[50] Lin CL, Huang LC, Chang YT, Chen RY, Yang SH. Under COVID-19 Pandemic: A quasi-experimental trial of observation on diabetes patients' health behavior affected by the pandemic from a coaching intervention program. Frontiers in Public Health. 2021;**9**:580032. DOI: 10.3389/fpubh.2021.580032

[51] Rosa WE, Karanja V, Kpoeh JDN, McMahon C, Booth J. A virtual coaching

workshop for a nurse-led community-based palliative care team in Liberia, West Africa, to promote staff well-being during COVID-19. Nursing Education Perspectives. 2021;**42**(6):E194-E196. DOI: 10.1097/01.NEP.0000000000000828

[52] Altunkurek ŞZ. The effect of online wellness coaching for nursing students during the COVID-19 lockdown on well-being: A qualitative study. IJMHP. 2021;**23**(4):577-588

[53] Tkacova R. Erickson health coaching: An innovative approach for weight management in obese patients with obstructive sleep apnoea? Medical Hypotheses. 2018;**120**:43-47. DOI: 10.1016/j.mehy.2018.08.012

[54] Stolk E, Ludwig K, Rand K, van Hout B, Ramos-Goñi JM. Overview, update, and lessons learned from the international EQ-5D-5L valuation work: Version 2 of the EQ-5D-5L valuation protocol. Value Health. 2019;**22**(1):23-30

Section 3

Uncovering Pandora's Box: Challenges for Health Systems and Society

Chapter 14

How COVID-19 Brought Medical Gaslighting to the Forefront and Made Invisible Illness Visible: Lessons from the BIPOC Long COVID Study

Margot Gage Witvliet

Abstract

Back in March 2020 I became ill with COVID-19. It almost killed me. My journey with the illness is documented publicly and I am featured in New York Times, USA Today, Washington Post and People Magazine to name a few publications. Health Magazine named me one of seven African American women unsung heroes of COVID-19. Last year in 2021 I was invited to address President Biden's COVID-19 Task Force Team. In the medical community, there is a pattern of treating people differently based on their gender, sexual orientation, age and disability status. COVID-19 shed light on the need for the medical community to shift to a modern outlook in the treatment of patients with invisible illnesses. In this chapter, I will discuss what is long COVID, findings from the BIPOC Long COVID Study, and how long COVID made invisible illnesses such as chronic fatigue syndrome, fibromyalgia, chronic Lyme disease and lupus visible. Recommendations are given on long COVID recovery.

Keywords: long COVID, medical gaslighting, invisible illness, African American, COVID-19, chronic fatigue syndrome, RECOVER, integrative medicine, health disparity

1. Introduction

Back in March 2020 I took one of the last flights allowed in from Amsterdam, The Netherlands to Houston, Texas. I was a perfectly fit, healthy young woman who did not smoke. I was an active social epidemiologist with a tenure-track assistant professorship at an American university with my entire life ahead of me. The idea that I could die from an airborne illness before I turned 40 was not in my reality. I had no autoimmune diseases. I am not someone who has struggled with a chronic illness, in fact I have rarely been sick with the common cold or flu. I have never broken a bone and I had no co-morbidities. I have two healthy children and before COVID-19, I was a hands-on active mother. Women in my family have consistently lived into triple digits.

By the second week of March all of that changed. For me, Covid-19 started out like the flu. Initially I did not think I had COVID-19, but rather that I was coming down with a bad cold. But my symptoms progressed quickly. By March 15, 2020, I had arrived home from a two-hour car drive, I sat outside to rest in my backyard, and I had an intense pain in my chest-- it felt like an elephant had sat on my chest. I stumbled inside and lay on my bed. I took deep breaths and waited for the pain to pass. At this point I knew something was terribly wrong, my heart had never felt like it would pop out of my chest in my entire life. The next day my symptoms worsened. I developed a slight cough, a headache and a sore throat—my sore throat has been ongoing for the past 2 years. To this day (June 2022), I still have a light sore throat, that intensifies after eating or talking for an extended period. My health rapidly declined after my heart issues arose. By mid-March I landed in the hospital because I could not breathe, and by the beginning of May, I had a seizure. Covid-19 almost killed me several times.

Doctors did not know what to do with me. I never had a fever, and I did not have a persistent dry cough, so even with my severe shortness of breath I did not present symptoms of how doctors expected COVID-19 patients to present. At that time, the American Centers for Disease Control (CDC) said that in order to have COVID-19, the patient had to have a fever. And so began my journey down the rabbit hole of the American healthcare system. I was not listened to by doctors, not taken seriously and infantilized. At one appointment, the doctor spoke the entire time with my husband, instead of speaking with me--the actual patient who was a 38-year-old woman with a PhD in social epidemiology and public health.

I joined a COVID-19 online support group, where I witnessed woman after woman, irrespective of their socioeconomic status, race or country location, share stories about how doctors were not believing them about their COVID-19 symptoms. Early in the pandemic, sharing your COVID-19 status publicly was taboo in the rural Southeast Texas town where I reside. But I decided that I would use the small platform that I had as an assistant professor to come forward about my health status and shed light on the fact that doctors were not believing women, and that women of color were having a particularly hard time being believed. Women of color were being drug tested and getting the police called on them at the hospital. In my own experience, when I presented at the emergency room with shortness of breath, I was always asked by hospital staff if I had "taken something." I would get asked repeatedly if I had used drugs. I was not treated with compassion until after my drug test came back clean.

My goal is to transform my negative experience with COVID-19 and the American healthcare system into a positive teaching moment. I was one of the first people in Texas to be interviewed by the local news about my COVID-19 symptoms lasting longer than a few weeks. Following this, I wrote an article in The Conversation about my COVID-19 experience [1]. That article received over 400,000 views. My video diary that I made documenting my trip from Amsterdam to Houston during the pandemic was re-published across several media outlets and received over 20,000 views [2]. It was unexpected, but my COVID-19 advocacy work led to me being named by Health Magazine as one of seven African American women unsung heroes of the COVID-19 pandemic [3]. I was featured in several American media outlets, some including MSNBC, People Magazine, Washington Post, New York Times, and in international media outlets in the UK, Indonesia, Korea, and New Zealand. I presented a TEDx Talk where I spoke about the problem with doctors not believing patients with chronic illnesses and how doctors need to treat patients with compassion and drop their biases at the door [4].

My TEDx Talk received over one million views. I started an online Facebook support group for BIPOC women with long COVID. The group was featured in the Washington Post in 2021 [5].

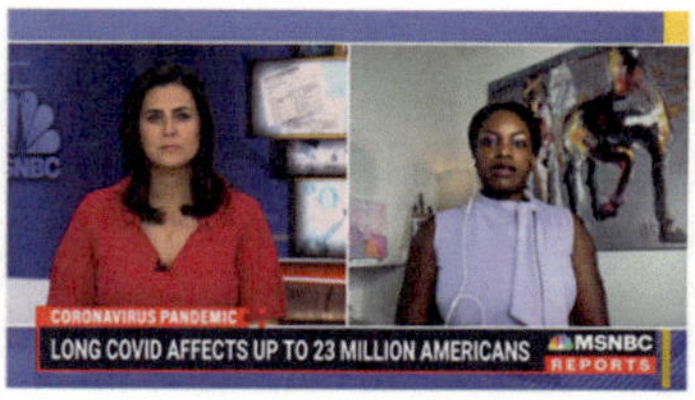
CORONAVIRUS PANDEMIC
LONG COVID AFFECTS UP TO 23 MILLION AMERICANS
MSNBC REPORTS

José Díaz-Balart Reports on Twitter

""I started seeing women, all women irrespective of color who were crying and telling stories about how doctors didn't believe them," @drgagewitvliet describes what drove her to create a group for Covid long-haulers. @LindseyReiser @MSNBC"

twitter.com

Today I am a COVID-19 survivor. It has been over 2 years and I am still in recovery [6]. I am not as sick as I once was, but I am not 100%. I have been diagnosed with post-acute sequelae of SARS-CoV-2 infection (or long COVID). It is estimated that half of the people who survive COVID-19 will get long COVID [7]. Long COVID is a chronic debilitating condition that effects multiple organs, including the brain [8]. People with long COVID develop symptoms that are similar to myalgic encephalomyelitis/chronic fatigue syndrome (ME/CFS) [8]. We also have chronic pain, and some develop renal, kidney and heart issues. Many continue to have pulmonary and gastrointestinal problems even after initial COVID-19 infection. The list of health problems caused by long COVID is wide ranging and diverse. Brain fog, mild dementia, pins and needle sensation, vision problems teeth and hair loss are just to name a few [8]. Long COVID is a debilitating health condition that severely impacts women more often than men [9]. Women aged 40–60 tend to experience more severe symptoms of long COVID [9].

I have been invited to address President Biden's COVID-19 Taskforce team [10] and I am on the Publications Oversight Committee of RECOVER, a 470-million-dollar long COVID research project funded by the American National Institute of Health (NIH) [11]. In July 2021, because of my advocacy efforts and that of many other COVID-19 patient advocates, President Joe Biden announced that long COVID could qualify as a disability [8]. In this chapter, I discuss medical gaslighting during the pandemic, findings from the BIPOC Long COVID Study, and explain how long COVID made invisible illnesses like ME/CFS, fibromyalgia, chronic Lyme disease, and Lupus visible.

2. Gaslighting during the pandemic

At the start of the pandemic in 2020 doctors knew very little about COVID-19. The CDC symptom guidelines were short. Doctors initially believed that a person with COVID-19 had to have a fever and a persistent cough to have COVID-19 [4]. Today we know that the list of COVID-19 symptoms is extensive [8]. We also know that a COVID-19 infection can cause post-COVID (also referred to as long Covid, chronic COVID, long-term effects of COVID, post-acute COVID-19), which is a post-viral condition where symptoms last 4-weeks or longer [8]. Currently there is no clear definition of long COVID, because COVID-19 is such a diverse illness, that manifests differently in each person, but researchers are working to change this [11]. Science has taught us that both adults and children can get long COVID [12]. The acute infection of COVID-19 does not have to be severe to get long COVID [13]. There are also people who have milder forms of long COVID and do not realize that they have long COVID [14]. For example, people who lost only their taste or smell, or people who only get headaches, and have no other health complaints. It is suspected that COVID-19 wreaks havoc in the mitochondria of immune cells and since mitochondria is paramount for cell survival this is one of the reasons why we can observe such devastating effects to health [15]. It is thought that long COVID patients have damage to blood vessels and nerve fiber damage [16], and this is harmful to all systems within the body, including the gastrointestinal and respiratory systems. It is also a possibility as to why in severe cases of long COVID exercise is excruciatingly painful. Science has found that long COVID causes brain inflammation, and it is one of the first viruses to break the blood brain barrier [17]. The neurological impacts of COVID-19 are profound, and it impacts cognitive ability. It is important to remember that people with long COVID have damage to their body that can cause unbearable pain even if medical tests or blood tests are not picking it up. The pain experienced by long COVID patients is unbearable. An increased risk of suicide exists in this population, and many have experienced psychosis [18].

When I became ill with COVID-19 during the first wave (March 2020), I never had a fever and never had a persistent cough. Given this, doctors did not initially believe that I had COVID-19. This made an already stressful medical situation even more horrendous. I was told by one doctor that my problems with breathing must be due to anxiety. Doctors tried to make me believe that my illness was all in my head. Since doctors could not ascertain what was wrong with me, they used mental health as a deflector instead of admitting that they did not have an answer for me on how to get well. In my case, it is true that I had anxiety, but my anxiety was not the reason I could not breathe. The fact that I could not breathe because my oxygen levels regularly dropped to as low as 60%, was the reason I had anxiety during my breathing attacks.

When COVID-19 raised my glucose levels, I was told by a doctor to watch my diet and exercise more. In essence I was blamed for my new-onset of high glucose levels, instead of the doctor connecting that the elevated glucose levels could be triggered by COVID-19. A few weeks later reports were published that COVID-19 can cause diabetes [19]. Further, the recommendation of a reformed diet and more exercise from the doctor was absurd, given that I was experiencing severe respiratory problems and post-exertional malaise. The doctor dismissed my issues and tried to make me believe that my health problems were my fault. The doctor assumed that I had a poor diet and did not exercise as the reason of why I now had elevated glucose levels. The doctor was treating me from a biased perspective instead of examining my entire patient history. What I experienced by this doctor and several other doctors both male and female from all varying racial and ethnic backgrounds is a term called medical gaslighting. Many people who initially became ill with COVID-19 during the first wave had an extremely hard time being believed by doctors when they presented with COVID-19 symptoms to emergency rooms. Unfortunately, dismissal and disbelief by doctors is still happening to this day. In some countries long COVID is not even recognized as an illness. A report out of Africa shows that even though doctors believe in COVID-19, patients and doctors are not recognizing the illness long COVID [20]. This is also happening in Trinidad and Tobago. Patients are being dismissed by doctors, and doctors are focused only on treating the symptoms without ever addressing the elephant in the room (i.e., long Covid).

When a person makes another person question their memory or perception of a given situation this is referred to as gaslighting. Internally I knew that prior to my COVID-19 infection I was a healthy person, and that my elevated glucose levels were not because of poor diet or lack of exercise, but that this doctor was attempting to make me doubt my own experience, which is a common characteristic of gaslighting [21]. Gaslighting is not just a medical phenomenon, it can occur anywhere and between anyone. Gaslighting is a form of psychological abuse that involves a power component, with people who use these tactics typically being in a position of power as compared to their victim [22]. The psychological impact left on the person who has experienced gaslighting can be profound [22]. Patients who experience medical gaslighting might start to question their own reality, especially if the person doing the gaslighting is a medical doctor [23]. Anxiety, hypertension and depression can develop in a person experiencing medical gaslighting, resulting in loss of patient-doctor trust, and in extreme cases, some patients might withdraw from social life [24, 25].

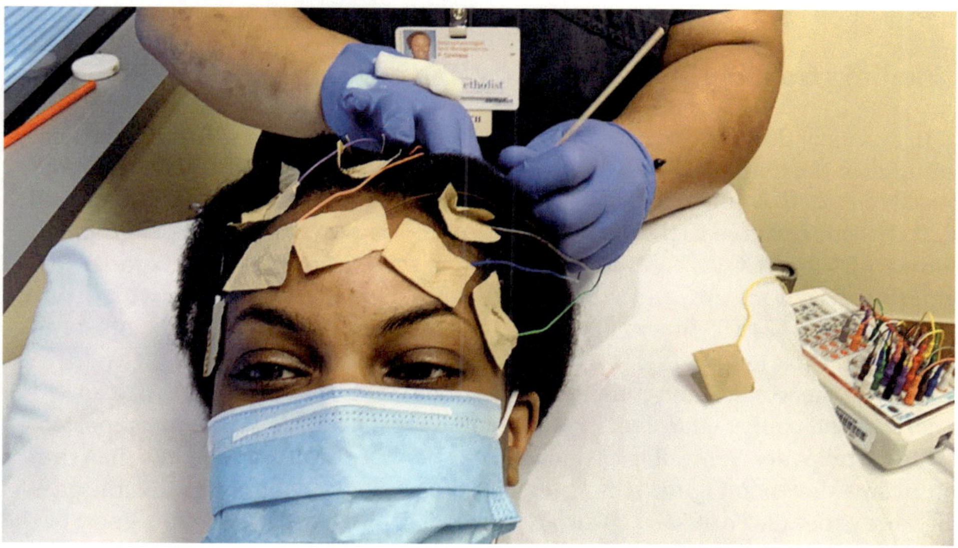

Medical gaslighting does not happen to everyone equally. It occurs most often to women and people of color. For illnesses where there is no clear test to ascertain if a person has the illness, medical gaslighting is a common occurrence. For example, a study found that women who present with symptoms of abdominal pain are not believed by doctors in the same way men are believed who report with the same type of pain [26]. Medical gaslighting is particularly a problem when there are no objective tests to diagnosis the health complaint. Patients in this "difficult to diagnose" category are often blamed and are not believed by doctors [25]. Doctors might dismiss difficult to diagnose patients with having a mental health issue, rather than having a physiological problem, which leads to devaluing of the patient [27, 28]. Disparity in treatment by doctors because of a patient's gender, race, sexuality, age or disability status has been a problem for people with chronic illnesses long before the COVID-19 pandemic [29–32]. Given that research has thoroughly documented bias in healthcare for decades, and little has been done to resolve this issue, the COVID-19 pandemic has highlighted that it is time for medical school curriculum to systematically address biases that doctors and other medical staff bring to the treatment room.

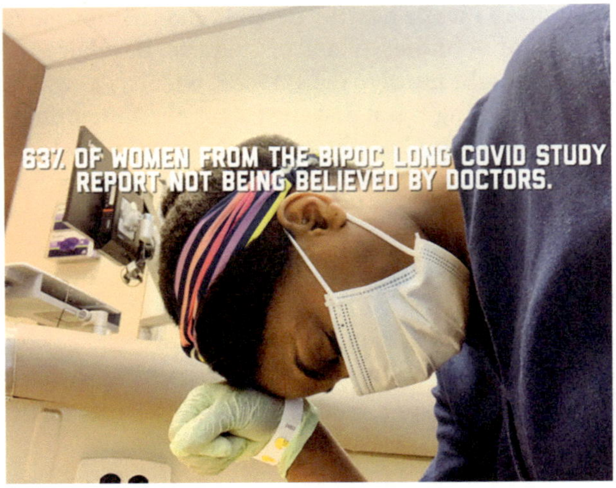

3. Findings from the BIPOC long COVID study

In Spring of 2022 I distributed an Intuitional Review Board (IRB) approved questionnaire to the online BIPOC women long COVID support group. The term BIPOC is used to refer to women of color. This group has been in existence since summer of 2020 and was featured in the Washington Post [5]. It is an online support group for women with long COVID. Women from around the world share their experience, symptoms, recovery tips, and support each other mentally as they deal with their newfound long COVID illness. The women in the group were asked to complete a study about their long COVID symptoms and experience.

Most of the women who completed the questionnaire (n = 46) were African American and college educated. **Figure 1** shows the top health complaints reported by the participants. Some of the women had even more health complaints then the complaints shown in **Figure 1**, but over 50% of the women who completed the questionnaire experienced at least 18 different health complaints. Despite this, most of the women (63%) report not being believed by their doctors about their health complaints. And of the 27 women who went to the hospital, 19.6% of them report being drug tested for narcotics when they went for medical assistance. More than half of the women (78.3%) report their trust in doctors has been lowered since contracting COVID-19.

The total devaluation by doctors during the COVID-19 pandemic happened to a lot of people, especially women and in particular women of color. The questionnaire asked women to report tips on what they did to find the right doctor. Many of the women reported never being able to find the right doctor. Others reported having an emotional breakdown in the office before being heard. Those with long time doctors reported that their doctors focused on treating their symptoms. **Box 1** highlights tips

Kept searching until I found someone who would listen.
Chose a DO instead of an MD.
After my positive antibodies test, my doctor took me seriously.
Research and read reviews. And have a doctor that is a black female.
I do not tolerate gaslighting.
My PCP referred me to the new Covid clinic within the hospital.

Box 1.
Select responses to question: what did you do to find the right doctor for you?.

extracted from the questionnaire that showed how some women handled navigating the health system, while dealing with medical gaslighting.

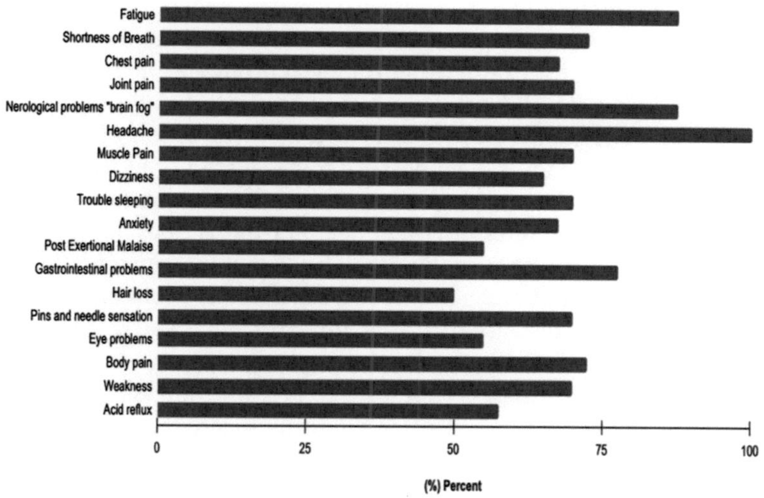

Figure 1.
Top Long COVID Health Complaints in BIPOC Women.

The sample size for the BIPOC Long COVID Study is small. However, results are consistent with news reports that highlight how doctors showed a pattern of dismissing long COVID patients [33–35]. The COVID-19 pandemic shed a huge spotlight on the sexism and racism prevalent in medical culture. As observed in **Figure 1**, the top three health complaints reported by BIPOC women with long COVID are headaches (100%), fatigue (87.5%) and neurological problems (87.5%). These symptoms are not typically ascertainable from a medical test, making them difficult to diagnosis by a doctor. Given past research, it is then not surprising that more than half of the women who completed the BIPOC Long COVID questionnaire reported experiencing medical gaslighting. Clearly, the findings from the BIPOC Long COVID Study highlight that it has been nearly impossible for many doctors to think outside of the box when it comes to diagnosing long COVID. The COVID-19 pandemic shed light on how the ridged frame of thinking can be disastrous during a pandemic when scientific information is rapidly changing and evolving.

4. Recognizing invisible illness

Before the pandemic, the world was not thinking about the nearly 17–24 million people around the world who have CFS/ME [36]. Nor were we thinking about the 2–4% of people around the globe with fibromyalgia [37]. Or the estimated 14% of the global population that has had Lyme disease [38], or the estimated five million people around the world with Lupus [39]. All four of these illnesses are chronic conditions that disrupt the immune system and are similar to long COVID [40–43]. The sheer volume of people who fell deathly ill with long COVID at once, and the relentless advocacy of patient-led groups, has led to a global movement that has commanded post-viral illnesses take center attention on the world stage. Long COVID patients taught the world to see invisible illnesses.

When our mind thinks of the word *disability,* most often it connects to a *visible* disability (such as someone who is in a wheelchair). We seldom think about *invisible* illnesses (also known as silent illnesses) that cause a person to be disabled. Invisible illnesses are wide ranging, for example neurological problems, mental health, digestive and addiction issues can all be classified as an invisible disability [44]. The main characteristic of an invisible illness is that the primary health complaint is not visible or easy to see, and for some invisible illnesses a medical scan or bloodwork cannot detect the health problem. Even though the invisible illness cannot be seen, and the person who has the invisible illness might appear normal, it does not mean the person living with the illness is making it up. Research finds that women with invisible disabilities often encounter microaggressions from medical professionals and are not believed or taken seriously because they appear healthy or are attractive [45]. Just because someone does not look sick and is smiling or having a good time does not mean that they are not disabled or do not have an invisible illness.

When people come to doctors complaining of unexplainable debilitating fatigue not explainable by another diagnosis, they are often diagnosed with ME/CFS. If the predominant problem is unexplainable pain on certain places on their body, then the patient is streamed into the fibromyalgia category. Similar to long COVID, ME/CFS is an invisible illness that causes extreme fatigue that is not resolved by rest [46]. People with ME/CFS can face a host of other symptoms some including headache, sleep disturbances, neurological issues and sore throat [47]. Severe ME/CFS can restrict a person to being bed bound because of the extreme pain that is caused by movement, light, and sound [47, 48]. Few fully recover from ME/CFS, and most patients only experience symptom reduction [48] ME/CFS can cause social isolation and job loss [47, 48]. Like ME/CFS, one of the main health complaints for fibromyalgia is fatigue [49]. However, with fibromyalgia, chronic pain tends to center around specific trigger points. Symptoms of fibromyalgia also include sleep problems, headaches, and gastrointestinal issues to name a few [50]. People with ME/CFS or fibromyalgia are often met with skepticism by their doctor, family or friends. Many people do not fully understand how debilitating ME/CFS or fibromyalgia can be for a person. Women are more often diagnosed with ME/CFS, and fibromyalgia as compared to men [50, 51] and people of color are often underdiagnosed by doctors, yet it has been identified that people of color have a higher prevalence of ME/CFS in the general population [51, 52].

Chronic Lyme disease and Systematic Lupus Erythematosus (lupus) differs from ME/CFS and fibromyalgia in that the doctors can identify a cause of the condition [53, 54]. Typically, if a patient has symptoms of immune system dysfunction and has been bitten by a tick, a doctor is able to treat the acute Lyme infection [54]. Chronic Lyme disease has a host of symptoms, some including extreme fatigue, chronic pain, and neurological problems to name a few [54]. For lupus the patient undergoes a series of major blood tests to identify if a patient has lupus. Nevertheless, even though there is a blood test for lupus, lupus is an autoimmune disease that is considered an invisible illness because some symptoms, for example extreme fatigue, are not visible [53]. Lupus can trigger many health complaints, some experience chronic pain, hair loss, cardiovascular problems, stoke, and rashes. Lupus occurs more often in women as compared to men [53]. In America, Lupus is more commonly seen in African Americans, followed by Latinx and Asian Americans [39]. Outcomes are often worse for African American women with lupus [55].

Long COVID is now part of the growing list of invisible illnesses. As evident in **Figure 1**, most of the women are experiencing health complaints that are invisible. As a bystander, you cannot see the pain from pins and needle sensations that 70% of women in the BIPOC Long COVID Study report having. The bystander can also not see the weakness and body pain reported by 70 and 72.5% of the women respectively. The joint pain (70%) and muscle pain (70%) is also invisible. This means that most of the women in the BIPOC Long COVID Study are in pain. In my personal experience, for the past 2-years, I have not awoken without a headache and have not experienced a day of being pain-free. As I sit here and write this chapter, I appear normal and healthy. However, I have ringing in my ears (tinnitus), a throbbing headache mostly contained to my left frontal lobe, sharp shooting pain on my right frontal lobe, a pins and needles sensation radiating through my arms and legs, I have chest pain and sensitivity to heat and external stimuli. I have joint pain that feels like arthritis, making every stroke of the keyboard painful. Despite the pain and extreme fatigue that I experienced for the past 2-years, my situation is improving and that gives me hope to a full recovery. Unfortunately, I cannot say the same for many women in the BIPOC Long COVID Study. About 70% of these women report that they do not believe they will ever get better.

People who have long COVID have been turning to the ME/CFS community for advice and guidance since people with ME/CFS have been dealing with the ramifications of chronic fatigue for decades. The world has largely ignored people with ME/CFS, but COVID-19 has helped bring their advocacy efforts to the forefront. Long COVID is an invisible illness that shares many similarities to ME/CFS. Many long COVID patients have learned from people with ME/CFS that pacing is important. Pacing is a technique to conserve energy to get the body through the day [56]. It is imperative that a person with long COVID learns to "pace" themselves. Unfortunately, even people with long COVID are still not aware of this powerful technique to help manage long COVID. In the BIPOC Long COVID Study, roughly 48% of women reported never having heard of pacing. Public health programs focused on long COVID recovery and treatment need to raise awareness about pacing, because many people with long COVID are going to have a problematic recovery process if they do not learn to appropriately manage their energy throughout the day.

5. Where do we go from here?

The BIPOC Long COVID Study shares similar findings as compared to other investigations that show people with long COVID report a multitude of health complaints simultaneously (some including fatigue, chest pain, headaches, and so on) [57–59]. At a certain point, doctors will need to accept that even though the scientific community has not identified a clear definition of long COVID, because it manifests and impacts each person differently, we cannot deny that people are experiencing health complaints. The first doctor who took my complaints seriously was my neurologist. He was the first person to identify that the symptoms I reported appeared to manifest in the same way as ME/CFS. I had never heard of ME/CFS before talking to him.

It is important to acknowledge that a questionnaire implemented in an online support group has its limitations. Nevertheless, the stories shared by these women show a pattern and can teach the medical community how to deal with patients with invisible illnesses. The questionnaire asked women: *What (if anything) do you think doctors or nurses could have done better when you came for medical help?* Two main themes were identified 1.)

patients wanted their doctors to listen to them, be patient, open minded, and compassionate 2.) patients did not want to be led to believe that their health problems were due to anxiety. One of the hardest things for a medical professional to have to admit is that they do not know how to help their patient. The findings from the BIPOC Long COVID Study highlight how it is imperative for doctors to have empathy with their patients, even for those patients who present with difficult to diagnosis illnesses.

Long COVID has affected millions of people at once, and because of our struggles, the people who have ME/CFS and those suffering from other post-viral illnesses have been brought to the forefront. The ME/CFS community has been largely ignored for far too long and research on post-viral illness deeply underfunded. According to research, ME/CFS impacts a great proportion of the population in the US as compared to HIV/AIDS and almost half that of cancer, yet ME/CFS research is one of the least funded research areas by the NIH [60]. Instead of starting from scratch, we should begin research investigations on treatment modalities for long COVID that is a continuation on the path that was already made by others who have been investigating post-viral illnesses like ME/CFS prior to the COVID-19 pandemic.

6. Treatment tips

We must acknowledge that we cannot fit long COVID symptoms into a box. Long COVID recovery will require an integrative medicine treatment approach. Integrative medicine focuses on whole body healing [61]. Integrative medicine increases quality of life in cancer patients and increases patient satisfaction [62]. Western medicine has been slow to adopt integrative medicine into the healthcare system, [62, 63] leaving people with chronic illnesses at a disadvantage because of not using a whole-body approach to recovery. In order to make solid advances on COVID-19 treatment and recovery we need to raise awareness and educate doctors about long COVID symptoms. In addition to this, long COVID recovery should focus on healing both mental and physical health.

The women in the BIPOC Long COVID Study report doing the recovery work to take care of their mental health. Alternative practices to manage symptoms are a widely used approach amongst the women. The main alternative practices reported were meditation, followed by art therapy, acupuncture and herbs. Two women report doing physical therapy. All but seven of the women report being on vitamins, supplements, and probiotics. More than half of the women were on medicines prescribed by doctors. Some of the medicines included those for respiratory symptoms (e.g., Albuterol inhaler, Breo inhaler, zyrtec), others for mental health (e.g., Gabapentin, Xanax, Cymbalta, Wellbutrin XL), high blood pressure (benazepril), heart and diabetes medication, and medication for pain and sleep aids were reported. Other personal recovery tips shared by the women in the study are shown in **Box 2**.

It should be noted that although the women share their experience and recovery tips, there is no cure for long COVID. None of the women in the sample were fully recovered. To improve quality of life I have found that targeted meditation helps manage symptoms. Everyone will not be able to complete physical activity, but as you progress in your recovery light low-intensity physical activity (such as a short slow walk, yoga or Tai Chi) might be possible. Listening to your body is important and can aid in the recovery process. Getting plenty of rest is necessary and monitoring vitals is useful along with drinking plenty of water and treating the symptoms. I also suggest doing intensive cognitive work for short periods of time (e.g., reading, writing or

"Never take antibiotics while having Covid it will not treat viral infection and could lead to severe gut complications as in my case even if your symptoms are mild stay rested do not work out and keep eating healthy."	*"Find at least one good support group. An online group is the best option for me. Stay current on new information. A good support group will provide information and links to studies and panel discussions. Be extra vigilant about what you put in your body. Start with one thing. I'm doing a deep dive into sugar. What it actually is and how it actually interrupts and eventually shuts down what our bodies are designed to do. Pay attention to what Covid is teaching you...."*
"Take Vitamin Supplements; focus on getting sleep."	*"Pay attention to your body and get emotional support!"*
"Ginger tea, sunlight, vitamins."	*"Rest a lot."*
"Surround yourself with people who are on the journey and who understand. Do not give up on yourself. Stay hydrated."	*"To get medical support quickly. I feel my body went through more damage because of the medical delay in treatment."*
"Listen to your body and rest, not everyone will believe you, seek support groups."	*"Get plenty of rest and drink water. These seem to make me feel better."*
"Try to avoid stressful situations if possible."	*"Be prepared for a battle, advocate for yourself and do not stop fighting, even when it seems no one is listening."*
"Get dental checkup."	*"Keep a personal medical journal."*
"Eat less processed foods. Rest, allow yourself to rest. Learn to listen to your heart rate. I use a Fitbit type of watch now, and any time my bp and heart rate starts to rise, it alerts me. I stop and force myself to breathe."	*"Do not give up on getting better: stay active and Prayful; Do online Bible study lessons; be an interchange of encouragement to someone daily. I have a young lady that calls me so much with her problems that I get a break from thinking about mine. More happiness in giving than there is in receiving; Be peaceful and stay calm remember "A calm heart gives life to the body." The Journal of the American Medical Association reports: "men who experience outbursts of anger have twice the risk of strokes as men who control their tempers." Get a hobby. I like fishing or watching others fishing now that I experience pain."*

Box 2.
Recovery tips from BIPOC women with long COVID.

puzzles) to exercise your brain. Strengthening the gut by eating healthy, adding a probiotic to your diet and taking vitamins and supplements is also important.

Another important aspect of my recovery process has been to try to minimize stress as much as possible and do an activity that brings me joy daily. Your body needs rest, but ultimately it needs to feel safe so that it can take the necessary time to heal from the trauma caused by COVID-19. It is important to keep in mind that recovery is not a sprint it is a marathon. I do not look at my progress each day, instead I examine the trend of my progress overtime. I am not in the same state that I was at 6 months, or at 12 months or at 18 months and so on.

7. Conclusions

The COVID-19 pandemic showed the world that we need to improve how medical doctors are trained. Medical gaslighting by doctors during the pandemic was a consistent pattern around the world. Medical gaslighting did not just happen to a few people, the blatant gaslighting happened to a substantial portion of the long COVID community. It has ruined patients trust in doctors. Medical school curriculum should be expanded to include formal training on how to recognize and reduce bias in health-care settings. It should also include making integrative medicine the norm, rather than the exception. Even though people with long COVID have a long way to go with recovery, it is possible that with the right treatment, quality of life can be improved. The first step in accomplishing this is to remove doctors from your healthcare team who do not take your health complaints seriously. The second step is tapping into the power of integrative medicine.

Acknowledgements

Thank you to the online BIPOC Women Long COVID Support Group for completing the BIPOC Long COVID Study. This research was funded by the Lamar University College of Arts and Science Dean's Summer Fellowship.

Author details

Margot Gage Witvliet
Lamar University, Beaumont, Texas, USA

*Address all correspondence to: mgage1@lamar.edu

References

[1] Gage WM. I'm a COVID-19 long-hauler and an epidemiologist – here's how it feels when symptoms last for months [Internet]. The Conversation. 2020. Available from: https://theconversation.com/im-a-covid-19-long-hauler-and-an-epidemiologist-heres-how-it-feels-when-symptoms-last-for-months-143676 [Accessed: June 25, 2022]

[2] Gage WM. Video diary [Internet]. 2020. Available from: https://youtu.be/NVb8LzlIoGU [Accessed: June 15, 2022]

[3] Peck P. These 7 black women are the unsung heroes of the COVID pandemic [internet]. Health 2021. Available from: https://www.health.com/mind-body/health-diversity-inclusion/these-7-black-women-are-the-unsung-heroes-of-the-covid-pandemic [Accessed: June 20, 2022]

[4] TedxMileHigh. I've had COVID-19 for a year. Here's what I've learned|Margot Gage Witvliet|TEDxMileHigh [Internet]. www.youtube.com. 2021. Available from: https://youtu.be/4LX_JRHZdkI [Accessed: June 20, 2022]

[5] Ables K. Covid "long haulers" have nowhere else to turn—So they're finding each other online. Washington Post. 2020. Available from: https://www.washingtonpost.com/technology/2020/10/01/long-haulers-covid-facebook-support-group/ [Accessed: June 20, 2022]

[6] Gage WM. My 15-month rollercoaster ride with COVID-19: A social epidemiologist's perspective. Scandinavian Journal of Public Health. 2022;**50**(1):1-3. DOI: 10.1177/14034948211067682

[7] Groff D, Sun A, Ssentongo AE, et al. Short-term and long-term rates of Postacute sequelae of SARS-CoV-2 infection: A systematic review. JAMA Network Open. 2021;**4**(10):e2128568. DOI: 10.1001/jamanetworkopen.2021.28568

[8] CDC. COVID-19 and Your Health [Internet]. Centers for Disease Control and Prevention. 2021. Available from: https://www.cdc.gov/coronavirus/2019-ncov/long-term-effects/index.html [Accessed: June 20, 2022]

[9] Torjesen I. Covid-19: Middle aged women face greater risk of debilitating long term symptoms. BMJ. 2021;**372**:n829. DOI: 10.1136/bmj.n829

[10] US Department of Health and Human Services. Health Equity Task Force Meeting Readouts – The Office of Minority Health [Internet]. 2021. Available from: https://www.minorityhealth.hhs.gov/omh/Content.aspx?ID=22546&lvl=3&lvlid=123 [Accessed: June 28, 2022]

[11] RECOVER. Researching COVID to Enhance Recovery [Internet]. 2022. Available from: https://recovercovid.org [Accessed: July 20, 2022]

[12] Kikkenborg Berg S, Palm P, Nygaard U, Bundgaard H, Petersen MNS, Rosenkilde S, et al. Long COVID symptoms in SARS-CoV-2-positive children aged 0-14 years and matched controls in Denmark (LongCOVIDKidsDK): a national, cross-sectional study. Lancet Child Adolesc Health. Sep 2022;**6**(9):614-623. DOI: 10.1016/S2352-4642(22)00154-7. Epub: 2022 Jun 23. PMID: 35752194; PMCID: PMC9221683

[13] van Kessel SAM, Olde Hartman TC, Lucassen PLBJ, van Jaarsveld CHM. Post-acute and long-COVID-19 symptoms in patients with mild diseases: A systematic

review. Family Practice. 2022;**39**(1):159-167. DOI: 10.1093/fampra/cmab076

[14] Ducharme J. You could have long covid and not even know it. Time. [Internet]. 2022. Available from: https://time.com/6191655/long-covid-under-diagnosed/ [Accessed: July 20, 2022]

[15] Miller B, Silverstein A, Flores M, et al. Host mitochondrial transcriptome response to SARS-CoV-2 in multiple cell models and clinical samples. Scientific Reports. 2021;**11**:3

[16] Oaklander AL, Mills AJ, Kelley M, Toran LS, Smith B, Dalakas MC, et al. Peripheral neuropathy evaluations of patients with prolonged long COVID. Neurology Neuroimmunology and Neuroinflammation. 2022;**9**:3

[17] Meinhardt J, Radke J, Dittmayer C, Franz J, Thomas C, Mothes R, et al. Olfactory transmucosal SARS-CoV-2 invasion as a port of central nervous system entry in individuals with COVID-19. Nature Neuroscience. 2021;**24**(2):168-175. DOI: 10.1038/s41593-020-00758-5

[18] Sher L. Are COVID-19 survivors at increased risk for suicide? Acta Neuropsychiatrica. 2020;**32**(5):270-270. DOI: 10.1017/neu.2020.21

[19] Sathish T, Kapoor N, Cao Y, Tapp RJ, Zimmet P. Proportion of newly diagnosed diabetes in COVID -19 patients: A systematic review and meta-analysis. Diabetes, Obesity and Metabolism. 2020;**23**(3):870-874

[20] Dalberg. Creating a Publicly-Led Long Covid research Agenda. [Internet]. 2021. Available from: https://wellcome.org/reports/creating-publicly-led-research-agenda-long-covid [Accessed: June 12, 2022]

[21] Dorpat TL. On the double whammy and gaslighting. Psychoanalysis & Psychotherapy. 1994;**11**(1):91-96

[22] Sweet PL. The sociology of gaslighting. American Sociological Review. 2019;**84**(5):851-875

[23] Fraser S. The toxic power dynamics of gaslighting in medicine. Canadian Family Physician. 2021;**67**(5):367-368. DOI: 10.46747/cfp.6705367

[24] McQuillan S. Gaslighting: What Is It? Psycom.net - Mental Health Treatment Resource Since 1986. [Internet]. 2022. Available from: https://www.psycom.net/gaslighting-what-is-it/ [Accessed: July 15, 2022]

[25] Sloan M, Naughton F, Harwood R, Lever E, D'Cruz D, Sutton S, et al. Is it me? The impact of patient-physician interactions on lupus patients' psychological well-being, cognition and health-care-seeking behaviour. Rheumatology Advances Practise. 2020;**4**(2):37

[26] Chen EH, Shofer FS, Dean AJ, Hollander JE, Baxt WG, Robey JL, et al. Gender disparity in analgesic treatment of emergency department patients with acute abdominal pain. Academic Emergency Medicine. 2008;**15**(5):414-418. DOI: 10.1111/j.1553-2712.2008.00100.x

[27] McManimen S, McClellan D, Stoothoff J, Gleason K, Jason LA. Dismissing chronic illness: A qualitative analysis of negative health care experiences. Health Care for Women International. 2019;**40**(3):241-258. DOI: 10.1080/07399332.2018.1521811

[28] Lapp CW. Initiating care of a patient with myalgic encephalomyelitis/chronic fatigue syndrome (ME/CFS). Frontiers in Pediatrics. 2019;**6**:415. DOI: 10.3389/fped.2018.00415

[29] Schieber A-C, Delpierre C, Lepage B, Afrite A, Pascal J, Cases C, et al. Do

gender differences affect the doctor-patient interaction during consultations in general practice? Results from the INTERMEDE study. Family Practice. 2014;**31**(6):706-713

[30] Gordon HS, Street RL, Sharf BF, Souchek J. Racial differences in doctors' information-giving and patients' participation. Cancer. 2006;**107**(6):1313-1320

[31] Bhugra D. Doctors' attitudes to male homosexuality: A survey. Sexual and Marital Therapy. 1990;**5**(2):167-174

[32] Chrisler JC, Barney A, Palatino B. Ageism can be hazardous to Women's health: Ageism, sexism, and stereotypes of older women in the healthcare system. Journal of Social Issues. 2016;**72**(1):86-104

[33] Fong A. "Medical gaslighting" harming long-COVID patients. Healthy Debate. [Internet]. 2022. Available from: https://healthydebate.ca/2022/07/topic/medical-gaslighting-long-covid/ [Accessed: July 21, 2022]

[34] Cooney E. From medical gaslighting to death threats, long covid tests patients [internet]. Stat 2021. Available from: https://www.statnews.com/2021/11/22/long-covid-patients-medical-gaslighting-death-threats/ [Accessed: July 21, 2022]

[35] Jason L, Perkins V. Long COVID and Gaslighting | Psychology Today [Internet]. 2022. Available from: https://www.psychologytoday.com/us/blog/the-mental-health-revolution/202204/long-covid-and-gaslighting [Accessed: July 21, 2022]

[36] Centers for Disease Control and Prevention. CDC Team Takes ME/CFS Around the World | [Internet]. 2020. Available from: https://blogs.cdc.gov/global/2020/05/12/cdc-team-takes-me-cfs-around-the-world/ [Accessed: July 20, 2022]

[37] Häuser W, Fitzcharles MA. Facts and myths pertaining to fibromyalgia. Dialogues in Clinical Neuroscience. 2018;**20**(1):53-62. DOI: 10.31887/DCNS.2018.20.1/whauser

[38] Dong Y, Zhou G, Cao W, et al. Global seroprevalence and sociodemographic characteristics of *borrelia burgdorferi sensu lato* in human populations: A systematic review and meta-analysis. BMJ Global Health. 2022;7:e007744

[39] Lupus Foundation of America. Lupus Facts and Statistics. 2018. Available from: https://www.lupus.org/resources/lupus-facts-and-statistics [Accessed: June 20, 2022]

[40] Mensah FKF, Bansal AS, Ford B, Cambridge G. Chronic fatigue syndrome and the immune system: Where are we now? Neurophysiologie Clinique/Clinical Neurophysiology. 2017;**47**(2):131-138

[41] Gur A, Oktayoglu P. Status of immune mediators in fibromyalgia. Current Science. 2008;**12**:175-181

[42] Bockenstedt LK, Wormser GP. Review: Unraveling Lyme disease. Arthritis & Rheumatology. 2014;**66**(9):2313-2323

[43] Askanase A, Shum K, Mitnick H. Systemic lupus erythematosus: An overview. Social Work in Health Care. 2012;**51**(7):576-586

[44] Ann DN. Invisible disability. Ethics. 2005;**116**(1):153-213

[45] Olkin R, Hayward H, Abbene MS, VanHeel G. The experiences of microaggressions against women with visible and invisible disabilities. Journal of Social Issues. 2019;**75**(3):757-785

[46] Fukuda K, Straus SE, Hickie I, Sharpe MC, Dobbins JG, Komaroff A. The chronicfatiguesyndrome:Acomprehensive approach to its definition and study. International chronic fatigue syndrome study group. Annals of Internal Medicine. 1994;**121**(12):953-959

[47] Assefi NP, Coy TV, Uslan D, Smith WR, Buchwald D. Financial, occupational, and personal consequences of disability in patients with chronic fatigue syndrome and fibromyalgia compared to other fatiguing conditions. The Journal of Rheumatology. 2003;**30**(4):804-808

[48] Dafoe W. Extremely severe ME/CFS-A personal account. Healthcare (Basel). 2021;**9**(5):504

[49] Vincent A, Benzo RP, Whipple MO, McAllister SJ, Erwin PJ, Saligan LN. Beyond pain in fibromyalgia: Insights into the symptom of fatigue. Arthritis Research & Therapy. 2013;**15**(6):221. DOI: 10.1186/ar4395

[50] Williams DA, Clauw DJ. Understanding fibromyalgia: Lessons from the broader pain research community. The Journal of Pain. 2009;**10**(8):777-791. DOI: 10.1016/j.jpain.2009.06.001

[51] Bhui KS, Dinos S, Ashby D, et al. Chronic fatigue syndrome in an ethnically diverse population: The influence of psychosocial adversity and physical inactivity. BMC Medicine. 2011;**9**:26. DOI: 10.1186/1741-7015-9-26

[52] Gage Witvliet M. Post-COVID Syndrome Is Real, And POCs are Disproportionately Losing the Battle. Blavity News & Politics [Internet]. 2020. Available from: https://blavity.com/post-covid-syndrome-is-real-and-pocs-are-disproportionately-losing-the-battle?category1=opinion [Assessed May 21, 2022]

[53] Pons-Estel GJ, Alarcón GS, Scofield L, Reinlib L, Cooper GS. Understanding the epidemiology and progression of systemic lupus erythematosus. Seminars in Arthritis and Rheumatism. 2010;**39**(4):257-268. DOI: 10.1016/j.semarthrit.2008.10.007

[54] Trevisan G, Bonin S, Ruscio M. A practical approach to the diagnosis of Lyme borreliosis: From clinical heterogeneity to laboratory methods. Frontiers in Medicine. 2020;**23**:7

[55] Somers EC, Marder W, Cagnoli P, Lewis EE, DeGuire P, Gordon C, et al. Population-based incidence and prevalence of systemic lupus erythematosus: The Michigan lupus epidemiology and surveillance program. Arthritis & Rhematology. 2014;**66**(2):369-378. DOI: 10.1002/art.38238

[56] Kos D, van Eupen I, Meirte J, Van Cauwenbergh D, Moorkens G, Meeus M, et al. Activity pacing self-Management in Chronic Fatigue Syndrome: A randomized controlled trial. The American Journal of Occupational Therapy. 2015;**69**(5):6905290020. DOI: 10.5014/ajot.2015.016287

[57] Davis HE, Assaf GS, McCorkell L, Wei H, Low RJ, et al. Characterizing long COVID in an international cohort: 7 months of symptoms and their impact. E. Clinical Medicine. 2021;**38**:101019

[58] Silva Andrade B, Siqueira S, de Assis Soares WR, de Souza RF, Santos NO, Dos Santos FA, et al. Long-COVID and Post-COVID Health Complications: An up-to-date review on clinical conditions and their possible molecular mechanisms. Viruses. 2021;**13**(4):700

[59] Seeßle J, Waterboer T, Hippchen T, Simon J, Kirchner M, Lim A, et al. Persistent symptoms in adult patients

1 year after coronavirus disease 2019 (COVID-19): A prospective cohort study. Clinical Infectious Diseases. 2022;**74**(7):1191-1198. DOI: 10.1093/cid/ciab611

[60] Mirin AA, Dimmock ME, Jason LA. Research update: The relation between ME/CFS disease burden and research funding in the USA. Work. 2020;**66**(2):277-282. DOI: 10.3233/WOR-203173

[61] Brown BI. Chronic fatigue syndrome: A personalized integrative medicine approach. Alternative Therapies in Health and Medicine. 2014;**20**(1):29-40

[62] Gannotta R, Malik S, Chan AY, Urgun K, Hsu F, Vadera S. Integrative medicine as a vital component of patient care. Cureus. 2018;**10**(8):e3098. DOI: 10.7759/cureus.3098

[63] Seetharaman M, Krishnan G, Schneider RH. The future of medicine: Frontiers in integrative health and medicine. Medicina (Kaunas, Lithuania). 2021;**57**(12):1303. DOI: 10.3390/medicina57121303

Chapter 15

Emotional and Psychological Impact of COVID-19 Induced Delay in Treatment of Medical Conditions

Harpreet Kaur and Asmita Kaundal

Abstract

COVID-19 pandemic significantly affected the physical, social, economical and mental health globally. Social distancing, quarantine and national wide lockdowns became new norm. Hospital emergencies and were flooded with patients diagnosed with COVID-19, Intensive care units were full with critically ill COVID-19 patients. Most of the health care facilities were diverted towards the management of COVID 19 patients. Majority of the manpower were involved in the screening, diagnosing and management with those infected with COVID 19. There was no arrangements for non COVID patients which lead to delay in diagnosis of new onset disease and cancellation of the previously planned appointments of those with chronic disease. Delay in treatment resulted in increased anxiety, stress, fear and emotional and psychological disturbances in many.

Keywords: Covid-19, psychological impact, fertility treatment, treatment

1. Introduction

Covid-19 pandemic caused by SARS-CoV-2 virus hit the world in December 2019 [1, 2]. Because of rapid rise in the cases worldwide it was declared as an international emergency by WHO on 30th January 2020. Social distancing, face mask, hand hygiene became the new norms. Public transport & travel restriction were implemented in most of the countries.

While all the efforts were made to curtail the transmission of the virus and management of those affected by the virus, a lot of routine procedures, treatment appointments were put on halt. Most of the hospitals both public and private were either managing COVID-19 patients or only those with emergency conditions. As a result, lot of patients suffering from diseases other then COVID-19 had to cancel their scheduled appointments indefinitely. Due to the uncertainty neither the doctor nor the patients were sure when will the routine care start again which leads to anxiety, frustration, fear of progression of disease or development of complications related to diseases and depression in many of the patients and health care providers as well.

According to a report published by WHO in June 2020, 94% of the member countries reported that all or some of the ministry of health staff with responsibility for non-communicable diseases were reassigned the duty for management of Covid-19. As per this report around 53% of the countries disrupted their medical services for hypertension, 49% for diabetes, 63% for rehabilitation services, 42% for cancer and nearly 31% for cardiovascular diseases [3]. Due to the delay in treatment many patients develop anxiety which also manifested as physical symptoms like palpitation, gastrointestinal disturbances, depression, substances abuse. Mental health of such patients waiting for procedures and treatment worsened.

2. Non-communicable disease

Nearly 70% of deaths in the developed nations and 80% in low & middle-income countries occur due to non-communicable disease every year [4].

Non-communicable disease include disease like hypertension, diabetes, coronary artery disease, cancers etc. Patient suffering from such conditions need repeated appointments to adjust their drug dose, check compliance to the drugs, follow improvement in the symptoms and to check for any further progression of the disease. Due to the closing of all non-emergency services during the pandemic resulted all routine appointments were postponed resulting in delayed treatment. Due to this sudden disruption in the existing health care system patients and health care professionals did not get time to discuss and plan their further management. This caused lot of anxiety and distress in many patients suffering from the any of the disease. Many patients experienced mental health problems, sleep disturbances, anxiety, mood disorders to add on to the existing symptoms but had no clue whom to seek clue from.

3. Cancer management

Being diagnosed to have cancer in itself is distressing for a patient and family. The anxiety levels are higher in newly diagnosed cases and new stressor can be difficult to manage for such patients [5–7]. Treatment delay due to COVID-19 pandemic and the fear associated with higher chances of acquiring infection due to week immune system lead to increased psychological issues in many cancer patients [8–10]. Many patients could not travel to hospitals on the scheduled appointments due to travel restriction and many of the hospitals temporarily suspended their services causing delay in treatment. Delayed treatment lead to progression of the disease and raised the mortality rate. A study done by Yingjun ye et al. found that psychological distress was significantly higher in the patient with cancer during COVID 19 as compared to the healthy volunteers [11].

4. Fertility treatments

Infertility i.e. not able to conceive is one of the most distressing diagnosis for a couple and is associated with lot of anxiety, depression and feeling of guilt.

Due to the advancement in the fertility services now many couple see ray of hope. Ovulation induction, intrauterine insemination, in-vitro fertilisation are some of the options which can be opted by the couple as per their medical needs decided after meticulous fertility workup. The whole work-up is itself time demanding and cycle dependent. Cycle cancellation of any reason can be distressing for a couple who is waiting to conceive for long [12, 13]. During the pandemic due to the restrictions and fear of contracting the disease lot of cycles needed to be cancelled and several couples kept waiting for their treatment. Due to the risk of exposure and conservation of resources on March 2020 American Society of reproductive Medicine (ASRM) and many other international societies recommended to suspend all kind of fertility treatments [14]. In a study published in 2020 by Kaur H et al. shows that 50% of the fertility treatment cycles were cancelled due to COVID-19 pandemic and 16.4% of the couples found it extremely upsetting. Around 10.9% experienced sleep disturbances, 14.15 were anxious, 18.4% had mood disturbances and 17.4 had disturbed thoughts [15].

5. Pregnancy and childbirth

Pregnancy and childbirth is one of the most joyful news for a couple. Lot of physical and hormonal changes takes place in the body to prepare for a growing baby and childbirth. Many women may experience mood swings, irritability and psychological issues like sleep disturbances, anxiety, fear and depression along with the other physical symptoms of pregnancy. These changes also make women more prone to infections due to decreased immunity. During the pandemic though the emergency obstetrics care were functional but routine ante-natal care were suspended. Routine antenatal care involves inquiry regarding any high-risk factor posing present pregnancy at higher risk of any adverse outcome, routine examination for maternal and fetal well-being, immunisation during pregnancy, investigations, ultrasound and childbirth preparedness. Due to the limited knowledge and evidence about the COVID-19 and its impact on pregnancy it was assumed that COVID-19 can cause a threat to the pregnant women and baby. Many pregnant women suffered anxiety because of the fear of contracting the disease. Antenatal women also suffered psychological issues in the absence of routine antenatal checkup and medical reassurance that everything is going fine. Women with early pregnancy were unsure about the risk of COVID-19 to the baby and experienced more psychological issues. Some even terminated the pregnancy. Women in advanced pregnancy were distressed because of the uncertainty of the place of delivery and limited options for transport in odd hours, fear of contracting COVID-19 on hospital admission for delivery. Many women even chose to deliver at home by female relatives and suffered complications like.

6. Postpartum care

Period immediately after delivery is very crucial. Women requires a lot of support emotionally and physically to handle the changes that occurred with the birth of the baby. Initiating breastfeeding could be a real stressor for women. Reassurance and support from family members can help them adjust. Due to social distancing and to avoid overcrowding in the hospitals women did not get enough support postpartum and they were left at there own to manage. Feeling of loneliness and fear of contracting COVID-19 by mother or baby added to the anxiety. Even at home due to lockdown and travel restriction many women lack support post-delivery because of which many women experienced anxiety, sleep disturbance, mood swings and agitation.

7. Contraceptive needs

Many couple could not access contraceptive services during the pandemic due to closure of many of the hospitals and medical stores. Due to lockdown and restrictions also many could not visit the nearby medical stores as per their convenience. Those who could not get the contraceptive of their choice either practiced temporary abstinence, natural methods or did not use any method. Unintended pregnancies resulting as a result of non use of contraceptives needed abortion services and resulted in unsafe abortion services or continued with unwanted pregnancy and delivered. Many children born as a result of such unwanted pregnancies were abandoned. Many women suffered anxiety disorders, sleep disturbances and feeling of guilt because of this.

8. Abortion care

Since all the efforts were made to tackle COVID-19 and related emergency many routine family planning suffered. One of such important services was abortion care. Abortion services are usually used by a women/couple in cases of unintended pregnancy due to contraceptive failure or non use of contraceptives or rape. Unintended pregnancy can be a cause of psychological issue in a couple if they are not prepared to have a baby, due to financial or personal reasons. During the pandemic many couples with unintended pregnancy could not avail medical abortion services within time as the out-patient/family planning departments were closed, patient were themselves also scared to visit hospital, medical stores could not dispense MTP kits due to unavailability of the prescription. As a result many couples had to keep the pregnancy and deliver at term which adversely affected the mental health of the mother and couple.

9. Adolescents health

Adolescent means between childhood and adulthood from age 10–19 years. This is the time when a person experiences physical, cognitive and psychosocial growth. Most of the habits related to diet, exercise, substance use and sexual activity are formed during this period. For a healthier development adolescents need information, opportunities, safe and supportive environments.

Though considered to be the most healthy phase of life adolescent also struggle through lot of medical and psychological issues which needs to be addressed. Certain conditions like Polycystic ovarian disease, Abnormal uterine bleeding, sexual concerns, sexually transmitted diseases and contraception could not be addressed due to lockdown during COVID. Due to the uncertainty regarding future mental issue further deteriorated. Cases of eating disorders, obesity and body image disorders rise but due to unavailability of the routine health care services the issues could not be addressed.

10. Mental disease

Patients already suffering from psychiatric diseases like depressive disorders, anxiety disorders, schizophrenia etc. faced major challenges due to the changes in brought about due to pandemic. Many of them on long term treatment and follow -up could not plan there scheduled appointments and hence missed the necessary treatments. Some of them experienced worsening of the existing symptoms while others found difficult to cope with the new stressor along with their existing symptoms.

11. Substance abuse

Social distancing, quarantine, limited travels are the measures used to prevent COVID 19 transmission however these measures resulted in negative emotions, boredome, worthlessness in many and specially those trying to abstain from the substance abuse. Outbreak resulted in relapse in many long-term abstainers due to missing of counselling and treatment sessions. Many suffered intolerable and life-threatening withdrawal symptoms. Due to lack of medical services to address the issues or inability to reach the facilities many found it difficult to cope with the situation resulting in increased relapse, irritability, domestic violence and suicidal attempts [16].

12. Preventing health service

Health services aimed at prevention of certain non-communicable disease, cancer screening like screening for cervical cancers were suspended and hence most of the patients missed the opportunity to be diagnosed for treatable pre-cancerous lesion.

13. Minor ailments

Apart from the chronic and existing disease there are certain acute conditions which does not require emergency management but certainly require treatment as the symptoms can be boresome to the patient. In the absence of an appropriate diagnosis patient feel scared about the new onset symptoms. Certain such symptoms like abnormal uterine bleedings, acute abdominal pain, new onset headaches, ear infections, trauma remained untreated in the absence of routine care. Postponement of appointments for these non COVID or non-emergency conditions cause frustration and unrest to many.

14. Neuropsychiatric sequelae of COVID-19

None of the countries were prepared for such pandemic. Even the countries with best of health care system faced shortage of beds, ventilators during the first and second peak. Millions of people died due lack of effective management. Fear, anxiety about contracting the disease, uncertainty about future, disruption in work and social isolation affected psychological wellbeing of people. Since SARS-CO -V-2 also affects the central nervous system many studies have shown acute neuropsychiatric symptoms like cerebrovascular accidents/stroke and encephalopathies [16]. Patients presented with symptoms like headache, dizziness, myalgia, loss of smell and loss of taste. A lot of people experienced mood changes, anxiety disorders and sleep disturbances because of it. Those who contracted COVID-19 also suffered post-traumatic stress disorder (PTSD) [17, 18].

COVID 19 Pandemic had a significant impact on the existing health care system. As per WHO dashboard around 564,126,546 patients have been infected and around 6,371,354 died because of COVID- 19 virus till 22nd July 2022. Since Majority of the health care system was over-burdened due to the COVID 19 cases there was no place and arrangements which were made for non COVID patients. COVID-19 pandemic brought major challenges to the existing health care system through-out the world. Countries with underdeveloped digital healthcare system suffered the most. Due to the delay in treatment for new onset medical conditions and follow up and continued management of those on long term treatment adversely affected patients existing medical condition. As a lot of patients developed psychological issue and sleep disturbances. While a lot of effort was being made to curtail the transmission of COVID-19 and prevention and management of the complications because of it no separate arrangements were made to manage the longstanding disease and no effort was made to address the mental health issues of such patients [19].

Author details

Harpreet Kaur* and Asmita Kaundal
Department of Obstetrics and Gynaecology, AIIMS, Bilaspur, H.P., India

*Address all correspondence to: drharpreetsidhu7@gmail.com

References

[1] Carlos WG, Dela Cruz CS, Cao B, et al. Novel Wuhan (2019-nCoV) coronavirus. American Journal of Respiratory and Critical Care Medicine. 2020;**201**(4): P7-P8. DOI: 10.1164/rccm.2014p7

[2] Wu F, Zhao S, Yu B, et al. A new coronavirus associated with human respiratory disease in China. Nature. 2020;**579**(7798):265-269. DOI: 10.1038/s41586-020-2008-3

[3] The Impact of the COVID-19 Pandemic on Noncommunicable Disease Resources and Services: Results of a Rapid Assessment. Geneva: World Health Organization; 2020

[4] Global Health Estimates 2016: Life expectancy, 2000-2019. Geneva, World Health Organization; 2018. Available from: http://www.who.int/gho/mortality_burden_disease/ife_tables/en/

[5] Linardos M, Carnevale S, Agostini L, et al. Multidisciplinary interview to assess distress in patients waiting for breast cancer treatments. Translational Cancer Research. 2018;**7**(S3):S266-S271. DOI: 10.21037/tcr.2018.02.17

[6] Hansen RP, Olesen F, Sørensen HT, et al. Socioeconomic patient characteristics predict delay in cancer diagnosis: A Danish cohort study. BMC Health Services Research. 2008;**8**(1):49. DOI: 10.1186/1472-6963-8-49

[7] Verna L, Cortellini A, Giusti R, et al. Cancer care after natural disaster: Different countries, similar problems. Journal of Global Oncology. 2019;**5**:1-2. DOI: 10.1200/jgo.19.00155

[8] Porzio G, Aielli F, Verna L, et al. Home care for cancer patients after an earthquake: The experience of the "L'Aquila per la Vita" home care unit. Journal of Pain and Symptom Management. 2011;**42**(3):e1-e4. DOI: 10.1016/j.jpainsymman.2011.06.004

[9] Tam CW, Pang EP, Lam LC, et al. Severe acute respiratory syndrome (SARS) in Hong Kong in 2003: Stress and psychological impact among frontline healthcare workers. Psychological Medicine. 2004;**34**(7):1197-1204. DOI: 10.1017/s0033291704002247

[10] Wu KK, Chan SK, Ma TM. Posttraumatic stress after SARS. Emerging Infectious Diseases. 2005;**11**(8):1297-1300. DOI: 10.3201/eid1108. 041083

[11] Ye Y et al. Psychological distress of cancer patients caused by treatment delay during COVID 19 pandemic in China: A cross-sectional study. Psycho-Oncology. 2022;**31**(9):1-9. DOI: 10.1002/pon.5946

[12] Farr SL, Anderson JE, Jamieson DJ, Warner L, Macaluso M. Predictors of pregnancy and discontinuation of infertility services among women who received medical help to become pregnant, National Survey of family growth, 2002. Fertility and Sterility. 2009;**91**(4):988-997

[13] Lawson AK. Psychological stress and fertility. In: Stevenson EL, Hershberger PE, editors. Fertility and Assisted Reproductive Technology (ART): Theory, Research, Policy and Practice for Healthcare Practitioners. 7th ed. New York City: Springer Publishing Company; 2016. pp. 65-86

[14] American Society for Reproductive Medicine. Patient Management and Clinical Recommendations During the

Coronavirus (COVID- 19) Pandemic. 2020. Available from: https://www.asrm.org/globalassets/asrm/asrm-content/news-and-publications/covid-19/covidtaskforce.pdf. [Accessed May 5, 2020]

[15] Kaur H, Pranesj GT, Rao. Ak. Emotional impact of delay in fertility treatment due to COVID-19 pandemic. Journal of Human reproductive sciences. 2020;**13**(4):317-321

[16] Mao L, Wang M, Chen S, He Q, Chang J, Hong C, et al. Neurological manifestations of hospitalized patients with COVID-19 in Wuhan, China: A retrospective case series study. medRxiv. 2020;**77**(6):1-9. DOI: 10.1101/2020.02.22.20026500

[17] Kang L, Li Y, Hu S, Chen M, Yang C, Yang BX, et al. The mental health of medical workers in Wuhan, China dealing with the 2019 novel coronavirus. Lancet Psychiatry. 2020a;**7**:e14. DOI: 10.1016/S2215-0366(20)30047-X

[18] Kang L, Ma S, Chen M, Yang J, Wang Y, Li R, et al. Impact on mental health and perceptions of psychological care among medical and nursing staff in Wuhan during the 2019 novel coronavirus disease outbreak: A cross-sectional study. Brain, Behavior, and Immunity. 2020b;**87**:11-17. DOI: 10.1016/j.bbi.2020.03.028

[19] Gagliardi AR et al. The psychological burden of waiting for procedures and patient-centred strategies that could support the mental health of wait-listed patients and caregivers during the COVID-19 pandemic: A scoping review. Health Expectations. 2021;**24**:978-990

Chapter 16

Effects of Covid-19 Pandemic on Women's Mental Health: A Critical Review of Literature

Chika Eze, Nneka Okafor, Emelda I. Emmanuel and Chinecherem Iloka

Abstract

Although COVID-19 has affected both men and women, it seemingly has impacted on women's mental health in peculiar ways, specifically in terms of varying forms of abuse such as increased gender-based violence (GBV), which dehumanizes women. Across the globe, women have been notable victims of gender-based violence, but the surge of COVID-19 has worsened the records of GBV. Therefore, this chapter provides a critical review of literature conducted through three database sites: Google Scholar, Research Gate, and Sage based on researches published across 2020–2022 (and other available data documents) in relation to the effects of COVID-19 on women's mental health. Based on the reviewed articles, recommendations were made for strategic adjustment, particularly for policy makers and for women themselves to be more proactive in being agentive toward self-protection and advocacy.

Keywords: COVID-19, women's mental health, gender-based violence, victims, strategic adjustment

1. Introduction

The COVID-19 pandemic has had a major impact on the mental health and well-being of many vulnerable groups [1] of which women are among those most heavily affected [2]. Although COVID-19 seems to hit men harder than women, based on the fact that fatality rate for men who have contracted virus is 60–80% higher than for women [3], its continual spread around the world has severely impacted on women [3–5]. This severe effect is largely manifested through lockdown situations, which apart from affecting women's employability, have also exacerbated risks of violence, exploitation, abuse, or harassment against women [6]. The assumption regarding the severe effect of the pandemic on women is based on the fact that any global/national/local emergence is a risk factor that tends to escalate gender-based violence (GBV) [1, 4, 5], of which COVID-19 is no exception. In this perspective, United Nations Population Fund [7] in conjunction with European Parliamentary Forum for Sexual & Reproductive Rights [8] projected that gender-based violence has increased due to COVID-19 lockdown making it difficult for women to have safe shelter and support.

Hence, the reality is that the restriction of movement as governments' containment measure to control the spread of the virus has compelled women/girls to spend longer period of time with their perpetrators, resulting in sustained experience of greater gender-based violence, exploitation, abuse, or harassment [3, 9]. Put in another form, the UNFPA has warned that women are more likely to face domestic violence behind closed doors during lockdown due to Government restrictions on movement, that is "the stay at home" measures to curb the spread of the disease, especially at a period when counseling and support services may be limited [10].

In this chapter, GBV is presented as the outcome of unequal and unjust social conditions based on gender relations [11], facilitated by the limited mobility during the COVID-19 safety protocol across the globe [9, 12–14]. Tentatively, the hub of the risk factor escalating the increased GBV experience for women is leveled on the nationwide lockdown safety protocol. Hence, this chapter focuses on exploring how confinement to the home environment has contributed to the increased gender-based violence that women encountered during the COVID-19 pandemic and its impact on their mental health.

As part of the presentation, the chapter makes some recommendations, proposing that women become more proactive in terms of self-protection. In addition, policy makers ought to device further ways of ensuring that perpetrators of GBV are re-oriented toward self-transformation in order to foster safer environment for promoting dignity for all.

2. The global narratives

Across the globe, there were increased narratives revealing incidences of GBV within the context of COVID-19 pandemic. The report from United States reflects that there was significant increase in gender-based violence and domestic violence during the period of COVID-19 lockdown. For instance, UN Women Australia global report emphasized that prior to the COVID-19 pandemic, one out of every three women/girls experienced gender-based violence, but during the pandemic, the situation worsened to one out of every two women/girls [15]. UN Women/UN Women Count report affirms such recordings indicating that women encounter GBV directly or indirectly during the COVID-19 pandemic [5]. Furthermore, UNFPA reported that although the lockdowns, curfews and other restrictions during the COVID-19 pandemic were measures taken to increase the safety of all, these measures were rather sources of increased risk of violence and death for women/girls [15]. The report went further to express that the number of women/girls aged 15–49 years who experienced sexual or physical violence by an intimate partner before the pandemic were 243 million across the globe [15]. But within the context of the pandemic, the figures have almost doubled [16, 17]. However, these figures may change after the pandemic, though that might not be certain.

The report emphasized that the exacerbating factors were due to security, health and money worries, cramped living conditions, isolation from abusers, movement restrictions, and deserted public spaces [15]. Whatever the reasons were, the essential fact is that women/girls' mental health was gravely impacted upon and such is worrisome. In a more recent document, UN Women and UNDP report stated that COVID-19 has deepened a trio of interlocking crises that threaten women and girls around the world [4, 5], as could be seen in spiking levels of gender-based violence, steep losses of employment, and unmanageable increase on unpaid work care. Interestingly, these three levels of threats are very important. But this chapter strictly addresses the issue of increased levels of gender-based violence in terms of reviewing published research that reports gender-based violence during the pandemic and its impact on women's mental health and what possible options women and the wider society ought to engage in, in order to tackle such a menace [18].

Focusing on global statistics, specific narratives across nations are not encouraging; for instance, the statistics from Brazil show an increased incidence of domestic violence to the tone of 40–50% during the pandemic period [19]. In France, in addition, the report says that there is a 30% increase, and the report from Spain indicates an 18% increase [20, 21]. Across the Arab world, it was noted that GBV rates increased during the COVID-19 pandemic in many Arabic countries such as Lebanon, Syria, Jordan and Iraq [22–24]. In the Palestinian context, it has been reported that 37% of women were exposed to violence, while 58.6% of them experienced psychological violence, 23.5% encountered physical violence, 11.8% had sexual violence, 54.8% encountered social violence, and 55.1% encounter economic violence [25]. For China, the police reports of domestic violence were three times higher in February 2020 compared to reports from the previous year [26]. In Africa, the story is not different, and the report expresses that there is increase in gender-based violence during the heat of the pandemic [12, 14, 27]. The situation in Nigeria reflects the global trend of increased gender-based violence. GBV is reported to have significantly increased since the lockdown began in the three most affected areas (Lagos State, FCT, and Ogun State) by March 30, 2020 [12]. The Lagos State Domestic and Sexual Violence Response Team [28] reported a threefold increase in the number of telephone calls received through their hotlines in 1 month. In particular, service providers have reported sharp increases in cases of intimate partner violence and domestic violence.

The reality is that, in the face of such daunting experiences, women/girls are caught in the continuous web of ever struggling for equity as expressed in SDG goals. Therefore, this chapter particularly focuses on exploring the different forms of gender-based violence women/girls encountered during the pandemic as reflected in published articles between the years 2020 and 2022. However, particular attention is paid to African context based on the author's research interest and location.

3. Method

This chapter conducted a critical literature review of articles published between 2020 and 2022 aimed at exploring effects of COVID-19 on women's mental health. Consequently, a systematic search was conducted across three databases, namely Google Scholar, Research Gate, and Sage using the search term COVID-19 and/or coronavirus or pandemic, women's mental health, and gender-based violence including Africa. The rationale for focusing on Africa was based on the authors' contextual location using index-term definitions, dwelling on the authors' knowledge of the topic under investigation. The time parameters of the search were January 2020 to August 2022. Research Gate like Google Scholar is an aggregator database, referring to the fact that it includes content from various publishers (referring to different journals and databases). Thus, the rationale to opt for these two databases was based on the fact that they provide access to a large scope of work, which might have been excluded in more focused databases. Sage journals were included as it is a database that covers

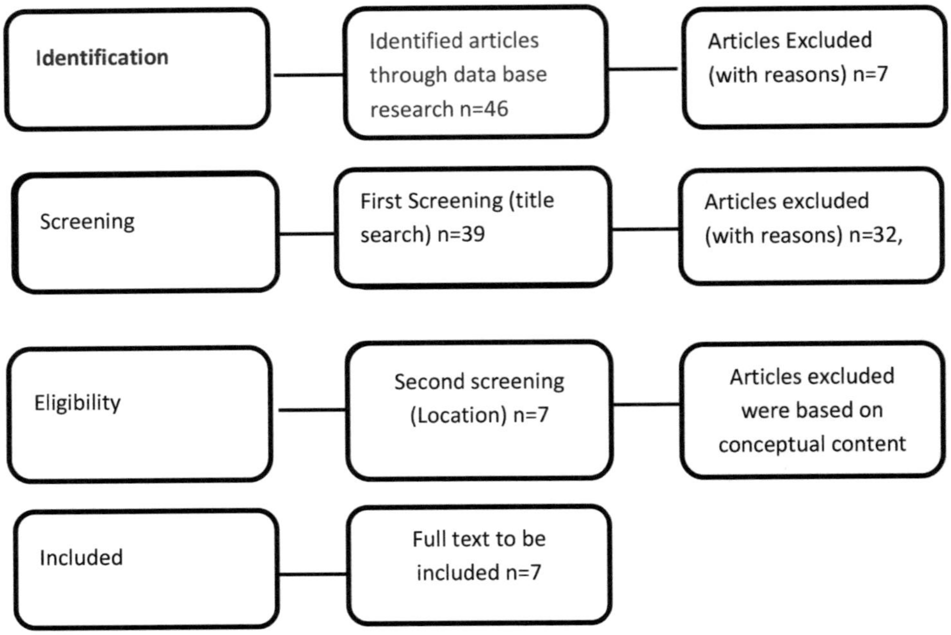

Figure 1.
PRISMA flowchart of reviewed articles.

social and behavioral sciences, including our interest on women's mental health and gender-based violence. We sourced 25 articles from Google Scholar, Research Gate had 13, and Sage had 8 articles. Articles were screened and only articles (and reports/ reviews) that had these keywords in their titles or abstracts were considered in the current chapter. Articles that were duplicated in terms of being published in more than one database were merged. In this context, we opted for one instead of reviewing the two. Articles selected for retrieval were independently assessed by two authors for conceptual rigor. Two reviewers were included to avoid bias. Working together in pairs enable verification and contributed to apt possible level of methodological rigor. Statistically, the review included seven published articles in relation to women's mental health and COVID-19, revealing how COVID-19 has facilitated varying degree of gender-based violence in Africa. The criterion for inclusion or exclusion of reviewed articles was based on content analysis of which article aligns itself with the thematic focus of the chapter. In addition, only articles focused on Africa were included (**Figure 1**).

Based on the thematic analysis, the review is presented in one key theme of COVID-19 movement restriction and its implication for heightened gender-based violence and impact on women's mental health. This one key theme is expressed *via* three sub-themes as follows: Women's emotional and physical abuse, sexual abuse, and economic challenges.

4. Review report of gender-based violence during the COVID-19 pandemic

As stated earlier, the review from previous literature is presented in one board theme: Women confinement and gender-based violence during COVID-19 pandemic,

S. No.	Authors	Title	Research design	Major findings	Sub-theme 1: Emotional abuse	Sub-theme 2: Economic	Sub-theme 3: Sexual	Intervention
1.	Ndlovu et al. (2022) [27]	COVID-19 impact on gender-based violence among women in South Africa during lockdown: a narrative review	Literature Review (Mini Review)	COVID-19 restricted movement heightened women's experiences of gender-based violence	Psychological distress among GBV victims is exacerbated mainly by social isolation during the pandemic lockdown	Other factors that aggravate violence are economic-related as women were forced to remain in abusive relationship due to economic dependence	Heightened sexual abuse as perpetrators and victims are forced to spend long period of time together	Need to develop strategies and measures to protect victims. Government should offer free mental health counseling to victims.
2.	Dlamini (2021) [29]	Gender-Based Violence, Twin Pandemic to COVID-19	Literature review (symposium paper presentation)	Gender-based violence increased significantly in the face of COVID-19 pandemic lockdown safety measures.	Women experience heightened emotional/ physical abuse in the face of lockdown measures to scrub further spread of COVID-19.	N/A	Equally women encounter greater sexual abuse during COVID-19 pandemic as they are forced to spend longer period of time with their perpetrators.	GBV requires multiprong/ multi-stakeholder solution such as gender-budgeting. E.G.: engaging fiscal policy to address gender inequality. Secondly, civil society should create awareness regarding gender inequality.

S. No.	Authors	Title	Research design	Major findings	Sub-theme 1: Emotional abuse	Sub-theme 2: Economic	Sub-theme 3: Sexual	Intervention
3.	Sediri et al. (2020) [14]	Women's mental health: acute impact of COVID-19 pandemic on domestic violence	Quantitative design, data collected from 751 Tunisian women	Increased GBV against women during the COVID-19 lockdown (from 4.4 to 14.8%; $p < 0.001$).	Psychological (emotional) abuse was the most frequent type of gender-based violence (96%)	Another form of violence that women experienced during this period was economic related (41%)	Physical abuse reflects 10%, which is linked to some kind of sexual abuse.	Strengthening strategies to protect women during periods of crisis, starting with family orientation to change mindsets for the perpetrators and victims of GBV.
4.	Allen (2021) [30]	COVID-19 and Sexual and Reproductive Health of Women and Girls in Nigeria	Literature review	Social distancing, self-isolation, quarantine and treatment had psychological outcomes that were not considered in the emergency response to the crisis in the case of Nigeria	Psychological (emotional) abuse for women and girls	Economic abuse surfacing in extreme hardship for girls and women	Sexual abuse that has resulted in unwanted pregnancies, particularly for girls.	Policy response to support/care for girls/women during crisis period.

S. No.	Authors	Title	Research design	Major findings	Sub-theme 1: Emotional abuse	Sub-theme 2: Economic	Sub-theme 3: Sexual	Intervention
5.	Groenewald et al. (2022) [31]	Adolescent sexual and reproductive health during COVID-19 pandemic: A mini review	Literature review focused on teenage pregnancy, sexual violence, abortion, and the barriers toward accessing SRH services during the pandemic (including contraceptives)	The literature highlighted increases in child sexual abuses in African countries during the pandemic.	Girls were emotional abused and exploited during the national lockdown restrictions.	Economic hardship arising from restricted movement left girls/women vulnerable to domestic violence, increased risk of sexual abuse and increased early marriages among girls.	Unwanted pregnancies as a result of sexual assaults on girls/ women	Policy engagement to protect girls/ women. Also, government to provide resources to care for teenage mothers
6.	Tadesse et al. (2020) [32]	Prevalence and Associated Factors of Intimate Partner Violence Among Married Women During COVID-19 Pandemic Restrictions: A Community-Based Study	Quantitative design, a community-base cross sectional study, sampling 617 Ethiopian women.	Findings indicate that the COVID-19 preventive measures, such as confinement have worsened the incidence of gender-based violence, particularly for women.	Results show that 22% of the participants have experienced heightened psychological (emotional) abuse emerging from GBV during the COVID-19 pandemic.	There was evidence of economic dependence, which makes women more prone to GBV abuses.	The participants have also encountered sexual abuse during the lockdown safety measures.	Government policy to promote gender equity aimed at eliminating violence against women beyond COVID-19 pandemic. In addition, accessibility of education for women should be promoted.

S. No.	Authors	Title	Research design	Major findings	Sub-theme 1: Emotional abuse	Sub-theme 2: Economic	Sub-theme 3: Sexual	Intervention
7.	Fawole et al. (2021) [12]	Home was not a safe haven: women's experiences of intimate partner violence during the COVID-19 lockdown in Nigeria	Qualitative design: Case reports of women's experiences of GBV during the COVID-19 pandemic lockdown measures.	The report identified that intimate partner violence (IPV) happened prior to COVID-19 pandemic but the severity increased during the lockdown.	Women were psychological (emotional) traumatized by their GBV abuses.	Women experienced untold economic deprivation that made them more vulnerable to GBV abuses.	Women also experienced sexual abuses.	Legal measures to prosecute the perpetrators Also societal response such as community involvement and advocacy are needed.

Table 1.
Reviewed articles.

reflecting women's emotional and physical abuse, sexual abuse, and financial abuse. Generally, these three sub-themes captured some of the contextual confinement experience that women across Africa encountered during the COVID-19 pandemic, which by extension could be similar to the experiences of women across the globe. The reviewed articles were from Ethiopia, Nigeria, South Africa, and Tunisian. The findings are presented in **Table 1**. Reviewed Articles, reflecting the thematic summary findings of the reviewed articles with emphasis on how the movement restriction has led to heightened increase of gender-based violence during the COVID-19 lockdown.

5. Brief discussion of the reviewed articles

Literally, all the reviewed articles engaged the discourse of confinement to the home environment to describe women's increased experience of gender-based violence during the COVID-19 pandemic [12, 14, 27, 29–32]. In unison, all the seven articles (including other related reports) claimed that the safety protocol of lockdown imposed by government compelled men and women to spend longer period of time together at home, which heightened the incidences of gender-based violence. The popular argument is that the lockdown protocol has dual effect. On the one hand, it helped to control the rapid spread of the virus, by reducing the frequency of contracting the virus. But on the other hand, the limited mobility skyrocketed women's experience of gender-based violence as men and women were forced to spend long hours together resulting to greater experience of GBV. Hence, the dominate reality is that women encountered an increased experience of GBV during the COVID-19 lockdown, which could have a lasting effect on their mental well-being. Accordingly, what follows is a summary of the predominate themes that the reviewed articles surfaced, reflecting psychological abuse embedded in emotional/physical abuses, sexual abuse and economic abuse, which all put together impacted on women's mental health and well-being.

6. Women's psychological abuse: emotional/physical abuses during COVID-19 lockdown safety protocol

Unanimously, all the reviewed articles affirmed that the COVID-19 safety protocol of restricted movement/lockdown worsen women's experience of GBV [12, 14, 27–32]. The argument is that COVID-19 pandemic and its associated safety protocol forced men and women to stay at home for longer period of time. In this context, the reality is that women who experienced violence of any kind could not even leave the house and/or seek support from others. One research narrative review based on exploring the impact of COVID-19 on South African women's experience of GBV stated that, at the start of the lockdown in March 2020, 87,000 cases of GBV and interpersonal violence were reported, reflecting a significant increase compared to pre-COVID-19 space [28]. Although the authors emphasized that the reports did not indicate what type of interpersonal relationships or who the perpetrators were, they argued that men are often noted as the aggressors. They backed up their argument with South African President Ramaphosa's concern during one of the COVID-19 progress report regarding seriousness of GBV and femicide, and his statement that at every three hours, a woman loses her life due to GBV in the country [28]. If a woman loses her life every three hours, such happening is horrendous and a pointer to the fact that COVID-19 has indeed facilitated heightened GBV experience for women, which no doubt impacts on their mental health and well-being. Another research finding focusing on Nigerian women's experience of GBV during the COVID-19 pandemic reechoed the same increased reality of violence, reaffirming emotional and physical abuses [12]. In this perspective, the report reflected cases of how women have been threatened by their partners to be banished from the house and/or ostracized by their children. Such threats are sources of emotional torture for some of the women [12]. Another corroborating research finding confirms that women/girls in Nigeria were emotional tortured in the face of national lockdown, and the report clearly indicated that women/girls who were abused could not seek for help/support from others [31]. Certainly, it was in this context that some researchers have described the home as no longer a safe place to be [12]. In addition, a research report from Tunis also presents similar findings, indicating that women experience emotional torture during COVID-19 pandemic [14], which they describe as having psychological impact. In fact, the researchers claimed that 78% of cases recorded during the lockdown were *de novo*, meaning that these women were assaulted for the first time [14]. Hence, the researchers expressed that in Tunisia, the Ministry of Women, Family and Childhood reported that GBV during the COVID-19 pandemic rose sevenfold. These narratives were indicative of the daunting GBV experiences women across African nations have encountered, and implications will reflect on their state of mental health.

7. Women's experiences of sexual abuse during the COVID-19 lockdown

Another devastating GBV experience that nearly all the reviewed articles reported were cases of sexual abuse during the COVID-19 lockdown. In most cases, the articles emphasized that incidences of sexual abuse arose as women encountered excessive sex demands from their partners based on the fact that they were confined to stay at home for long period of time. In regard, a sensational case report was made of a woman, who was sighted running away from her house onto the street nearly naked in the bid to escape from her husband, who according to her has had sex all night yet wanted some more [12]. The woman in her own views expressed that she has to run onto the empty street despite the lockdown restrictions because she did not want her husband to snuff out all the life in her. Furthermore, the same research reported that some women who resisted their husband's excessive sex demands often times encounter physical beating [12]. Similar cases of sexual abuses were reflected in a mini-research review focusing on adolescent sexual and reproductive health during COVID-19 pandemic [29]. Hence, there is strong affirmation that sexual violence was on the increase across African nations during the lockdown restrictions and not only for women but also for girls and children [30]. In this regard, they reported that in Uganda, sexual violence was the "third most reported form of abuse contributing 20.1% of all the cases" [31]. Equally, their report indicated that Kenya had witnessed a significant increase of more than 80% in teenage pregnancies in 2020 compared to 2019 (Kenya Situation Report. Nairobi: UNOCHA Kenya, 2020 cited in [31]). Similarly, in Malawi, in 2020, an approximately 35% rise was noted in the number of teenage pregnancies among adolescent girls (Davies, 2020 cited in [31]).

In addition, they stated that sexual violence against girls had been reported across West of Africa including Benin, Cameroon, Côte d'Ivoire, Gambia, Ghana, Guinea, and Sierra Leone (Commonwealth Foundation [31]. In general, the dominant argument is that prevalence of sexual violence is associated with unwanted pregnancies including ever raising demand for abortion, and all of these impact on mental health and wellness of life [30]. Another study reported 22% prevalence of intimate partner sexual violence among Ethiopian women during the COVID-19 pandemic lockdown [30]. Therefore, there is evidence-based speculation regarding the risk factors associated with COVID-19 pandemic and increased incidences of GBV, and what is more worrisome is the type of impact such experiences make on women's mental health.

8. Women's economic abuse during the COVID-19 lockdown

Women economic abuse has been concurrently alleged to by all the reviewed articles, pointing to the fact that COVID-19 pandemic demean women's economic power further than it used to be. In this context, a good number of the articles argued that women who used to struggle to run small entrepreneur business scales such as selling bean cakes and water among many others, suddenly discovered that the lockdown protocol prevented them from doing so [12, 29], which for some women has led to excessive financial dependence on their partners [28]. The resultant effect is that women were emotional and physically abused when they ask for resources that they partners could not afford to supply [12, 29].

One of the research projects reviewed narrated how the "stay at home" restriction order had forced a woman to remain in her boyfriend's house for a long period of time and eventually there was shortage of food and the boyfriend locked up the woman in the house [12]. The boyfriend went out for hours, only to return in the evening drunk and physically attacked her. She sustained injury from the violence. Similar cases were reported by [12, 14] claiming that financial stress is one of the facilitating factors for increased GBV experiences for women. Other scholars argued that informal traders who depend on their partners for financial support have no alternative than to remain in abusive relationship in order to secure their daily bread [6, 27]. Hence, financial stress is represented through reduced income and bleak future because of restricted movement and retrenchment are potential catalyst flaming violence against women.

In the same vein, a case study report of a woman who during the pandemic lockdown asked the husband to collect N30,000 that a friend had sent to her from abroad but her husband after collecting the money, refused to relinquish the money to her [12]. Although the woman insisted amidst verbal insults from her husband to retrieve the money from him, that led to her leaving the house with her children in seek of safety in a relative's house. Thus, she and her children became internally displaced for a time being and such is another form of emotional torture, directly or indirectly impacting on mental health. Consequently, it can be argued that economic stress forms part of the reason for further GBV experience during the COVID-19 pandemic. And in most cases, women/girls are always at the receiving end of being victims.

9. Recommendations

This chapter makes only two recommendations based on the vital issues raised within the reviewed articles: one for women to improve their level of proactiveness in the face of any adversity, particularly in sustaining a viable economic strength. The act of achieving proactiveness should be done through advocacy, which ought to promote self-efficacy and assertiveness. In addition, some form of psycho-education ought to be conducted while carrying out the advocacy programs. In order to achieve a viable level of proactiveness, women in particular need to be involved in conducting the advocacy process, wherein they (women) ought to create the awareness for and with themselves. Such advocacy can be championed by Ministry of Women Affairs (including women's organizations) through media and faith-based channels.

The key aim of the awareness creation will be focusing on facilitating women's ability to treasure the need to be resilient, which will include the act of self-efficacy, assertiveness, and independent, which can be achieved through psycho-education. This is based on the notion that depending on their partners for sustenance has resulted in varying abuses: be it emotional, physical, and/or sexual. It does not mean that women could end GBV by just being economic independence but rather such a stance will minimize the GBV abuses. In all, women may not be able to achieve much on their own without the help of men; therefore, the awareness creation ought to include soliciting the cooperation of men. Thus, the advocacy process has to factor in men as active participants (reflecting the act of communal (collective) involvement, which is usually Africa's strategic step reflecting interdependence). The involvement of men could be achieved through media/faith-based channels, wherein men should be encouraged to appreciate women and perceive them as valued.

The second recommendation relates to policy makers, which strongly laid emphasis on the fact that women should be more agentic in protecting themselves from abuse by voicing out the experiences. In this stance, existing policies ought to be reviewed to include clauses that advocate for women's proactiveness toward self-protection and economic independence. To achieve this stance, women in carrying out the advocacy process ought to continue to include aspects of creating the awareness that speaking out matters. In addition, policy makers should device means to ensure that the perpetrators of GBV are re-oriented toward self-transformation to promote a safer environment for all. Below is a diagram indicating the channel through which the intervention process could be achieved.

10. Intervention process

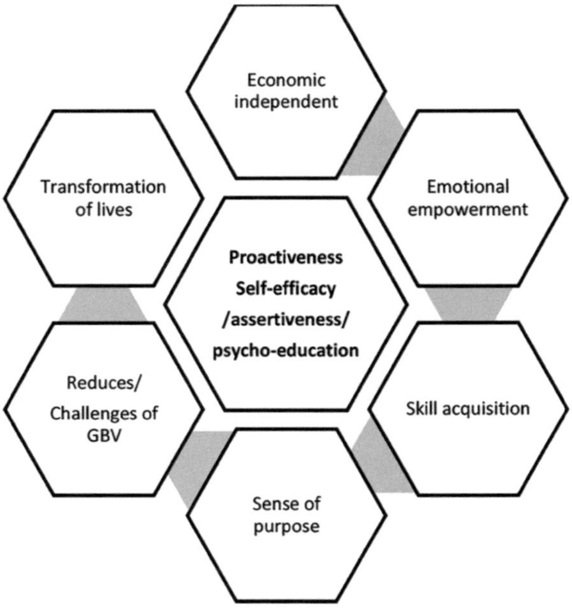

11. Conclusion

The effects of COVID-19 have impacted on women's mental health due to an increased number of GBV during the national and international lockdown. It has impacted on women's mental health in peculiar ways as varying forms of abuses such as increased gender-based violence (GBV), which dehumanizes women. Across the globe, women have been notable victims of gender-based violence, but the surge of COVID-19 has worsened the records of GBV, particularly in the face of home confinement. The chapter provides a critical review of literature based on published research across 2020–2022 (and other available data documents) in relation to the effects of COVID-19 on women's mental health. Based on the reviewed articles, recommendations were made, reflecting the need for strategic adjustment, particularly for policy makers and for women themselves to be more proactive in being agentive toward self-protection.

Authors' report

A total of seven articles were reviewed for analysis out of the 46 initially sourced articles. The delimiter for such choice was based on the chapter thematic focus of exploring COVID-19 pandemic and its associated impact on women's mental health, particularly in Africa. The reviewed articles have been asterisked in the reference list. However, all the work as reflected in the reference list contributed vital information toward the chapter's formulation and presentation.

Author details

Chika Eze[1]*, Nneka Okafor[2], Emelda I. Emmanuel[3] and Chinecherem Iloka[4]

1 Veritas University Abuja, Abuja, Nigeria

2 University of Nigeria, Nsukka, Nigeria

3 Ibrahim Badamasi Babangida University, Lapai, Nigeria

4 Compact Impact Foundation, Abuja, Nigeria

*Address all correspondence to: chikashcj@gmail.com

References

[1] Cowie H, Mayer C. The Impact of the COVID-19 Pandemic on the Mental Health and Well-Being of Children and Young People 2020. Children & Society. DOI: 10.1111/chso.12430

[2] Marshall L, Bibby J, Abbs I. Emerging Evidence on COVID-19's Impact on Mental Health and Inequalities, in Health Foundation. 2020. Available from: https://www.health.org.uk/news-and-comment/blogs/emerging-evidence-on-covid-

[3] OECD. Women at the Core of the Fight against Covid-19 Crisis, in OECD Policy Responses to Coronavirus (COVID-19). 2020. Available from: https://www.oecd.org/coronavirus/policy-responses/Women-at-the-core-of-the-fight-against-COVID-19-crisis-553a8269/

[4] UNFPA. Covid-19: Reporting on Gender-Based Violence during Public Health Crises. 2020. Available from: https://www.unfpa.org/resources/covid-19-reporting-gender-based-violence-during-public-health-crises

[5] UN Women. UN Women and UNDP Report: Five Lessons from COVID-19 for Centring Gender in Crisis. 2020. Available from: https://www.unwomen.org>feature-story>2022/06

[6] Mittal S, Singh T. Gender-based violence during COVID-19 pandemic: A mini-review. Front Global Women's Health. 2020;**1**(4):1-7

[7] United Nations Population Fund. Impact of the COVID-19 Pandemic on Family Planning and Ending Gender-based Violence, Female Genital Mutilation and Child Marriage. 2020. Available from: https://www.unfpa.org/sites/default/files/resource-pdf/COVID19_impact_brief_for_UNFPA_24_April_2020_1.pdf

[8] European Parliamentary Forum for Sexual & Reproductive Rights, International Planned Parenthood Federation. Sexual and Reproductive Health and Rights during the COVID-19 Pandemic. 2020. Available from: https://www.ippfen.org/sites/ippfen/files/202004/Sexual%20and%20Reproductive%20Health%20during%20the%20COVID-19%20pandemic.pdf

[9] Du Q. Chinese families see surge in domestic violence amid Covid-19 lockdown. Global Times. 2020. Available from: www.globaltimes.cn›content

[10] World Economic Forum. The COVID-19 Pandemic Could Have Huge Knock-On Effects on Women's Health, Says the UN. 2020. Available from: https://www.weforum.org/agenda/2020/04/covid-19-coronavirus-pandemic-hit-women-harder-than-men

[11] Parkes J, Heslop J, Oando S, Sabaa S, Januario F, Figue A. Conceptualizing gender and violence in research: Insights from studies in schools and communities in Kenya, Ghana and Mozambique. International Journal of Educational Development. 2020;**33**(6):546-556

[12] Fawole OI, Okedare OO, Reed E. Home was not a safe haven: women's experiences of intimate partner violence during the COVID-19 lockdown in Nigeria. BMC Women's Health. 2021;**21**:32. DOI: 10.1186/s12905-021-01177-9

[13] Mahamid F, Veronese G, Bdier D. Gender-based violence experiences among Palestinian women during the

COVID-19 pandemic: Mental health professionals' perceptions and concerns. Conflict and Health. 2022;**16**:13. DOI: 10.1186/s13031-022-00444-2

[14] Sediri S, Zgueb Y, Ouanes S, Ouali U, Bourgou S, Jomli R, et al. Women's mental health: Acute impact of COVID-19 pandemic on domestic violence. Archives of Women's Mental Health. 2020;**23**:749-756

[15] UNDP. Gender-Based Violence and Covid-19. 2020

[16] UN Women Australia. The Shadow Pandemic: Violence against Women during COVID19. 2020. Available from: https://unwomen.org.au/the-shadow-pandemic-violence-against-women-during-covid-19/

[17] UN Women | UN Women Count. Measuring the Shadow Pandemic: Violence against Women during COVID-19. 2021. Available from: https://data.unwomen.org/publicatios/vaw-rga

[18] UN Women. COVID-19 and Violence against Women: What the Data Tells Us. 2022. Available from: https://www.unwomen.org/en/news-stories/feature-story/2022/11/covid-19-and-violence-against-women-what-the-data-tells-us

[19] Bastos G. Addressing Violence against Women (VAW) under COVID-19. 2020. Available from: https://documents1.worldbank.org›curated›pdf

[20] Boserup B, McKenney M, Elkbuli A. Alarming trends in US domestic violence during the COVID-19 pandemic. The American Journal of Emergency Medicine;**38**(12):2753-2755. DOI: 1016/j.ajem.2020.04.077

[21] Campbell AM. An increasing risk of family violence during the Covid-19 pandemic: Strengthening community collaborations to save lives. Forensic Science International: Reports. 2020;**2**:100089. DOI: 10.1016/j.fsir

[22] Abuhammad S. Violence against Jordanian women during COVID-19 outbreak. International Journal of Clinical Practice. 2021;**75**(3):e13824. DOI: 10.1111/ijcp.13824

[23] Diab JL. Pandemic-linked vulnerabilities for forced migrants: The increasein gender-based violence in the Arab world. Journal of Migration Affairs. 2020;**3**(1):90-98. DOI: 10.36931/jma.2020.3.1.90-98

[24] Mahmood KI, Shabu SA, M-Amen KM, Hussain SS, Kako DA, Hinchliff S, et al. The impact of CoViD-19 related lockdown on the prevalence of spousal violence against women in Kurdistan region of Iraq. Journal of Interpersonal Violence. 2021;**37**:13-14, NP11811–NP11835. DOI: 10.1177/0886260521997929

[25] Bdier D, Mahamid FA. The association between gender-based violence, wellbeing, and mental health outcomes among Palestinian women. Journal of Concurrent Disorders. 2021:87-104. https://concurrentdisorders.ca/2021/05/27/

[26] Axios J. China's Domestic Violence Epidemic. 2020:1-19. Available from: https://www.axios.com/china-domestic-violence-coronavirusquarantine-7b00c3ba-35bc-4d16-afdd-b76ecfb28882.html

[27] Ndlovu S, Mulondo M, Tsoka-Gwegweni J, Ndirangu J. Covid-19 impact on gender-based violence among women in South Africa during lockdown: A narrative review. African Journal of Reproductive Health. 2022;**26**(7):71

[28] United Nations Nigeria. Gender-Based Violence in Nigeria during the

Covid-19 crisis: The Shadow Pandemic. 2020. Available from: https://www.unwomen.org/en/news/stories/2020/4/statement-ed-phumzile-violence-against-women-during-pandemic

[29] Dlamini NJ. Gender-based violence, twin pandemic to Covid-19. Critical Sociology. 2021;**47**(4-5):583-590

[30] Allen F. Covid-19 and sexual reproductive health of women and girls in Nigeria. Cosmopolitan Civil Societies: An Interdisciplinary Journal. 2021;**3**(2): 1-11. DOI: 10.5130/ccs.v13.i2.7549

[31] Groenewald C, Isaacs N, Isaacs D. Adolescent sexual and reproductive health during the COVID-19 pandemic: A mini review. Frontiers in Reproductive Health. 2022;**4**:794477. DOI: 10.3389/frph.2022.794477

[32] Tadesse AW, Tarekegn SM, Wagaw GB, Muluneh MD, Kassa AM. Prevalence and associated factors of intimate partner violence among married women during COVID-19 pandemic restrictions: A community-based study. Journal of Interpersonal Violence. 2020:1-9. https://www.researchgate.net/publication/346719446

Chapter 17

Conflict Settings and COVID-19's Effects on Psychological Health

Derebe Madoro

Abstract

The COVID-19 epidemic's ongoing effects on the conflicted, disturbed environment tend to exacerbate mental health issues. People from areas afflicted by conflict are put under double stress as a result. The majority of displacement due to conflict has occurred in Ethiopia. Mental disturbance among those affected by conflict has been recognized as a significant public health issue. Therefore, this study's objective was to assess how the COVID-19 outbreak in Ethiopia's conflict-affected population affected people's mental health and its correlates. Mental distress was reported at about 49.4% with a 95% CI of 47 to 52.9%. Being female gender (AOR = 3.01, 95% CI 1.61, 5.44), fired house materials when present (AOR = 3.49, 95% CI 1.61, 5.44), Living in a host community (AOR = 1.8, 95%CI 1.97, 3.35), living alone (AOR = 3.57, 95%CI 2.06, 6.19), and sexual assault (AOR = 4.1, 95% CI 2.37 to 6.94) were found to be substantially correlated. Conflict-affected people have a high risk of mental distress during COVID-19 era. Therefore, the ministry of health and humanitarian organizations should work collaboratively in providing consistent; psychosocial support and appropriate intervention for conflict-affected people.

Keywords: psychological health, conflict, setting, COVID 19, Ethiopia

1. Introduction

In order to address the health and development catastrophe brought on by the virus, low- and middle-income countries get assistance from the UN COVID-19 Response and Recovery Fund [1]. The COVID-19 conference took place in Eastern Africa while the region's governments struggled with a number of problems. Millions of people have been compelled to leave their homes due to protracted hostilities, droughts, and insecurity [2]. Millions more have fled to neighboring countries where they live in makeshift refugee camps. The majority of the countries in the region are in some type of fragile and conflict-prone state (for example, Somalia and South Sudan) and/or are undergoing political reform (for example, Sudan and Ethiopia). They have a very low capability to contain the COVID-19 pandemic and lower the ensuing unemployment, poverty, and hunger [2].

Some of the most significant political, security, and conflict developments related to COVID-19 and its effects on neighboring nations include the postponement of Ethiopia's August 2020 elections and the declaration of a state of emergency by the government. Given that many of Ethiopia's most potent opposition groups and one of its most potent regional governments (Tigray) have voiced their opposition to these changes, this might be a significant source of conflict. If COVID-19 spreads widely across the nation, the mounting costs of the disease could cause significant socio-political instability. COVID-19's rising economic expenses could become sources of serious socio-political instabilities if it spreads broadly across the country. Since November 4, 2020 war has been started following Ethiopian Northern Command attack by Tigray People Libration Front (TPLF). A millions were displaced, thousands massacred, all public and private infrastructures destroyed in the conflict setting, children were raped in group, thousands killed [3, 4]. This in turn highly influences the mental well-being of conflict-affected people in Ethiopia during COVID-19 era.

"One in five persons in conflict zones lives with some type of mental disease, ranging from mild sadness or anxiety to psychosis," was according to WHO data from 2019. To contain the COVID-19 epidemic and reduce the accompanying unemployment, poverty, and starvation, it is also stated that "almost one in ten people live with a mild or severe mental disorder [5]." Despite the fact that there was limited research among students from conflict-affected areas, various research on the impact of the pandemic on individuals' mental and psychological well-being, notably at the college and university level, were undertaken during COVID-19 in Ethiopia. In the Benchi Sheko zone, for instance, the prevalence of sadness, anxiety, and stress was 21.2%, 27.7%, and 32.5%, accordingly [6], while the psychological impact of COVID-19 was 16.2% among college students [7]. According to another study, 22.2%, 39.6%, and 40.2% of graduating class members, respectively, suffered from stress, anxiety, or depression [8]. In a related study, depression was shown to be widespread in 46.3% of participants, anxiety in 52%, and stress in 28.6% [9]. The prevalence of depression, anxiety, and stress among university students in Addis Abeba was 51%, 51.6%, and 11.1%, respectively [10].

Students are subjected to both direct and indirect repercussions of violence during armed conflict, including erroneous military enlistment, murders, gender-based violence, trafficking, illegal detentions, and family separation [11]. Schoolchildren who have experienced conflict are more likely than those who have not to experience post-traumatic stress disorder, sadness, or anxiety [12]. Direct and indirect exposure to traumatic events, as well as increased levels of daily stressors, are suggested to be the causes of these effects [13]. There are not many mental health therapies available for conflict-affected students, and treatment disparities between adults and primary school students in low-resource settings are even worse [14].

People who have had to move frequently have gone through various traumas, acts of violence, wounds, and economic crises, making them more vulnerable to psychiatric issues [15–17]. The following issue is likely to get worse as a result of the COVID-19 epidemic's ongoing spread. Despite this, there are no reports on the influence of the pandemic and the conflict environment on the mental health of those affected by the conflict in Ethiopia. For people affected by armed conflict, mental anguish has been identified as a key public health concern and has been connected to social network alterations, poverty, unemployment, community violence, and unsecured living situations. Therefore, even when the hostility has subsided and the crisis has passed, emotional distress is substantially associated with a lower quality of life [18, 19]. Additionally, mental trauma can affect anyone and have a detrimental effect on everyday activities, sleep quality, productivity, and job performance [9]. Their long-term academic, social, and mental health results may be significantly impacted by their capacity to manage the epidemic and to effectively and correctly regulate their emotions and behavior during the pandemic [20].

The prevalence of mental disorders appears to be significantly higher than the general population in post-conflict and conflict-ridden cultures, including student populations [21]. Statistical estimates from a number of general population studies indicated that the prevalence of mental distress ranges from 1% to 5% [22, 23], and for high-risk populations such as displaced people [24, 25], it ranges from 3% to 58%. When COVID-19 was in effect, it was anticipated that mental anguish would increase in a conflicting environment [26]. To the best of the investigators' knowledge, Ethiopia has not had any particular published studies. As a result, this study aimed to close that gap by generating new knowledge regarding the mental health of conflict-affected people in Ethiopia during the COVID-19 era.

2. Methods

From April 1 to April 30, 2021, a community-based cross-sectional survey was undertaken. During the mid-COVID-19 outbreak in south Ethiopia, the survey was done in conflict-affected areas. In which more than a million were displaced in year 2018 due to inter-communal violence and conflict between Gedeo and Guji zone in south Ethiopia [27]. The respondents were chosen using a systematic random selection procedure. Because the conflict-affected people resided in different sites, proportional allocation to the number of household in each site was used to ensure that the sample was representative. The study covered all houses in the conflict-affected area of south Ethiopia that are situated on the border between the Gedeo and West Guji zones, as well as those that were accessible during the data collection period. Seriously ill people were not allowed to participate in the study.

According to a study conducted in Adama, Ethiopia, the sample size was calculated using the single population proportion technique, with a 3% margin of error (d), a 95% confidence interval of certainty (alpha = 0.05), and a 10% non-response rate, assuming p = 21.6% [28]. A total of 795 people were chosen as a representative sample size. Mental distress was the study's dependent variable. Conflicted- and trauma-related factors, clinical-related factors (history of mental illness, family history of mental illness, pre-existing medical illness), COVID-related factors (suspected/confirmed for COVID-19, knowledge about COVID-19), and social support were all independent variables. Using pretested questionnaires, data was collected by six Bsc nurses and routinely monitored by three psychiatry professionals. The questionnaire was translated into Amharic and then back to English to verify uniformity. Data collectors were taught how to conduct interviews with respondents and how to clarify any ambiguous questions as well as the study's goal. They were also taught about ethical principles and how to gain informed consent from respondents.

Mental distress was measured using the Kessler Psychological Distress Scale (K-10, [29]). The K10 scale, which consists of 10 questions on emotional states and a five-point rating scale for each response, is an easy way to gauge psychological distress. The K10 scale is a 10-item survey that asks respondents to score their recent 30-day anxiety and depressive symptoms on a five-point Likert scale. Participants in this study were classified as normal if they received a score of 20 or less, whereas those who had a score of 20 or more were identified as experiencing emotional distress [30]. It was validated with a consistency of 0.93, sensitivity of 84.2%, and specificity of 77.8% at a cut-off point of 6/7. It was reasonable as a result [31].

The Oslo-3 social support scale, which goes from 3 to 14, is used to assess social support. According to this scale, those who score between 3 and 8 are considered to have insufficient social support, those who score between 9 and 11 have moderate social support, and those who score between 12 and 14 have high social support [32]. According to this study's findings, pupils who scored below the minimum requirements during the study's conduct had lower law achievement. Data on sociodemographics, drug use history, clinical variables, COVID-19-related characteristics, and conflict and trauma-related events were gathered using yes/no response questionnaires and operationalized in accordance with a number of academic works.

Epidata version 4.2 was used to clean, code, and enter data, which was subsequently exported to SPSS Data was cleaned, coded, and entered using Epidata version 4.2 before being exported to SPSS version 24 for descriptive methods analysis and data summarizing. Logistic regression analysis was used to establish links between mental anguish and related factors. In bivariable logistic regression, variables with a P value of less than two were included in the multivariable logistic regression model. An adjusted odds ratio (AOR) with a 95% confidence interval was used to assess the strength of associations, and a P value of less than 0.05 was considered statistically significant (CI).

3. Results

A total of 795 participants participated in the study, and all of them responded. Men made up the majority of the 412 responders (51.8%). The responders were, on average, 21.98 (2.22) years old. Urban areas produced the bulk of responses (517, or 65.1%) (**Table 1**).

Variables	**Frequency(n)**	**Percent (%)**
Age		
15–19 years old	403	50.6
20–24 years old	238	29.9
≥25 years old	154	19.3
Gender		
Male	412	51.8
Female	383	48.2
Religion		
Orthodox	117	14.7
Protestant	588	73.9
Catholic	74	9.3
Muslim	11	1.4
Other*	5	0.6
Perform less well than anticipated		
Yes	354	44.5
No	441	55.4

Variables	Frequency(n)	Percent (%)
Living area		
Urban	517	65.1
Rural	278	34.9
Living with		
Alone	185	23.3
With single parents	166	20.9
With friends/relatives	67	8.4
With both parents	377	47.4
Financial constraint		
Yes	496	62.4
No	299	37.6
Living in host community		
Yes	431	54.2
No	364	45.8

**others: only Jesus, Jehovah witness.*

Table 1.
Description of socio-demographic factors among people from conflict affected setting in South Ethiopia, 2021 (n = 795).

Regarding the COVID-19-related factors, 93(11.5%) of respondents had a history of possible or proven positive for COVID-19. Out of the total respondents, 17(2.1%) had experienced death in the household and most of the respondents 598(75.2%) had Sufficient familiarity with COVID-19. With regard to clinical characteristics, 122 (15.3%) of the respondents had ever been treated for a known psychiatric illness. Of a total study participants, 150(18.9%) were khat users within 3 months. With respect to psychosocial characteristics of respondents, more than one-third of respondents 306(38.5%) had a poor social assistance (**Table 2**).

Out of the total participants, 461(57%) of participants reported aversion to safety and 358(45%) observe firing house materials around them. Whereas, more than one-third (68%) of participants family's houses were destroyed during conflict (**Table 3**). The prevalence of mental distress among conflict-affected people from conflict-affected settings were determined to be 49.4% in this study, with a 95% confidence interval of (47–52.9%). Multivariate logistic regression revealed significant correlations between respondents' mental distress and sexual assault, house fires when present, female gender, residing in the host community, and living alone, all with a P value of 0.05.

Sexual assault victims were 4.1 times more likely than their peers to experience mental distress (AOR = 4.1, 95% CI 2.37–6.94). When compared to their counterparts, people who had their homes fired upon during hostilities or war had a 3.49 higher risk of developing mental distress (AOR = 3.49, 95% CI 1.61, 5.44). Females were 3.01 times more likely than males to experience mental distress (AOR = 3.01, 95% CI 1.61–5.44). Those living in the host community were 1.8 times more likely to have mental distress (AOR = 1.8, 95%CI 1.97, 3.35), and participants living alone were 3.57 times more likely to have mental distress (AOR = 3.57, 95%CI 2.06, 6.19) (**Table 4**).

Variables	Frequency(n)	Percent (%)
Possible or proven positive for COVID-19		
Yes	93	11.7
No	702	88.3
I read about COVID-19 for the majority of the time		
Yes	128	16.1
No	667	83.9
Known mental illness		
Yes	122	15.3
No	673	84.7
Psychiatric problem in the family		
Yes	92	11.6
No	703	88.4
Health issue that was present before		
Yes	168	21.1
No	627	78.9
COVID death in the household		
Yes	17	2.1
No	778	97.9
Sufficient familiarity with COVID-19		
Yes	598	75.2
No	197	24.8
Received education on COVID-19		
Yes	205	25.8
No	590	74.2
Social assistant		
Low	306	38.5
Medium	352	44.3
High	137	17.2
Alcohol use in the past 3 month		
Yes	39	4.9
No	756	95.1
Khat use in the past 3 month		
Yes	150	18.9
No	645	81.1
Tobacco use in the past 3 month		
Yes	21	2.6
No	774	97.4

Table 2.
Description of COVID related, psychosocial, clinical and behavioral factors of participants from conflict affected setting in South Ethiopia, 2021 (n = 795).

Variables	Percent (%)
Childhood abuse	15
Family tragedy	17
Injury	19
Engaged in the conflict	22
Abducting	25
Split from family	27
Torture	30
Sexual assault	32
Absence of shelter	39
Observe firing house materials	45
Food security	55
Aversion to security	57
Assets devastation	68
Imprisonment	27
Being in war	21
Childhood abuse	39

Table 3.
Trauma and conflict related events from conflict affected setting in South Ethiopia, 2021 (n = 795).

Explanatory variables	Mental distress		COR(95%CI)	AOR(95%CI)
	Yes	No		
Gender				
Male	185	227	1	1
Female	275	108	3.12 [1.84, 4.37]	3.01 [1.61, 5.44]***
Age				
15-19	318	85	3.55 [1.32, 3.99]	2.9 [0.17, 3.4]
20–24	166	72	2.1 [2.18, 4.33]	1.9 [0.89, 3.1]
> = 25	79	75	1	1
Living area				
Urban	329	185	1.58 [1.18, 2.14]	1.41 [0.56, 3.04]
Rural	147	131	1	1
Social support				
Poor	102	204	4.1 [2.49, 6.29]	3.33 [0.95, 5.70]
Moderate	56	296	1.54 [0.87, 2.50]	1.34 [0.76, 2.38]
Strong	15	122	1	1
Health issue that was present before				
Yes	111	57	1.45 [0.95, 2.25]	1.26 [0.76, 2.08]
No	359	268	1	1

Explanatory variables	Mental distress		COR(95%CI)	AOR(95%CI)
	Yes	No		
Sexual assault				
Yes	74	99	3.26 [2.05, 5.04]	4.06 [2.37, 6.94] **
No	116	506	1	1
Sufficient familiarity with COVID-19				
Yes	122	476	0.68 [0.55, 2.64]	1.1 [0.87, 2.19]
No	54	143	1	1
Fired house martials when present				
Yes	292	66	3.69 [2.54, 5.39]	3.49 [2.7, 5.89]**
No	238	199	1	1
Living in host community				
Yes	145	286	2.12 (1.95,4.15)	1.8 [1.97, 3.35]*
No	70	294	1	1
Living with				
Alone	70	114	2.87 (2.03, 5.31)	3.57 [2.06, 6.19] **
With single parents	29	137	0.98 (0.51, 1.86)	1.19 (0.62, 2.26)
With friends/relatives	11	55	0.92 (0.71, 2.19)	1.46 (0.80, 2.68)
With both parents	67	311	1	1

$^{*}p < 0.05$.
$^{**}p < 0.01$.
$^{***}p < 0.001$.

Table 4.
Multivariable logistic regression analysis showing an association between factors and mental distress among people from conflict affected setting in South Ethiopia, 2021 (n = 795).

4. Discussion

The prevalence of mental distress was found to be 49.4% in this study, with a 95% confidence interval of (47–52.9%) among conflict-affected people, according to the findings of this study. The prevalence found in this study resembles that found in Saudi Arabia (58.1%) [9], and Pakistan 57.6% [33]. On the other hand, the results of the present investigation were lower than those of a Pakistani study, which registered 68.4 [34]. The gap may be because of different methodologies utilized in Pakistan to conduct an online cross-sectional survey, which could have produced results that were more subjective and biased than those acquired through the in-person interviews used in this study. Financial, cultural, or environmental disparities could also have a role. Nevertheless, the prevalence found in this study was higher than that seen in earlier studies conducted in Canada 39.5% [35, 36], Malaysia 30.7% [34], China 27% [37], Croatia 19.4% [38], and Ethiopia 21.2% [6] 51.3% of the students at Addis Ababa were from Ethiopia [9], followed by Gondar 46.3% [39], 47% from students in Europe [40], and Pakistan 48% [41]. This study was conducted in a conflict-affected environment during the COVID-19 era, however, specific participants from conflict-affected environments were not included in the earlier investigations. Each country may have a distinct level of understanding and perception of COVID-19, which measures people's capacity to cope with stress.

Participants who experienced firing house materials when present were 3.49 times more likely than those who did not experience firing household materials during the conflict/war to experience emotional distress. People, like other creatures, become anxious or terrified when exposed to or seeing a terrible scenario. The possible reason might be, the participants feel that those types of losses will be difficult, if not impossible, to replace, resulting in increased psychological distress. Also following a traumatic event like the destruction of personal property, acute stress is a typical response, if this problem persists may become a risk to develop PTSD. This finding is supported by a study done in northwestern Nigeria [42–44].

Being a female was found to be one of the strongest predictors of mental distress. Mental distress was three times more common in females than in males. According to the report, girls suffer more harm than boys because they are more likely to experience sexual assault on school property or because their parents keep them at home when the security situation deteriorates. According to research, girls usually quit school after it is full, and their educational outcomes in countries afflicted by violence are frequently worse than boys'. One of the reasons is a fear of sexual assault in the classroom [45]. During times of war, gender inequality is entrenched and women are disproportionately disadvantaged in terms of personal safety, resource access, and human rights. Girls who live in a nation that is experiencing conflict are about 2.5 times more likely to be out of school, and adolescent girls are almost 90% more likely to have dropped out of secondary school [46]. This collectively worsens people's mental health in a situation of conflict.

When compared to their counterparts, those who were living alone were 3.57 times more likely to have mental distress. These findings are in line with the studies done in Arbaminch town, Ethiopia, in Harar, and southeast Nigeria [47–50]. The answer could be that parents are more concerned about their daughters than their friends and relatives, which can reduce the likelihood of sexual abuse which in turn influences the mental health of thechildren who live with them in conflict areas during the era of COVID-19.

The odds of having mental distress among participants living in a host community due to internal displacement were 1.8 times higher as compared to their counterpart. Sexual abuse followed by mental distress in the past year and throughout the course of one's lifetime is strongly correlated with displacement. Those who have experienced displacement and living in a host community are 9–10% more likely to experience sexual violencewhich negatively influences their mental health at some point in their lives and 6–8% more likely to experience past years sexual violence [51–53].

When compared to counterparts, those who had sexual assault were 4.1 times more likely to have mental distress. The disparity could explain the observed disparities in tool, socioeconomic, environmental, and study design (in Croatia, for example, an 8-wave longitudinal study was used). In addition to the prevalence of wartime rape and sexual violence committed by people outside the home, rates of intimate partner violence are significantly higher in conflict settings [54]. For survivors of sexual and other gender-based violence, there can be a number of detrimental effects, including social ramifications and poor health [55]. A study found a considerable frequency of psychological distress and other mental issues among survivors of sexual and gender-based violence in areas of armed conflict. Anxiety disorders (including Posttraumatic

Stress Disorder (PTSD), major depressive disorder, medically unexplained problems, substance use disorders, and suicidal ideation are among the mental disorders reported [56].

5. Conclusion

High rate of mental distress was found from conflict affected setting. Being female, fired house materials when present, sexual assault, living host community, and living alone were all significant indicators of mental distress. As a result, the ministry of health and humanitarian organizations should collaborate to provide persons living in conflict-affected areas with constant psychosocial assistance and appropriate intervention. To reducethe double burden of COVID-19 and conflict on mental health, special attention is needed.

6. The Study's strengths and limitations

First, this is the first research of its kind in Ethiopia, involving peoples from conflict-affected areas. Second, it included key variables that had previously been overlooked in previous research. One of the study's strengths was that it measured the outcome variable with an updated standardized and validated instrument. Only students from conflict-affected parts of south Ethiopia were included, which was one of the disadvantages.

Ethical approval

All data collection methodologies, as well as the Helsinki Declaration, received ethical approval from Dilla University's college of health science and medicine's ethical review board under the number DU/225/7/111. Following a brief description of the study's purpose, we obtained written informed consent from those aged 18 and up, as well as assent (parental informed consent) from those under 18. The information was kept completely confidential.

Acknowledgements

The author of this chapter would like to express his gratitude to all of the university administration's personnel. Dilla University's Department of Psychiatry, College of Health and Medicine, merits our gratitude. Finally, I want to express my gratitude to all of the participants for their cooperation and assistance in gathering the essential information.

Author's contribution

The author participated in the article's drafting, revision, or critical review, gave final approval of the version that would be published, agreed on the journal to which the article would be submitted, and agreed to take responsibility for all aspects of the project. The author made a significant contribution to the work reported, whether it was in the conception, study design, execution, data acquisition, analysis, and interpretation, or all of these areas.

Funding

Non applicable.

Statement on data sharing

On reasonable request, the corresponding author made the data for this study available.

Author details

Derebe Madoro
Department of Psychiatry, College of Medicine and Health Science, Dilla University, Dilla, Ethiopia

*Address all correspondence to: derebemd@gmail.com

References

[1] Hezam IM. COVID-19 global humanitarian response plan: An optimal distribution model for high-priority countries. ISA Transactions. 2021;**124**:1-20

[2] Megersa K. COVID-19 in Eastern Africa: Impact Analysis on Conflict and Security.K4D Helpdesk Report 847. Brighton, UK: Institute of Development Studies; 2020

[3] Yusuf S. COVID-19 and Political Stability in Ethiopia. Ethiopia: Institute of Peace and Security Studies, Addis Ababa University; 2020

[4] Østebø MT, Østebø T, Tronvoll K. Health and politics in pandemic times: COVID-19 responses in Ethiopia. Health Policy and Planning. 2021;**36**(10):1681-1689

[5] Charlson F, van Ommeren M, Flaxman A, Cornett J, Whiteford H, Saxena S. New WHO prevalence estimates of mental disorders in conflict settings: A systematic review and meta-analysis. The Lancet. 2019;**394**(10194):240-248

[6] Aylie NS, Mekonen MA, Mekuria RM. The psychological impacts of COVID-19 pandemic among university students in bench-Sheko zone, south-West Ethiopia: A community-based cross-sectional study. Psychology Research and Behavior Management. 2020;**13**:813

[7] Tadesse W, Mihret S, Biset G, Muluneh A. Psychological impacts of COVID-19 among college students in Dessie town, Amhara region, Ethiopia; cross-sectional study. Research Square. 30 Jun 2020. DOI: 10.21203/rs.3.rs-38100/v1 PPR: PPR181928

[8] Mekonen EG, Workneh BS, Ali MS, Muluneh NY. The psychological impact of COVID-19 pandemic on graduating class students at the University of Gondar, Northwest Ethiopia. Psychology Research and Behavior Management. 2021;**14**:109

[9] Simegn W, Dagnew B, Yeshaw Y, Yitayih S, Woldegerima B, Dagne H. Depression, anxiety, stress and their associated factors among Ethiopian university students during an early stage of COVID-19 pandemic: An online-based cross-sectional survey. PLoS One. 2021;**16**(5):e0251670

[10] Sahile AT, Ababu M, Alemayehu S, Abebe H, Endazenew G, Wubshet M, et al. Prevalence and severity of depression, anxiety, and stress during pandemic of COVID-19 among college students in Addis Ababa, Ethiopia, 2020: A cross sectional survey. International Journal of Clinical Experimental Medical Sciences. 2020;**6**(6):126

[11] UNICEF. Children UNOotSRotS-Gf, Conflict a: Machel Study 10-Year Strategic Review: Children and Conflict in a Changing World. New York, USA: UNICEF; 2009

[12] Slone M, Mann S. Effects of war, terrorism and armed conflict on young children: A systematic review. Child Psychiatry & Human Development. 2016;**47**(6):950-965

[13] Miller KE, Rasmussen A. War exposure, daily stressors, and mental health in conflict and post-conflict settings: Bridging the divide between trauma-focused and psychosocial frameworks. Social Science & Medicine. 2010;**70**(1):7-16

[14] Lee C, Nguyen AJ, Russell T, Aules Y, Bolton P. Mental health and psychosocial

problems among conflict-affected children in Kachin State, Myanmar: A qualitative study. Conflict and Health. 2018;**12**(1):1-11

[15] Murthy RS, Lakshminarayana R. Mental health consequences of war: A brief review of research findings. World Psychiatry. 2006;**5**(1):25

[16] Hasanović M. Psychological consequences of war-traumatized children and adolescents in Bosnia and Herzegovina. Acta Medica Academica. 2011;**40**(1):45-66

[17] Roberts B, Ezard N. Why are we not doing more for alcohol use disorder among conflict-affected populations. Addiction. 2015;**110**(6):889-890

[18] Akinyemi OO, Owoaje ET, Ige OK, Popoola OA. Comparative study of mental health and quality of life in long term refugees and host populations in Oru-Ijebu, Southwest Nigeria. BMC Research Notes. 2012;**5**(1):1-9

[19] Priebe S, Gavrilovic J, Bremner S, Ajdukovic D, Franciskovic T, Neri G, et al. Course of post-traumatic stress disorder following war in the Balkans: 1-year follow-up study. Psychological Medicine. 2013;**43**(9):1837-1847

[20] Kazmi SSH, Hasan DK, Talib S, Saxena S: COVID-19 and lockdwon: A study on the impact on mental health. 15 Apr 2020. Available at SSRN: https://ssrn.com/abstract=3577515

[21] Farhood L, Dimassi H. Symptom Prevalence of PTSD, Anxiety, Depression, Effect of Exposure and Mediating Factors on a Population from Southern Lebanon. LEBANON: AMERICAN UNIV BEIRUT; 2006

[22] Browne G, Hemsley M. Consumer participation in mental health in Australia: What progress is being made? Australasian Psychiatry. 2008;**16**(6):446-449

[23] Hobfoll SE, Canetti-Nisim D, Johnson RJ, Palmieri PA, Varley JD, Galea S. The association of exposure, risk, and resiliency factors with PTSD among Jews and Arabs exposed to repeated acts of terrorism in Israel. Journal of Traumatic Stress. 2008;**21**(1):9-21

[24] Fortes S, Lopes C, LAB V, Campos MR, Gonçalves DA, Mari JJ. Common mental disorders in Petrópolis-RJ: A challenge to integrate mental health into primary care strategies. Revista Brasileira de Psiquiatria. 2011;**33**(2):150-156

[25] Steel Z, Chey T, Silove D, Marnane C, Bryant RA, Van Ommeren M. Association of torture and other potentially traumatic events with mental health outcomes among populations exposed to mass conflict and displacement: A systematic review and meta-analysis. JAMA. 2009;**302**(5):537-549

[26] Seidi PA, Ardebil MD, Jaff D. COVID-19 pandemic: New challenge to securing mental well-being in conflict settings. Asian Journal of Psychiatry. 2020;**51**:102151

[27] Yigzaw GS, Abitew EB. Causes and impacts of internal displacement in Ethiopia. African Journal of Social Work. 2019;**9**(2):32-41

[28] Dessie Y, Ebrahim J, Awoke T. Mental distress among university students in Ethiopia: A cross sectional survey. Pan African Medical Journal. 2013;**15**(1):95

[29] Andersen L, Grimsrud A, Myer L, Williams D, Stein D, Seedat S. The psychometric properties of the K10 and K6 scales in screening for mood and

anxiety disorders in the south African stress and health study. International Journal of Methods in Psychiatric Research. 2011;**20**(4):215-223

[30] Kessler RC, Andrews G, Colpe LJ, Hiripi E, Mroczek DK, Normand S-L, et al. Short screening scales to monitor population prevalences and trends in non-specific psychological distress. Psychological Medicine. 2002;**32**(6):959-976

[31] Tesfaye M, Hanlon C, Wondimagegn D, Alem A. Detecting postnatal common mental disorders in Addis Ababa, Ethiopia: Validation of the Edinburgh postnatal depression scale and Kessler scales. Journal of Affective Disorders. 2010;**122**(1-2):102-108

[32] Abiola T, Udofia O, Zakari M. Psychometric properties of the 3-item Oslo social support scale among clinical students of Bayero university Kano, Nigeria. Malaysian Journal of Psychiatry. 2013;**22**(2):32-41

[33] Kumar B, Shah MAA, Kumari R, Kumar A, Kumar J, Tahir A. Depression, anxiety, and stress among final-year medical students. Cureus. 2019;**11**(3):e4257

[34] Okafor N. Socio-Demographic Characteristics and Other Factors Associated with Depressive Illness among Medical Students at. Nigeria: The University of Port Harcourt; 2020

[35] Othman N, Ahmad F, El Morr C, Ritvo P. Perceived impact of contextual determinants on depression, anxiety and stress: A survey with university students. International Journal of Mental Health Systems. 2019;**13**(1):1-9

[36] Hamaideh SH. Alexithymia among Jordanian university students: Its prevalence and correlates with depression, anxiety, stress, and demographics. Perspectives in Psychiatric Care. 2017;**54**(2):274-280

[37] Li Y, Wang Y, Jiang J, Valdimarsdóttir UA, Fall K, Fang F, et al. Psychological distress among health professional students during the COVID-19 outbreak. Psychological Medicine. 2020;**51**:1-3

[38] Vulić-Prtorić A et al. "The psychological distress in students during the COVID-19 crisis: An 8-wave longitudinal study." PsyArXiv, 29 Aug 2020

[39] Akalu TY, Gelaye KA, Bishaw MA, Tilahun SY, Yeshaw Y, Azale T, et al. Depression, anxiety, and stress symptoms and its associated factors among residents of Gondar town during the early stage of COVID-19 pandemic. Risk Management and Healthcare Policy. 2021;**14**:1073

[40] Habihirwe P, Porovecchio S, Bramboiu I, Ciobanu E, Croituru C, Cazacu I, et al. Depression, anxiety and stress among college students in three European countries. European Journal of Public Health. 2018;**28**(suppl_4) cky214:26

[41] Syed A, Ali SS, Khan M. Frequency of depression, anxiety and stress among the undergraduate physiotherapy students. Pakistan journal of medical sciences. 2018;**34**(2):468

[42] Paolini A. School shootings and student mental health: Role of the school counselor in mitigating violence. Vistas Online. 2015;**90**:1-15

[43] Metzl JM, MacLeish KT. American Journal of Public Health. 2015;**105**(2):240-249

[44] Sheikh TL, Mohammed A, Agunbiade S, Ike J, Ebiti WN, Adekeye O.

Psycho-trauma, psychosocial adjustment, and symptomatic post-traumatic stress disorder among internally displaced persons in Kaduna, northwestern Nigeria. Frontiers in Psychiatry. 2014;**5**:127

[45] Ferris E, Winthrop R. Education and Displacement: Assessing Conditions for Refugees and Internally Displaced Persons Affected by Conflict. Background paper for the EFA Global Monitoring Report 2011. Paris: The hidden crisis: Armed Conflict and Education; 2010

[46] Ossiannilsson E. Challenges and opportunities for active and hybrid learning related to UNESCO post 2015. In: Handbook of Research on Active Learning and the Flipped Classroom Model in the Digital Age. Hershey, Pennsylvania: IGI Global; 2016. pp. 333-351

[47] Chinawa JM, Aronu A, Chukwu B, Obu H. Prevalence and pattern of child abuse and associated factors in four secondary institutions in Enugu, Southeast Nigeria. European Journal of Pediatrics. 2014;**173**(4):451-456

[48] Markos J, Semahegn A, Berhanu B. Assessment of sexual violence and associated factors among high school students in Harari regional state, Harar town. East Ethiopian Science Research. 2014;**2**(5):91-97

[49] Mekuria A, Nigussie A, Abera M. Childhood sexual abuse experiences and its associated factors among adolescent female high school students in Arbaminch town, Gammo Goffa zone, southern Ethiopia: A mixed method study. BMC International Health and Human Rights. 2015;**15**(1):1-9

[50] Abera L, Aliye A, Tadesse K, Guta A. Magnitude of child sexual abuse and its associated factors among high school female students in Dire Dawa, eastern Ethiopia: A cross-sectional study. Reproductive Health. 2021;**18**(1):1-12

[51] Kelly JTD, Holmes M, Gibbons N, Matabaro A, Voors M. Conflict, Displacement and Overlapping Vulnerabilities : Understanding Risk Factors for Gender-Based Violence among Displaced Women in Eastern Democratic Republic of Congo. Policy Research Working Paper; No. 9819. Washington, DC: World Bank; 2021. Available from: https://openknowledge.worldbank.org/handle/10986/36470 License: CC BY 3.0 IGO

[52] Akinsulure-Smith AM. Displaced African female survivors of conflict-related sexual violence: Challenges for mental health providers. Violence Against Women. 2014;**20**(6):677-694

[53] Stark L, Landis D. Violence against children in humanitarian settings: A literature review of population-based approaches. Social Science & Medicine. 2016;**152**:125-137

[54] Kelly JT, Betancourt TS, Mukwege D, Lipton R, Vanrooyen MJ. Experiences of female survivors of sexual violence in eastern Democratic Republic of the Congo: A mixed-methods study. Conflict and Health. 2011;**5**(1):1-8

[55] Sherrer MV. The role of cognitive appraisal in adaptation to traumatic stress in adults with serious mental illness: A critical review. Trauma, Violence, & Abuse. 2011;**12**(3):151-167

[56] Johnson K, Asher J, Rosborough S, Raja A, Panjabi R, Beadling C, et al. Association of combatant status and sexual violence with health and mental health outcomes in postconflict Liberia. JAMA. 2008;**300**(6):676-690

Chapter 18

Perspective Chapter: Decompression as a Safety Valve during Pandemic

Samir Rawat, Abhijit P. Deshpande, Ole Boe, Andrzej Piotrowski and Priya Joshi

Abstract

Under circumstances such as the COVID-19 pandemic, decompression is essential to slowly overcome the lockdown stressors as a transition period between lockdown and resuming work in a manner that is no longer going to be 'business as usual'. Firstly, we examine what is decompression in the context of reducing overwhelming and unwanted pressure emanating from the pandemic. Secondly, we reiterate the objectives and goals of decompression. Thirdly, we list ways in which one can decompress as a suitable way of endowing us with better psychological and much needed emotional support in pandemic times. Finally, the chapter offers guidelines for future research as this aspect has not been researched much and opens up new avenues in the field of psychosocial research in civilian as well as military contexts which brings the need for psychological debriefing to the forefront. The results of psychological disaster research to foresee, reduce and soothe the psychological effects of mass disasters – in this case, the global COVID-19 pandemic, maybe reconstructive.

Keywords: decompression, post-traumatic growth, pandemic, reconstruction, third-location decompression

1. Introduction

"Decompression fosters a means of progressively adjusting to a new normal, by allowing us to take a step back and reflect on the recent past before we leap ahead into unchartered waters of the future." - Lt Col Dr Samir Rawat

Life is tough at Siachen glacier, in the Himalayas, India, the highest altitude battle zone in the world. A vast land spread over approximately 75 km, the glacier is deadly, because of sub-zero temperatures, frequent avalanches, high-altitude weather uncertainties, crevasses which go unnoticed, almost unimaginable and scary conditions for even soldiers to be. Soldiers deployed at the glacier typically spend three to four months in extreme conditions, highly vulnerable to fatal high altitude ailments like frost bites, chill blains and hypothermia. When soldiers return from active service in operational zones, they may find it difficult to immediately adapt to what seems to be a new reality now, they need some 'time-off' to adjust and acclimatize to out-of-operations

IntechOpen

conditions. Military psychologists [1], recommend a period of decompression- a release from compression, for soldiers returning from operational duties.

Given the adversity, the globe experienced in 2020, a global crisis of COVID-19 which ravaged the world order, destroyed poor and developed economies alike, exerted immense pressure on the mental health of people across the globe and pushed a whole civilization into nothing less than a warlike zone. The battle was with an unknown enemy- a virus that caught nations, societies and communities off-guard and thrust them into battle of survival. Traditional systems of social support, interpersonal relationships, easy access to resources became, which served as buffer to problems earlier, were challenged with most nations calling for lockdowns and social distancing as immediate strategies to curb the spread of the virus. This period has resulted in people losing control over their actions and emotions because of the suddenness and magnitude of change that the pandemic has brought in. Now, though the battle against the virus is far from over, we must move forward to normalcy, roll up our sleeves and put together strategies to bounce back- be adaptively resilient. Nearly a year long lockdown has exhausted our mental capacities, has been additionally difficult due to multiple roles that some of us are expected to take on, has changed how we approach life in general. For economies, global markets and multi-national organization, it has been a tough time and getting back to relative state of normalcy is a task that requires planning and organisation. Just as soldiers, when returning from the operational duties are allowed a period of decompression, a populace that has been wrecked by the pandemic be allowed a period of decompression.

2. Definitions

Emotional decompression: **Consists of working on emotions, paying attention to mental schemas,** and releasing what's not useful to you, leaving space for well-being to enter.

De-acclimatise: The process of training the soldiers to be prepared for the volatility, vigilant, intense, sometimes dramatic nature of the battlefield and that soldiers unlearn some of the approaches to resilience and vigilance required during wartime and adapt to new realities and approaches for non-combat functioning.

Psychological debriefing: An intervention immediately following a traumatic event (e.g., a disaster) that aims to mitigate long-term distress and prevent the emergence of posttraumatic stress disorder in those exposed to the event.

Post-traumatic growth: A concept describing positive psychological change experienced as a result of struggling with highly challenging, highly stressful life circumstances.

9-R model of decompression: A nine-component model of decompression aiming to be a start point for future research and development into strengthening the understanding of how to manage the effects of combat and war fatigue.

3. Decompression: an ally in reconstruction

In this article, we will introduce to the readers the concept of *decompression*, its relevance in the pandemic times especially in managing post-traumatic stress and other psychological issues which come part and parcel with the pandemic. Borrowing from their own experiences in the highly-dramatic theatre of war, and the potential benefits of decompression, will guide us in how this can be used as a strategic approach as we move toward post-pandemic reorganization. The authors propose the '*9-R Model of Decompression*' [1], which provides insight into decompression aims to reduce the unsolicited pressures emanating from the pandemic, how decompression can result in better psychological well-being; backed with empirical data. Lastly, in concluding remarks, the authors throw light on the direction for further psychosocial research in the military and non-military contexts.

A conceptual understanding of psychological decompression finds most mention in military literature; it refers to a process that allows soldiers returning from theatre of military operations and duties in war zones, to adapt to the home environment gradually, in a systematic manner with the aim to reduce the potential for maladaptive psychological well-being [2, 3]. Decompression is viewed as a period of transition between high-stress operational environment and home environment perceived to be relatively less stressful [3]. This organised period of transition is also known as third location decompression or TLD [4].

Psychological health issues experienced by soldiers returning from combat zone are well researched and documented. Highly volatile, ambiguous environments that theatre of operations are, exert mental pressure and stress on soldiers in spite of being trained in the use of arms and technological advances of militaries. Whether returning home victorious or mere deployment under volatile uncertain conditions or even peace-keeping operations, some amount of stress is innate and places them at higher risks for post-traumatic stress disorder, depression, alcohol or drugs abuse, and other co-morbidity conditions [5–10]. Thus, with high vulnerability to post-traumatic stress disorders and related adjustment issues it seems reasonable that there is a period of relative adjustment to reduce the risks of full-scale disorders.

A period of psychological decompression with a focus on rest, cognitive and emotional reappraisal may a-part solution for soldiers after deployment along with psycho-educational interventions. In one of the studies [11], it was found that soldiers returning from war who got little time to decompress between off-operational duties and enrollment into inherently stressful academic environments, showed higher levels of academic stress than soldiers who got plenty or enough time to 'get back to the center'. Shea [11] noted that soldiers who did not get time to adjust to roles like that of a parent, husband, kin in their families, if were put through additional pressures of academic stress, would experience stress the most and not perform as per expectations. In another study, [though not documented as an empirical study] of how decompression got charted into after-deployment or homecoming programs for militaries across the globe, is after the Falklands War in 1982, British military personnel reached back home by either of two ways—entirely by sea, meant an additional week to return home or they ferried their journey by sea and air. Press reports of the time suggested that the soldiers who travelled by sea route, and spent more time between the war and homecoming had better psychological health than those who made the trip in a shorter time [12].

3.1 Value of decompression

While engaging with the enemy on the ground, in the skies or even at sea are challenging environments, where military personnel go through immense psychological and mental changes, what could be as challenging, is to transition to environments that place different needs on their mental and psychological resources- like playing different roles, being available for their families, adjusting to non-combat environment. To successfully tread, they must bring about physical and psychological changes [13]. A line of thought also suggests that personnel returning from operational environments may in fact be happy about being home right after, however, at the cost of signs of mental health symptoms getting masked [14].

Though there is perhaps no absolute consensus on definitions of decompression and what comprises decompression programs, there is a general understanding that this period consists of rest, and restoration and should have psychologists or trained mental health professionals conduct psychological debriefing. There is a general belief that decompression should be closer or in close proximity to the unit or teams that were together in the operational tasks. We will discuss some of the aims of decompression in this section, namely, providing opportunity for emotional settling, a safe place to de-acclimatise, and an opportunity for structured debriefing to release tension.

1. Emotional decompression: combat or operational environments are marked by exposure to deprivation from resources, isolation and oftentimes, no communication with families for long spells, exposure to war atrocities that may result in acute or chronic psychosocial issues irrespective of the consequences of the operations [5, 15, 16]. The guilt of surviving when their colleagues suffered injuries or lay dead on the battlefield, anxiety about being away from the high-tension, sorrow could be some of the general emotional reactions. Some of these may go unnoticed or un-reported during or after deployment mainly because of the notions of military being a profession where emotions are not exhibited openly [17]. Similarly, emotions resulting from fear of being killed or due to degree of sustained injury [18] could also place individuals at higher risks of developing post-traumatic stress disorder or other adjustment issues [like substance abuse, depression, insomnia, cognitive overload, etc.]. Negative emotions are known to be detrimental to motivation, performance and sense of achievement not just in military but also in non-military environments [19, 20]. Thus, it becomes imperative that the negative emotions are acknowledged and strategies to manage these negative emotions such that these do not interfere with wellbeing, or spillover/displace to other areas of one's functioning are made available. Third-location decompression is likely to provide with such much needed opportunities.

2. De-acclimatise: APA defines acclimatisation as adjustment or adaptation to new circumstances or environmental conditions, particularly the physiological changes that improve an individual's ability to tolerate environmental alterations [21]. Extending on the element of adjustment or adaptation, we propose that decompression allows for de-acclimatization, which is to suggest that as the military or operational training trains the soldiers to be prepared for the volatility, vigilant, intense, sometimes dramatic nature of the battlefield; it is also, imperative that when the battle is over, soldiers unlearn some of the approaches to resilience and vigilance required during wartime and adapt to new realities and approaches for non-combat functioning.

3. Psychological debriefing: Research in the area of trauma and stress suggest that psychological debriefing has positive therapeutic effects for people with exposure to trauma and volatile conditions [22–25]. Bartone and Adler [26] define debriefing [event-oriented after action debriefing] as a factual review of events, and reaction to events by the individual involved or the group/unit engaging in the events. In their classic research paper, they indicate the goals of debriefing to

be—identification of lessons learned during operations which can direct actions in the future, resolve any misconceptions there could be, help soldiers paraphrase their battle experience positively, reduce sense of isolation and also make soldiers better aware of possible psychological symptoms resulting from stressful battle conditions.

Similar directions for the use or structure of debriefing are found in the work of Everly and Mitchell [2], who coined the term 'critical incident stress debriefing'. According to CISD model [2], debriefing promotes emotional wellbeing by allowing opportunities for dialog to the soldier, where they can vent and work on their emotions, perceptions and appraisals of the critical events in the theatre of war. However, it is important to acknowledge that such expression of emotions can be overwhelming to soldiers, perhaps risking them to relive the events. Thus, the aim of psychological debriefing should be established and affirmed by psychologists and team leaders [or those who are close to the trauma context] before use to prevent this technique from being detrimental [27]. Post-mission debriefing sessions typically involve talking about critical or traumatic incidents during tour of duty [4]. While psychological debriefing may be seen as a viable technique for emergency responders, caregivers especially in the COVID times, the authors recommend the use of debriefing under strict vigilance and with caution, simply because pandemic has resulted in limited or depleted resources and the technique could in fact prove to be detrimental if missed shot. Debriefing could perhaps well be replaced with more effective techniques like cognitive therapy, mindfulness training [28, 29].

4. Fostering post-traumatic growth attitude: Decompression period can also be looked as a window of opportunity to foster growth-attitude among soldiers. Post-traumatic growth defined as positive and meaningful psychological change that an individual can experience after they have experienced a traumatic incident or event and are coping from it [30]. Though events like wars, or even calamities get associated with negative consequences, and changed worldviews, some may see these as opportunities to review their perceptions of world view before and after the events, restructure their thoughts and emotions and direct their action in order to grow, revitalize their self-concepts and relationships with others, from having experienced the events [31]. Thus, post-traumatic growth is essentially moving away from the baseline and toward growth in refurbishing the worldview, sense of control over what the future holds [31]. Research suggests that post-traumatic growth thoughts and attitudes are inversely related to post-traumatic stress symptoms [32, 33]. Decompression thus can be an important period when psychologists or professionals or team leaders can facilitate development of post-traumatic growth attitudes and cognitions. Post-traumatic growth perspective could prove useful in the post-COVID times with the virus having caused loss of enthusiasm and change in worldview with prolonged experiences of isolation, social distancing and uncertainty. For example, recent studies suggest emotional creativity, may result in post-traumatic growth attitude, thereby reduces the chances of full-blown post-traumatic stress disorder [34].

COVID-19 pandemic has brought about tectonic changes beyond the realm of imagination of most of societies, even for those who have experienced WW II, which so far was thought to be the most ravaging event of the century. Other epidemics [like SARS, plague, Ebola] and calamities have not had the magnitude of impact and consequences that COVID-19 has caused. Thus, it becomes essential that the available knowledge of the past from crisis management experiences be remodeled, reinvented and re-adapted to suit what may fit the bill for reconstruction post-COVID crisis.

3.2 Psychological consequences of covid-19 pandemic

Why a discussion on decompression becomes important lies in the spectrum of psychological, social and interpersonal impact COVID-19 virus has brought about. COVID-19 presents before us the most-multifaceted crisis the human race has seen, a battle where the enemy is unknown and unseen. No amount of intelligence and force mobilization can fully avert the mayhem that the virus resulted in. With some common knowledge or best described as available knowledge of how spread of the virus can be curtailed, governments across the world imposed lockdown of economies, restrictions on movement, curb of social and interpersonal interactions and what seemed to be business as usual was no longer the same. Medically, the rapid infection and contagion resulted in strained medical systems. Economically, it meant businesses were thrown into fiscal deficits and societies were propelled into threats of destabilisation and loss of normalcy. Beyond the socio-economic disaster that the pandemic has been, psychological impact has been beyond comprehension and indisputable [35, 36]. Research suggests that fear of the pandemic and its uncertain nature could be a precursor to stress disorders, anxiety and other related problems, depression and even substance abuse [37]. With businesses being affected, it has resulted in people losing their source of livelihood and thereby adds to the stress of managing families. These could have potentially triggered related problems of substance abuse and panic disorders [38]. For emergency responders, this has been a period of turmoil, both professionally and personally. Long working hours, limited resources, worries about those affected, fear of being infected, inadequate access to basic resources, not being allowed to meet own families, being continuously in the line of action, suddenly being forced into harm's way has all resulted in psychological distress [39].

A general environment of despair and loss of hope has resulted from the experience of loss of loved ones or witnessing death in close proximity or sense of being lost. Being home bound or quarantined has resulted in sense of loneliness and isolation and curtailed scope of human-to-human interaction or social support. Measures put in place as first reaction to curb spread of virus like lockdown and social distancing are likely to result in far-reaching psychological problems which may keep brewing on the inside and erode the very fabric of human civilisation more than the damage caused by the virus itself. Thus, it has been nothing short of a psychological warfare.

Yet, in all this, it is important to acknowledge that survival instinct is innate in the human race and while the pandemic might have bogged down the spirit, the ability to bounce back higher and with far greater strength also are innate. Further to the discussion on post-traumatic growth, the application of the same may be exemplified in times to come. New learning gathered from the pandemic can be put to use to develop habits and systems which are resilient as well wean off behaviors (like addictions, behaviors detrimental to general hygiene, burnout at work, pollution, etc.) which are detrimental in survival of the species.

4. 9-R model of decompression for war-at-hand

Most of decompression programs, as they exist in military organisations, agree on some of the core fundamentals like—belief that soldiers need some time-off after high-tension deployment, having collective decompression opportunities for those who experience challenging operations, providing for individual and group unwinding–rewinding sessions and focus of relaxation and rest. The aim of decompression programs is to restore and regain resilience in soldiers, authors of this article seek to provide and facilitate movement of societies, communities and organisations toward post-pandemic resilience and remodeling of mental capacities. The authors of this article, from their own experience of serving in the high-emotions theatre of war, volatile and uncertain battle grounds, as well as detailed research and empirical data (both internet data and personal communication) propose a nine-component model or 9-R model of decompression, see **Figure 1**. Authors also state firmly that an individual's willingness and urge to change the status quo, resources available, learn new coping and adapt with resilience lie at the centre or core of any effective program.

1. Rest: Rest which can be understood as ceasing of any movement or activities in order to recover strength, especially after stressful event. Rest is a vital for better mental and physical health and people recovering from strains and illnesses are advised to observe period of rest to reinstate health and wellbeing [40–42]. Human downtime, is important not just for survival, but also for creativity and innovation. A period of rest could help individuals to break the chain of negative thoughts and habits they may have developed during the pandemic and develop new ways to move into new reality with a sense of growth and resilience [43].

2. Relaxation: relaxation defined as an emotional state of low tension, marked by absence of arousal [resulting from anger, fear, anxiety] is much researched and approved technique in stress management [44, 45]. Relaxation if practised consciously or mindfully is likely to result in reduction of physical and psychological stress. Empirical data suggest that relaxation- physical and mindful mental relaxation results in lowered anxiety levels during pandemic [36]. Relaxation can have benefits like normalizing heart rate, better sleep, lower fatigue, reduce muscle tension, most of which could be the result of heightened levels of anxiety for soldiers after deployment in warzone or COVID warriors with changes in their life circumstances.

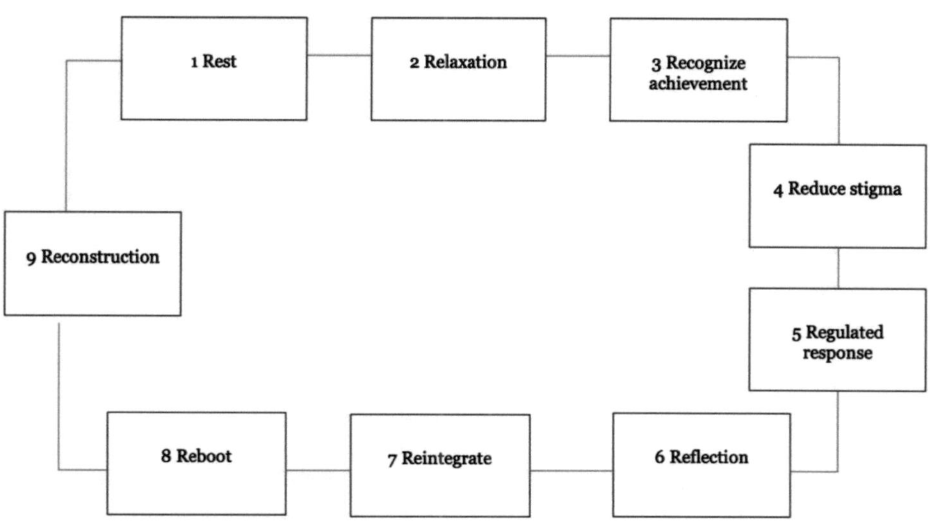

Figure 1.
9-R model of decompression.

3. Recognize achievement: Recognize one's own and other's achievement: In times like the pandemic or even battles, sense of self-worth and self-concepts may go through a sort of shift because the outcomes, personal loss, depletion of resources, and isolation. Dolan and Sanchez [46] suggest that in such times, being overly critical of oneself or others may be detrimental. A soldier who may have lost some of his fellow colleagues in the battle could already be struggling with guilt of survival or loss of a dear family member, may result in self-doubt of the caregiver. In such times, appreciation of their effort, could help in reinstating their belief in self-worth.

4. Reduce stigma: Stigma as defined by Goffman [47] is an attribute, of discrediting, reducing a person from a whole and usual person to a tainted, discounted one. By and large, intense situations like fighting a war or being involved in high-tension situations may be associated with a sense of bravado, valour and grit, there are certain inherent expectations especially and traditionally of how soldiers need to be—not come across as ones exhibiting emotions, being a team player. While most of these expectations may be occupational requirement, any deviation in following the same may have stigma attached to it. Decompression should be viewed as a period when such soldiers are provided with assistance to overcome fear of being stereotyped and steer clear any such detrimental thoughts they may have. In 2020, when most of the nations experienced the wrath of the virus, emergency first responders like medical professionals, doctors, police, pharmacos were the first to respond, which also placed them at a higher risk of infection and the risk of infection may get associated with stigma [48]. For instance, since the epicenter of the virus was located in one of the Asian countries, there were cases of discrimination being reported against foreigners of Asian origin [49, 50]. The debilitating effects of stigma place patient or affected groups of people at risk of being discriminated and isolated and thus lead to more psychological concerns. Now that societies take time to reflect before plunging into the future, measures should be taken to reduce the stigma and make available psychological assistance for people who could be at higher risks or being discriminated.

5. Regulated response: the pandemic has posed unique and unexpected challenges and health risks that place additional pressure on our coping resources. Collective restraint and control will enable our ability to curb the spread of the infection. The self-regulatory approach includes cognitive and emotional skills that allow us to intentionally control thoughts, emotions, and behavior [51]. A soldier's ability to regulate during operations and even peace-keeping operations [which partly comes from military training], is critical to in sustaining military prudence and conforming to military norms and standards [52]. Decompression could be viewed as a period to strengthen self-regulatory habits such that soldiers restrain or control any spillover of negativity or other emotions like performance anxiety, extreme caution from highly charged combat environments into relatively docile family, interpersonal and social environments. Just like how soldiers are expected to observe restraint in their reactions, emotions, the pandemic has placed a demand on the civilian societies to control and manage their actions- like restrained movement, measures of hygiene, controlling substance abuse, etc. When working professionals return to workplace, it could be required of them to continue to observe limited interactions with

their colleagues and also follow protocols such that they do not place themselves or others in the harm's way.

6. Reflection: self-reflection is defined as an ability to willingly learn more about one's fundamental purpose and to willingly exercise introspection [53]. As the world witnesses, almost a full range of change for example reorganization of lifestyle during and after the pandemic an ability to reflect on one's thoughts, feelings and actions would be imperative [54]. During the decompression phase, reflection can help, steer clarity about the perceptions of the situation and how one approaches the change process. Reflection could be effective especially after a critical incident when certain milestones have been achieved or when one is trying to make sense of available information. A simple reflection of which habits [like social distancing, no smoking] helped in minimizing the effects of the virus or for soldiers reflecting on how training worked effectively during operations could go a long way in directing actions and thoughts for the future.

7. Reintegrate: any crisis brings with it some degree of loss of equilibrium. Golan [55] refers to a crisis as a sequence of events leading the movement from lack of equilibrium or disequilibrium to the state of equilibrium. Right after a war is fought or in this case a psychological war which is far from over, the definition of reality which existed has been challenged. Thus, as we take some time out, it is important that we re-assess the meaning and purpose of new reality and how best we respond to the changes that are resulting from a fairly long period of disruption. Reintegration would likely require making conscious changes in self and environment, organizations and communities. For example, organizations are putting together robust rehabilitation plans for employees coming back to work, religious communities which provided assistance to their members through meetings and congregations are moving to online modes of communication, etc.

8. Reboot: Albert Einstein exclaimed that in the midst of every crisis lies great opportunity. This crisis though has been an unsolicited one, has brought to the fore that issues like climate change, global healthcare systems, medical and scientific advances, need to dealt with foremost priority and shared responsibility among nations and global institutions which were caught off guard. Just as when soldiers return from theatre of war, can use their experience—how they survive with limited resources, how they follow a disciplined life, being vigilant; these life skills could be most beneficial to the non-military world which is dealing with the crisis. The pandemic with its mulling consequences of loss, grief and negative emotions has changed behaviours and thoughts which could be detrimental, for example, loss of a family member could make an individual overly cautious or being isolated could result in an individual showing asocial traits and other altered behaviors. These consequences may go unnoticed, however, could covertly damage the fabric of human interactions. It is a right time to slam hard on the reset/reboot button and aim at building conducive transition models holistically.

9. Reconstruction: Reconstruction in Myer and Zunin's 'Phase of Disaster' theory [56] marks the stage of new beginning. This phase according to the theory is marked by individual and community effort to rebuild their lives while continuing to grieve the losses. Reconstruction particularly is the phase of recovery or

conscious effort to move toward state of recovery. Most of the nations have now begun their journey of recovery, a pandemic-like crisis, which requires collective force mobilization efforts on the part of developed nations- in form of providing the necessary resources and developing nations and poorer economies to use this time to build stronger and sustainable systems for better future.

The authors hope and assert that the model will prove a new direction in our endeavour to move toward re-integration and reconstruction of what lay in front of us as a new reality now that it becomes evident that moving to relative normalcy as a necessity for sustenance of the civilization. The 9-R decompression model aims to be a start point for future research and development into strengthening our understanding of how to manage the effects of combat and war fatigue. The period of decompression may vary from person to person and like in counselling, eclectic or customized approach may be an apt pick to deal with individual's socio-economic and psychological build.

5. Conclusion

In conclusion, the authors of the article promote the benefits of having a period of transition, between the social isolation that people around the globe have been forced to and going back to work or new reality. However, as psychologists and responsible leaders, it is also important to create awareness of the nature and the process of decompression, for it to be effective. Some research results suggest that if this transition is considered prolonged, this could have a negative impact on health and well-being of the individuals [57], thus caution and communication should be prioritized for decompression to be effective.

Decompression seems to be a viable solution given the necessity to tread being well and with relatively less damage to the foundation of the societies, organizations and communities. Thus, decompression programs need to be tailored to suit the requirements and could be coupled with other effective techniques and approaches—like post deployment longitudinal screening [58, 59], trauma-focused cognitive therapy [60] which have proven as if not more effective in managing psychological and physical wellbeing in the aftermath of a crisis.

Finally, the authors also acknowledge that thriving through calamities and disasters perhaps is partly innate. As a civilization, even when we face catastrophe like COVID-19 of sorts we are engineered in a way to sustain and thrive and some of us are likely to show exceptional courage and grit to turn a tragedy into testimony of progress and success and show the lead to way into a new future.

Author details

Samir Rawat[1], Abhijit P. Deshpande[1], Ole Boe[2]*, Andrzej Piotrowski[3] and Priya Joshi[4]

1 Symbiosis International University, Pune, India

2 University of South-Eastern Norway, Drammen, Norway

3 University of Gdansk, Gdansk, Poland

4 Military Mind Academy, Pune, India

*Address all correspondence to: ole.boe@usn.no

References

[1] Piotrowski A, Boe O, Rawat S, Bergh J. Significant value of decompression on lifting of lockdown during pandemic—Follow 9 R's. In: Military Psychology Response to Post-Pandemic Reconstruction. Jaipur, India: Rawat Publications; 2020. pp. 498-516

[2] Everly GS, Mitchell JT. A primer on critical incident stress management (CISM). The International Critical Incident Stress Foundation; 2003

[3] Hacker Hughes JGH, Earnshaw NM, Greenberg N, Eldridge R, Fear NT, French C, et al. The use of psychological decompression in military operational environments. Military Medicine. 2008;**173**(6):534-538

[4] De Soir E. Psychological adjustment after military operations: The utility of postdeployment decompression for supporting health readjustment. In: Bowles SV, Bartone PT, editors. Handbook of Military Psychology: Clinical and Organizational Practice. Cham: Springer International Publishing; 2017. pp. 89-103. DOI: 10.1007/978-3-319-66192-6_7

[5] Fear NT, Jones M, Murphy D, Hull L, Iversen AC, Coker B, et al. What are the consequences of deployment to Iraq and Afghanistan on the mental health of the UK armed forces? A cohort study. Lancet. 2010;**375**(9728):1783-1797

[6] Dedert EA, Green KT, Calhoun PS, Yoash-Gantz R, Taber KH, Mumford MM, et al. Association of trauma exposure with psychiatric morbidity in military veterans who have served since September 11, 2001. Journal of Psychiatric Research. 2009;**43**(9):830-836

[7] Adamson DM, Burnam MA, Burns RM, Caldarone LB, Cox RA, D'Amico EJ, et al. Invisible wounds of war: Psychological and cognitive injuries, their consequences, and services to assist recovery. RAND Corporation. 2008. Available from: https://www.rand.org/pubs/monographs/MG720.html

[8] Grieger TA, Cozza SJ, Ursano RJ, Hoge C, Martinez PE, Engel CC, et al. Posttraumatic stress disorder and depression in battle-injured soldiers. The American Journal of Psychiatry. 2006;**163**(10):1777-1783 quiz 1860

[9] Stimpson NJ, Thomas HV, Weightman AL, Dunstan F, Lewis G. Psychiatric disorder in veterans of the Persian Gulf War of 1991. Systematic review. The British Journal of Psychiatry. 2003;**182**:391-403

[10] Kelsall H, Sim M, Forbes A, Glass D, McKenzie D, Ikin J, et al. Symptoms and medical conditions in Australian veterans of the 1991 Gulf War: Relation to immunisations and other Gulf War exposures. Occupational and Environmental Medicine. 2004;**61**(12):1006-1013

[11] Shea KP. The effects of combat related stress on learning in an academic environment. 2010. Available from: https://krex.k-state.edu/dspace/handle/2097/6683

[12] Schell TL, Farris C, Miles JNV, Sloan J, Scharf DM. The Air Force Deployment Transition Center: Assessment of Program Structure, Process, and Outcomes. Rand Health Q. 2017;**7**(1):7

[13] Zamorski M, Britt TW. The psychology of transition: Adapting to home after deployment. In: Adler AB, editor. Deployment Psychology: Evidence-Based Strategies to Promote Mental Health

in the Military. Washington, DC, USA: American Psychological Association; 2011. pp. 153-174

[14] Bliese PD, Wright KM, Adler AB, Thomas JL, Hoge CW. Timing of postcombat mental health assessments. Psychological Services. 2007;**4**(3):141-148

[15] Allison-Aipa TS, Ritter C, Sikes P, Ball S. The impact of deployment on the psychological health status, level of alcohol consumption, and use of psychological health resources of postdeployed U.S. Army Reserve soldiers. Military Medicine. 2010;**175**(9):630-637

[16] Vasterling JJ, Proctor SP, Friedman MJ, Hoge CW, Heeren T, King LA, et al. PTSD symptom increases in Iraq-deployed soldiers: Comparison with nondeployed soldiers and associations with baseline symptoms, deployment experiences, and postdeployment stress. Journal of Traumatic Stress. 2010;**23**(1):41-51

[17] Hoge CW, Castro CA, Messer SC, McGurk D, Cotting DI, Koffman RL. Combat duty in Iraq and Afghanistan, mental health problems, and barriers to care. The New England Journal of Medicine. 2004;**351**(1):13-22

[18] Hoge CW, Terhakopian A, Castro CA, Messer SC, Engel CC. Association of posttraumatic stress disorder with somatic symptoms, health care visits, and absenteeism among Iraq war veterans. The American Journal of Psychiatry. 2007;**164**(1):150-153

[19] Pekrun R, Goetz T, Daniels LM, Stupnisky RH, Perry RP. Boredom in achievement settings: Exploring control–value antecedents and performance outcomes of a neglected emotion. Journal of Educational Psychology. 2010;**102**(3):531-549

[20] Zeidner M. Anxiety in education. In: International Handbook of Emotions in Education (Educational Psychology Handbook Series). New York, NY, USA: Routledge/Taylor & Francis Group; 2014. pp. 265-288

[21] American Psychological Association. Acclimatization—APA Dictionary of Psychology [Internet]. 2020. Available from: https://dictionary.apa.org/acclimatization

[22] Auxéméry Y. Treatment of post-traumatic psychiatric disorders: A continuum of immediate, post-immediate and follow-up care mediated by specific psychotherapeutic principles. Clinical experience in French-speaking countries. Encephale. 2018;**44**(5):403-408

[23] Campfield KM, Hills AM. Effect of timing of critical incident stress debriefing (CISD) on posttraumatic symptoms. Journal of Traumatic Stress. 2001;**14**(2):327-340

[24] Dolan N, Tedeschi C. A qualitative study of psychological outcomes in avalanche first responders. High Altitude Medicine & Biology. 2018;**19**(4):344-355

[25] Smith MH, Brady PJ. Changing the face of Abu Ghraib through mental health intervention: U.S. Army Mental Health Team conducts debriefing with military policemen and Iraqi detainees. Military Medicine. 2006;**171**(12):1163-1166

[26] Bartone PT, Adler AB. Event-Oriented Debriefing Following Military Operations: What Every Leader Should Know. Europe: US Army Medical Research Unit; 1995 Report No.: WRAIR/TR-95-0017

[27] van Emmerik AAP, Kamphuis JH, Hulsbosch AM, Emmelkamp PMG. Single session debriefing after psychological trauma: A meta-analysis. Lancet. 2002;**360**(9335):766-771

[28] van der Riet P, Levett-Jones T, Aquino-Russell C. The effectiveness of mindfulness meditation for nurses and nursing students: An integrated literature review. Nurse Education Today. 2018;**65**:201-211

[29] Ghawadra SF, Abdullah KL, Choo WY, Phang CK. Mindfulness-based stress reduction for psychological distress among nurses: A systematic review. Journal of Clinical Nursing. 2019;**28**(21-22):3747-3748

[30] Zoellner T, Maercker A. Posttraumatic growth in clinical psychology—A critical review and introduction of a two component model. Clinical Psychology Review. 2006;**26**(5):626-653

[31] Tedeschi RG, Calhoun LG. Target article: "Posttraumatic growth: Conceptual foundations and empirical evidence". Psychological Inquiry. 2004;**15**(1):1-18

[32] Dunigan JT, Carr BI, Steel JL. Posttraumatic growth, immunity and survival in patients with hepatoma. Digestive Diseases and Sciences. 2007;**52**(9):2452-2459

[33] Iversen AC, van Staden L, Hughes JH, Greenberg N, Hotopf M, Rona RJ, et al. The stigma of mental health problems and other barriers to care in the UK Armed Forces. BMC Health Services Research. 2011;**10**(11):31

[34] Zhai H-K, Li Q, Hu Y-X, Cui Y-X, Wei X-W, Zhou X. Emotional creativity improves posttraumatic growth and mental health during the COVID-19 pandemic. Frontiers in Psychology. 2021;**3**(12):600798

[35] Fagiolini A, Cuomo A, Frank E. COVID-19 diary from a psychiatry department in Italy. The Journal of Clinical Psychiatry. 2020;**81**(3):20com13357

[36] Ozamiz-Etxebarria N, Idoiaga Mondragon N, Dosil Santamaría M, Picaza GM. Psychological symptoms during the two stages of lockdown in response to the COVID-19 outbreak: An investigation in a sample of citizens in Northern Spain. Frontiers in Psychology. 2020;**18**(11):1491

[37] Shigemura J, Ursano RJ, Morganstein JC, Kurosawa M, Benedek DM. Public responses to the novel 2019 coronavirus (2019-nCoV) in Japan: Mental health consequences and target populations. Psychiatry and Clinical Neurosciences. 2020;**74**(4):281-282

[38] Qiu J, Shen B, Zhao M, Wang Z, Xie B, Xu Y. A nationwide survey of psychological distress among Chinese people in the COVID-19 epidemic: Implications and policy recommendations. Gen Psychiatr. 2020;**33**(2):e100213

[39] World Health Organization. Mental health and psychosocial considerations during the COVID-19 outbreak [Internet]. Report No.: WHO/2019-nCoV/MentalHealth/2020.1. World Health Organization; 2020. Available from: https://apps.who.int/iris/handle/10665/331490

[40] Svenson BE. Identification and elucidation of fields of research within health and social training courses of medium length. Interdiciplinaria. 1990;**9**:41-53

[41] Asp M. Rest. Global Qualitative Nursing Research. 2015;**2**: 2333393615583663

[42] Han B-C, Wallin O. Trötthetssamhället. Stockholm: Ersatz; 2016

[43] Chawla N, MacGowan RL, Gabriel AS, Podsakoff NP. Unplugging or

staying connected? Examining the nature, antecedents, and consequences of profiles of daily recovery experiences. Journal of Applied Psychology. 2020;**105**(1):19-39

[44] Corliss J. Six relaxation techniques to reduce stress. Harvard Health. 2016. Available from: https://www.health.harvard.edu/mind-and-mood/six-relaxation-techniques-to-reduce-stress

[45] Yanilov E, Boe O. Krav Maga: Combat Mindset & Fighting Stress: How to Perform under Alarming and Stressful Conditions. London: Meyer & Meyer Sports Ltd; 2020

[46] Dolan SL, Sanchez SG. Covid-19, stress, self-esteem, values, and psychological well-being: How to assess risks of becoming depressed, anxious, or suicidal? The European Business Review. 2020. Available from: https://www.europeanbusinessreview.com/covid-19-stress-self-esteem-values-and-psychological-well-being-how-to-assess-risks-of-becoming-depressed-anxious-or-suicidal/

[47] Goffman E. Stigma: Notes on the Management of Spoiled Identity. Reissue ed. New York: Touchstone; 1986 168 p.

[48] Abdelhafiz AS, Mohammed Z, Ibrahim ME, Ziady HH, Alorabi M, Ayyad M, et al. Knowledge, perceptions, and attitude of Egyptians towards the novel coronavirus disease (COVID-19). Journal of Community Health. 2020;**21**:1-10

[49] Coste V. Coronavirus: France faces "epidemic" of anti-Asian racism [Internet]. Euronews. 2020. Available from: https://www.euronews.com/2020/02/03/coronavirus-france-faces-epidemic-of-anti-asian-racism

[50] Haynes S. As coronavirus spreads, so does xenophobia and anti-Asian racism [Internet]. Time. 2020. Available from: https://time.com/5797836/coronavirus-racism-stereotypes-attacks/

[51] Boud D, Keogh R, Walker D. Promoting Reflection in Learning A Model. Reflection Turning Reflection into Learning. London: Routledge; 1985 References - Scientific Research Publishing [Internet]. Available from: https://www.scirp.org/%28S%28czeh2tfqyw2orz553k1w0r45%29%29/reference/referencespapers.aspx?referenceid=1434298

[52] Carver CS. Self-awareness. In: Handbook of Self and Identity. New York, NY, USA: The Guilford Press; 2003. pp. 179-196

[53] Blair C, Raver CC. Individual development and evolution: Experiential canalization of self-regulation. Developmental Psychology. 2012;**48**(3):647-657

[54] Rawat S. COVID-19: Showing resilience through self-regulation [Internet]. https://www.outlookindia.com/. 2020. Available from: https://www.outlookindia.com/newsscroll/covid19-showing-resilience-through-selfregulation/1785928

[55] Golan N. Treatment in Crisis Situations (Treatment Approaches in the Human Services). Bradford, UK: Stephen White Books; 1978. Available from: https://www.abebooks.co.uk/9780029120606/Treatment-Crisis-Situations-Approaches-Human-0029120608/plp

[56] Myers D, Zunin L. Phases of disaster. In: Training Manual for Mental Health and Human Service Workers in Major Disasters. Washington, DC: DHHS Publication, Department of Health and Human Services; 2000

[57] Buckman JEJ, Sundin J, Greene T, Fear NT, Dandeker C, Greenberg N, et al. The impact of deployment length on the health and well-being of military personnel: A systematic review of the literature. Occupational and Environmental Medicine. 2011;**68**(1):69-76

[58] Dunt D. Review of Mental Health Care in the Australian Defence Force and Transition Through Discharge. Department of Veterans' Affairs; 2019. Available from: https://www.dva.gov.au/documents-and-publications/review-mental-health-care-australian-defence-force-and-transition

[59] Hoge CW, Auchterlonie JL, Milliken CS. Mental health problems, use of mental health services, and attrition from military service after returning from deployment to Iraq or Afghanistan. JAMA. 2006;**295**(9):1023-1032

[60] Bisson JI. Post-traumatic stress disorder. BMJ. 2007;**334**(7597):789-793

Section 4

Daily Life, Work and Well-Being: Impact, Resilience and Adaptation

Chapter 19

A Way Forward: Psychological Adaptation and Transformation of Life Post COVID-19

Kanwar Hamza Shuja, Arfa Mubeen, Sania Mazher and Shazia Tariq

Abstract

This chapter focuses on the exclusive and social experiences of people in post-COVID-19 life. As it can be observed from the current scenario how people have already accepted COVID-19 as a part of their daily routine. That is from wearing masks to using hand sanitizers and other precautionary activities. Based on these observable changes and adaptation of habits, the current chapter will delve into the psychological causes based on various theoretical concepts and the present literature on how humans use varied mechanisms to adapt to aversive situations and emerge by transforming themselves to be more resilient than before. Likewise, the chapter will also focus on individual and social strategies that can be employed to further strengthen the resilience of people post COVID-19.

Keywords: post COVID-19, social experiences, psychological adaptation, transformation, theoretical concepts, resilience

1. Introduction

Coronavirus-19 (COVID-19) began as a viral pneumonia in China in late 2019. By March 2020, it has attained pandemic proportions as it transmitted rapidly throughout most of the world. The ease of transmission, lack of population immunity, as well as delayed responses in testing, lack of equipment, and the challenges in implementing community-based measures to limit contact were all taking an unprecedented toll on our collective health care, political, economic, and social-welfare systems [1]. COVID-19 has hitherto led to the sickening and loss of life for thousands of people (**Figure 1**). As initial evidence already indicates [2], it contains the potential of leaving deep psychological scars on many. With its unpredictability and the need for distance and isolation, COVID-19 has caused a tear in the fabric of our most fundamental methods of coping and calls for novel ways of adapting to and thinking about crises. In this chapter, we will discuss numerous theories and mechanisms of psychological adaptation to life after COVID-19. Life after COVID-19 is peculiar from the life before COVID-19. The mental health of people all over the globe has been affected. But now people are coping and adapting to COVID-19.

 IntechOpen

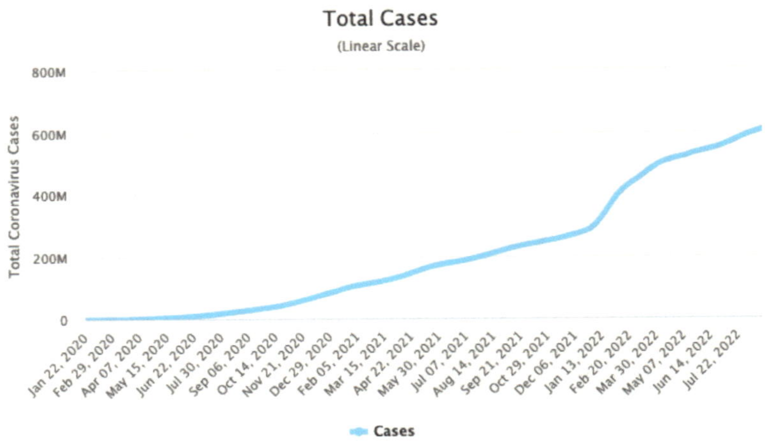

Figure 1.
Worldwide cases of coronavirus.

The COVID-19 epidemic led to a significant shift in how individuals embark on their routine lives and projects. To control the transmission of the virus, the triple shock of proclaiming a national health emergency, enforcing an economic shutdown, and combining social isolation and temporal distance became the conventional reaction, all of which produced long-term effects on how people perceive and perform social behaviors. From working to learning, from amusement to purchasing, from socializing to family life and love connections, from the meaning of home and living environments to our ideas and expectations of citizenship, nearly every sphere of practice has been impacted [3].

Sustainability experts refer to the epidemic as a possible catalyst for change in the direction of a more ecologically sound, socially just, and ethical future [4]. The crisis presents a once-in-a-lifetime chance to design a long-term transition depending on individual lifestyle changes, as well as a multi-stakeholder strategy build-up of systemic-institutional changes toward a larger, low-carbon arrangement [5]. The COVID-19-related watershed of changes provides both horror and promise to groups working to promote sustainable development.

It was evident from the start of the epidemic that individualism was one of the numerous ways the crisis manifested in our society. People raced to purchase products that they deemed essential. Grocery stores and supermarkets immediately ran out of toilet paper rolls and hand sanitizers, owing to some people buying far more than they needed and therefore exhibiting blatant contempt for the needs of others. Individualism, on the other hand, indicates governments' failure to care for citizens during challenging times [6].

The shutdown caused everyone's house the center of their existence, making it the distinct location for a variety of functions that were not initially envisioned. Excluding the populations like the elderly, few people would have expected to experience a life that was so physically and socially secluded. Isolation became the current social norm overnight. These trends predict that previously out-of-home activities will presently be exclusively conducted at home and that social relations and social life will be limited to a smaller and more intimate circle of trusted (clean-reliable) contacts. Accelerated trends allude to pre-COVID-19 initiatives that were scaled up and amplified during the epidemic, achieving mainstream status [7]. These things collectively induced a high level of mental distress and anxiety among people as was observed in several studies [8].

The digitization and remote involvement of both functional and emotional aspects of life, for example, have forced an internet-mediation of activities, which has pushed online navigation from the periphery to the center. Work, recreation, study, commerce, and love were all taking place in internet-enabled contexts, with the qualities of remoteness and multi-functionality established. Simultaneously, gamification of material from the entertainment, social, and academic sectors grew in popularity, combining virtual socializing and remote learning with immersive technology.

In the same way, wearing a mask was found to remain a visual feature that established temporal separation as a public health strategy in a recent study done in the Italian Venice metropolitan region [9]. Distances were measured by an operator operating a unique sensor-based "social distancing belt" between February 24 and April 29, 2020. "Unmasked," "masked," "do it yourself (DIY) masked," "goggles masked," and "goggles DIY-masked" were all used interchangeably. People tended to stay closer to an uncovered individual, but wearing a mask tended to increase the substantial distance between them. This contradiction can be answered by considering humans' inherent social nature, which promotes social over antisocial activity. Wearing a mask might transform unintentional social conduct into intentional antisocial behavior [10].

Mask-wearing and social distance restrictions may be eased in the near future, depending on danger levels. COVID-19 mitigation techniques might rapidly be adopted to combat outbreaks and subsequently withdrawn after the threat has passed—this would involve excellent communication. Without regulations, vulnerable or risk-averse individuals may continue engaging in pandemic behaviors such as wearing masks, particularly in congested areas like movie theatres and concert venues. The most draconian COVID-19 methods, like school closures, lockdowns, and travel restrictions, may no longer be acceptable to the public [11].

The instability of the contemporary globalized capitalist system, with its reliance on transnational financialized trades, just-in-time manufacturing, and lengthy, carbon-intensive international supply chains, has been revealed by COVID-19. It has also demonstrated how small economies are often more robust to massive shocks and can provide for themselves effectively and efficiently during a crisis. Economies based on mutualism and solidarity, which are embedded, inclusive, frequently informal, and turbulent, have thrived. For example, there has been a notable increase in solidarity and grassroots engagement in the domain of food provisioning, ranging from widespread food donations to the poor in India and Pakistan to the supply of mobile meals to disadvantaged groups in the United States and Canada [12].

Communities have bonded together to fill up holes in the system and assist people in need, with civil-society organizations collaborating with concerned governmental actors on occasion. In India's largely decentralized system, the state of Kerala, for example, has taken the lead in responding to COVID-19 by providing food distribution through free community meals organized by women's networks [13]. Such examples are suggestive of the communal bonds that arose and facilitated resilience in the aftermath of previous tragedies [14]. The question is whether such solidarity is limited to the specific environment of an emergency, or whether it hints at future potential economies.

COVID-19 risk reduction led to significant social isolation and loneliness, as shown by increased anxiety, sadness, drug misuse, and suicide ideation. Sheer pleasures, such as hugging family or friends, dining out, or seeing a grin that is not disguised behind a protective mask, appeal to the public. Humans are sociable creatures by nature. The United States began extensive socializing not long after the 1918 epidemic, with the Roaring Twenties bringing people together in crowded dance halls, movie palaces, and speakeasies. If there is social utility, some epidemic behaviors may survive, at least in part. A hybrid working (both remote and in-person) may outlive the epidemic, providing many people with a better work-life balance and more housing options. For the time being, air travel may also remain stationary. International traffic was 72 percent lower in December 2021 than in December 2019, and it may not rebound until 2024 [11].

2. Psychological adaptation after COVID-19 through the lens of evolutionary psychology

According to evolutionary psychology, evolutionary changes shape not only the physique but also the mind, where psychological systems are triggered, which are thought to be psychological modifications meant to handle issues that previously aided to survival and growth. Natural selection represents a crucial principle that Darwin offered that underlies much of current psychology study. It directs psychologists to groupings of evolutionary issues associated with survival and development.

Evolutionary theory, according to Wiles [15], explains "the diversity of species that has arisen through descent and adaptation from a distinguished ancestor." It refers to variations in life forms of living creatures over time as a result of inherent differences and organic selection processes that contribute to more egregious preservation and fertility rates of those better adapted to their surroundings, striving to increase the frequency of unique characteristics in the inhabitants. Whereas it is commonly believed that variance occurs at random intervals, natural selection guides the process and leads to the formation of multiple stressors that influence people differently, like access to food, global warming, and other types of competitions between organisms in the similar area [16].

Exclusion of population groups due to location or biological constraints might cause them to follow divergent evolutionary pathways, resulting in differentiation. Furthermore, the evolutionary theory contends that the existing variety of living species arose from a limited number of ancient predecessors [17]. The concept of evolution, as distinct from abiogenesis, thereby describes the cycle of exchange associated with every species, like the era of modern humans and our evolution from universal ancestors with other primates [18].

During the coronavirus epidemic in 2020, there will be significant variations in how people experience their lives. Teaching and learning processes in academic environments have evolved from conventional tactics such as face-to-face exchanges to digital training, in which students utilize technology and computer devices to communicate with online content. Many businesses have failed as a result of lockdowns. Those who can adjust to such alterations more rapidly and easily, on the other hand, will attend more competition. Furthermore, social relationships have shifted in so many aspects that the phrase "new normal" has become commonly used to characterize new appropriate behaviors that individuals have developed in response to the epidemic. In this chapter, we discuss psychological features thought to indicate traits of persons who can successfully adjust to challenges.

3. Resilience: the psychological trait of being able to bounce back

For an exceptionally extended period, the word "resilience" has been hotly disputed in psychology since it has diverse, complicated meanings depending on a person, a community, and a country, if they designate it as a feature, a practice, or a result. There are several ways to describe resiliency. The term "resilience" is derived from the Latin word "Resilens," which indicates "the elastic property of a material" [19]. The capacity to "come back from hardship, disappointment, and misfortune" [20] is equally described as a talent that will later "advance in self-responsibility" [21]. Another description of resilience represents the capacity to respond to stress-related situations calmly [22], like the capacity to restore instantly from traumatic circumstances [22, 23]. Furthermore, resilience is determined by whether people permit themselves to be overpowered by pressure and hardship or if they endure and adapt to obstacles [24]. Nevertheless, resilience can alter as a result of a person's development and interaction with the world [25]. Individuals may be more resistant at points in their life and less resilient at others [23].

In terms of cultural ramifications, the notion of resiliency varies according to a person's surroundings and mastery expertise. Face-to-face conversations with Afghans on their own meaning of the word "resilience" were utilized by researchers who conducted research in Afghanistan [26]. The research demonstrated resilience, which indicates "faith." They found that the Afghan people prioritized the future above the past since it dictated their current problems and well-being because what happened in the past could not be reversed. Similarly, as per the study of Michel Ungar, which was undertaken in various nationalities, resilience can vary substantially depending on cultural and contextual factors [27]. As a consequence, instead of concentrating on individual resilience, we should improve people's levels of resilience to boost resilience capacity in each person. This will lead to more possibilities for them to maintain a livelier life [28]. This refers to the concept of systemic resiliency, or the provision of excellent education and resources so that individuals may recognize their capability [29].

Resilience training may help with both therapeutic and preventative strategies for approaching problems. To begin, "the challenge model" proposes that if people encounter the danger of a non-tragic exposure occurrence, they will enhance their knowledge and manage it in the future [30]. For example, when teens are confronted with a modest degree of risk variables, they can benefit from it and practice what they have acquired when confronted with the same desperate circumstance in the future. Children are prepared for emergency response procedures and how to respond to a house fire during fire drills. Furthermore, "the compensating model" defines resilience as a strategy for avoiding traumatic experiences [31]. This is reinforced by studies on teenage alcohol withdrawal, which will reduce the risk of suicide in teens [32]. Inexorably, "the protective factor model" proposes that if dangers are minimized, the likelihood of a bad result decreases [30]. According to Andersson and Ledogar's [32] research, when young individuals are not introduced to substances, they are less prone to consume alcoholic beverages; consequently, reducing the risk for suicide.

Nevertheless, resilience exhibits some unique traits that set it apart from positivity, faith, and other attributes [33]. For example, being "proactive and reactive" in the face of overwhelming odds is a resiliency attribute. It is also defined as "the ability to come back" from traumas and life-altering situations [22, 34]. As a result, resilience may be defined as positive attitudes on risk variables that may be identified as risks that increase the likelihood of a poor consequence or decrease the likelihood of an optimistic one [35]. Put differently, resilience entails doing something and responding to adversity. Optimism and hope, on the other hand, represent solely optimistic states of thought. Briefly expressed, hope and optimism are best applied to events that may occur with a plan and can be described using identifiable variables, whereas resilience includes the need to be flexible, adjustable, and improvable in specific conditions [36].

Keeping everything discussed above in mind, resilience may be acquired by putting things in context and recognizing unreasonable thinking. It is eminent to recognize a transformation is unavoidable to develop adaptability. Being both positive and adaptable will aid a person in coping with adverse conditions. Lastly, learn from history and improve the future [33]. There are several daily steps that everyone may undertake to improve their resistance. For instance, individuals can go for a stroll to nourish their bodies moving and generate endorphins into their bodies. People can equally strike up conversations with someone they are familiar with and can have a general discussion. Gathering a deep breath every time they are anxious may also be beneficial. People who acquire this personality feature are more likely to reinforce their "self-responsibility," allowing them to study more effectively and develop in a vigorous manner since they have conquered challenges [37]. To explain the psychological effect of resilience, we can look at a recent ecological model that was suggested by researchers based on resilience including various resources that were found to be directly associated with resilience and non-resilience [38].

4. Agility: the psychological trait of adapting to changes

Many individuals have explored the word "agility" or "learning agility" and attempted to define it. The capacity to retain from experience shows people's capacity to control the changing requirements of their employment, according to the definition of "agility" [39]. It was equally described as "a person's capacity to study consists of a broad and varied number of characteristics and proficiencies, including but are not restricted to persons' intellectual ability [40, 41], eagerness to study and active pursuit of educational possibilities [42, 43], and personal characteristics such as openness to experience [44]."

The potential to do so rapidly and in a variety of circumstances was also termed agility [45, 46]. In their search for a more precise definition of the term, DeRue et al. [47] revealed that learning agility has been predominantly associated with the capacity to learn. They then defined academic agility as "the aptitude to rapidly absorb a situation and move between ideas flexibly in service of knowledge inside and between interactions." They also established a scheme of learning agility based on the findings of Eichinger and Lombardo [48], which imply there are two essential elements of learning agility: speed and flexibility.

According to the work of Eichinger and Lombardo [48], agility is essential for the implementation of this psychological structure, as "the building of learning agility originated from the need to produce considerable numbers of competent workers capable of performing successfully in a changing situation." The research by Neubert et al. [49] additionally notes that "the association between learning agility and the trend for no routine and dynamic workplace features is evident." For instance, it is crucial to select a worker with high agility so that he or she can adapt to or respond to a variety of unforeseen situations. On a broader scale, Baran and Bible's [50] study propose, "At the group level, agility extends on what we know about high-performance groups by adding behaviours and mindsets that facilitate insight making and swift decision making." Additionally, as a business attribute, agility may benefit the company in a variety of ways. Gligor et al. [51] provide six elements of the qualities of agility that contribute to the growth of a business, including the ability to quickly change course, speed/accelerate processes, monitor the environment, encourage the client, modify strategies and processes (versatility), and integrate processes across firms.

5. Identification and training of possible vulnerable population

Psychologists have various tools that they have used to identify vulnerable populations and individuals who were affected by COVID-19 pandemic. The most common factors that were identified and linked with the pandemic were anxiety, stress, depression, and suicidal ideations [52]. Training should be given to hospital staff, and more psychological trainees must be hired to increase the reach of identifying possible cases. Additionally, online resources can be of great help as there are several studies that used online survey methods for the collection of data from individuals for connecting and associating possible linkages between COVID-19 and psychological issues [53]. With the help of such tactics, training of other medical staff can be of great use.

Moreover, resilience itself is a natural phenomenon that each human uses to a varied extent on daily basis. If psychologists can use mediums like social platforms to outreach to people and communities they can easily deliver their message across, teaching people how to use the resources they have to overcome their distress and fears and use their own capabilities and strengths in these times of need to emerge into a better-transformed version of themselves.

5.1 Post—COVID-19 as new era

The post—COVID-19 epidemic period became known as the "new normal." It is a time of hardships and insecurity. Flexibility, inquiry, risk minimization, education by investigating, education by doing, and attention are all highly valued in today's world [54]. All conceptions would be undergoing metamorphosis in this new normal. As the globe continues to confront socioeconomic challenges that highlight the need for reform, these notions will become more innovative. The kind and direction of change in the new normal would be determined by the type and quantity of programs evaluated during the society's crisis or stability state. More inventive strategies are anticipated to manage the constantly volatile market in this period. Many unique sorts of obstacles are foreseen in every industry throughout the new normal. This should increase the likelihood of creativity as a consequence of possibilities that come with the obstacles, as well as resilience, which represent a necessary attitude for existence during times of upheaval. This is essential as studies conducted during and post—COVID-19 pandemic suggested distress of varying degrees, while stating the distress flow to be continuous at the highest [55].

5.2 Importance of inspiration and resilience during times of transformation

The new normal necessitates effective alternatives that in turn can utilize and spread to several domains of life. At this pivotal juncture, it is vital to incorporate epidemic measures into routine lives. Concludingly, it is a period for creativity and endurance, which increases confidence in people and allows them to implement change [56].

The extreme turmoil caused by the COVID-19 epidemic generated unique possibilities that can currently be observed in medical and social progress and undiscovered financial concepts. With the rise of both dire moments and hazards, there are also concealed possibilities. For instance, as the duration of the lockdown increased, individuals began to experience worry or stress as a consequence of their concerns about their ultimate possibilities, as a consequence of the volatility and unpredictability that impacted their employment, educational ambitions, and overall life path. As a result, health officials and other state authorities must implement more involvement and participation programs to guarantee each individual has a supervisor to assist him or her in coping with the devastating repercussions of the post—COVID-19 overflow. The advisor's duty is to investigate the origins and attitude of motivation of the community engaged to promote their resilience [57].

5.3 A new journey of life and livelihood

More than ever before, this new normal is dictating how we live and earn a living. For example, we must wholly, at present, live with and fix the underlying factors that caused the disaster. Isolation difficulties, as well as taking and dealing with all safeguards, are becoming the standard. The COVID-19 epidemic is even shifting our criteria of life happiness away from cash and goods and toward capability, which contributes to the transformation. This requires a shift in attitude that recognizes the significance of having "life business strategies" that maintain enjoyment without being constrained by "what happens to you," but by "what occurs from you" [57].

While adjusting to the "New Normal," supplemental programs are required to alleviate the sensation and worry of the "BIG changes" arriving so quickly, which would have an instantaneous psychological effect like job insecurity, according to Buheji and Sisk [56]. Working from home is getting increasingly difficult, with many people and even organizations struggling to survive, competing for such scarce positions. As a result, every one of us must identify our novel regular function as a game while attempting to manage the unpredictable 3 Fs surrounding us: family, finance, and freedom.

People would be facing more constrained freedom of many activities that they did not anticipate to occur in their life during the transition to the new normal, particularly when the majority of this liberty is tied to the reason of preserving lives. As a result, it is time to reconsider our options for reorganizing. This resetting changes our mentality and forces us to reconsider what we desire from our lives and the courses we will follow. This is a watershed moment in our lives, therefore let us seize it.

5.4 Career resilience

After COVID-19, nearly every day, we overhear accounts of how this condition has tested people's resiliency or inspired them to persevere. Whether it is people handling telecommuting, health workers risking their personal safety by continuing to perform their responsibilities in close interaction with each other, or others suffering unemployment, resilience, and employment are intrinsically linked to the coronavirus discourse.

Modern scholars disagree on whether career resiliency (CR) is a trait, a skill, or a behavior. CR has been described in numerous ways [58, 59]. Yet the majority concur it is about adapting and enduring in the face of shocks or hardship, and they recognize its value while considering professions in today's fast-changing economy. Rochat et al. [60] outlined a procedure for determining the "fundamental elements of professional adaptability," which contains (1) Evaluating scenarios that may present threats to employment — in this case, COVID-19; and (2) Identifying related "risk and protective variables" to establish effective, adaptable results. They assert that CR functions as a mediator between unpleasant professional situations and potential rewards.

Most research on CR agrees that both personal and situational factors influence a person's career adaptability [59, 61, 62]. Personal characteristics, abilities, attitudes, and actions have been shown to cause favorable or negative effects on a person's resilience. Considerable implications for CR also include environmental elements such as welcoming workplaces, occupational characteristics, and supportive families [59]. These personal and situational traits are the "risk and protective components" described by Rochat et al. [60], particularly essential for occupational resilience. Therefore, a lack of resources renders people in danger and can adversely affect their resistance capacity, but personal resources can produce favorable outcomes.

Despite the indisputable significance of CR, one of the critical provisions of the endeavor to develop worker resiliency is the emphasis on transforming individuals instead of the environment, which frequently serves as the source of the problem [60, 63]. However, a lack of resilience is commonly perceived as a "personality defect" [64] and firms would prefer to recruit for resiliency and provide resistance training than adjust the organizational conditions that may be causing the problem. As organizations plan for a post-pandemic era, we have reached a critical point. How can institutions that invest in sustaining a competent workforce establish resilient cultures, and how might HRD assist?

5.5 Sustainability and careers after COVID-19

The requirements for successful professions include four factors: longevity, social space, action, and relevance. In practice, this means that sustainable jobs encompass the entirety of a person's life, including both paid and unpaid work. They acknowledge the confluence of several life contexts, such as social, professional, and familial, and accommodate the needs of each. Ultimately, they are assisted by professionally created options that prioritize both significance and utility [65]. Increased acknowledgment of collective responsibility among employees and their employers is a fundamental notion. Although these characteristics were not created for the COVID-19 era, they are well-suited for the future of professions.

Unexpected benefits of hiding in place have included the ability to reflect on one's professional past, present, and future, which has sometimes led to a re-evaluation of life and accomplished goals. It has fostered a revitalized awareness of social connectedness, highlighting the more congenial environment in which we live and work, and has enhanced the ties between work, social, and family life on an unprecedented scale. As individuals and organizations exit the first phase of COVID-19 adaptation, the experience will have transformed how we think about and conduct future work.

To develop a successful career post coronavirus, it will be essential to learn from this occurrence and utilize the knowledge gained. Being in a learning mode is a meta-competency in the quest of occupational longevity, according to Heslin et al. [66]. The McKinsey Institute [67] echoed this conclusion, but from a systems perspective, reckoning that "innovation, expertise, and adaptability" will likely be necessary to successfully emerge from this disaster.

Chudzikowski et al. [68] provided a further dimension to the sustainable link to the post-COVID study, adding extra layers of difficulty on how an environment affects professional choice. People make career decisions on the basis of how they value individual desires in combination with the needs of their communities, and these goals may change with professional phases, leading to numerous decisions at diverse career stages. Companies committed to retaining talent and developing a durable environment can assist in this endeavor by providing guidance and studying ways to maintain people participating and progressing over time [68]. As we progress, we have the opportunity to establish and strengthen workplaces that adhere to the triple bottom line of profits, planet, and people. This is an opportunity to begin again.

5.6 The conservation of resources (COR) theory

These many profession elements use Hobfoll's Conservation of Resources (COR) theory as a theoretical model to illustrate how professions are maintained, the potential implications of profession interruptions, and how assets can influence professional resiliency [61, 69, 70]. The COR idea was developed to help comprehend what occurs when individuals are exposed to distress [71]. Humans, according to Hobfoll [72], seek to develop and conserve resources and will endeavor to minimize the erosion of these resources when pressured. COR theory emphasizes the importance of the environment in the stress reaction and how it might diminish or enhance people's resources. COR theory highlights the significance of the environment in the stress response and how it can deplete or boost people's resources [73]. Therefore, this concept of gathering and keeping resources can characterize and aid in the management of professional disruptions, the development of resilience, and the maintenance of careers.

However, what happens to persons with meager resources? According to Hobfoll [72], resources are undistributed evenly, and those without resources are most exposed to increased losses. In addition, Hobfoll [73] hypothesized situations can threaten a person's resource capacity, with these occurrences offering greater problems for "less resource-endowed persons of financially affluent nations and for developing and financially distressed nations." This occurrence, COVID-19, has exacerbated the widening gaps between those with and without in recent years. COVID-19 has worsened disparities between populations within nations (like low-income and marginalized groups) and between nations [74]. Many individuals will lack the resources essential to remain resilient in the face of this career setback.

Consequently, what can be done to ensure that people have the essential skills and resilience components to enhance their resilience throughout this crisis? Clearly, this requires more than a singular, temporary solution. On the contrary, it involves constant efforts by organizations, authorities, and societies to examine a variety of techniques to aid individuals in amassing and maintaining riches. The importance of a holistic strategy that acknowledges the interconnection of business, government, and society. The coronavirus has deepened these links, extending across borders and requiring coordinated efforts or failure. As we advance in our rehabilitation, we must be determined not to abandon vast segments of the population.

6. Conclusions

Conclusively, humans have a great capacity for adaptability in adverse situations. History is filled with such evidence of how humans have survived and triumphed over such difficult situations. Currently, humans have already developed habits such as using face masks and sanitizers as part of their daily routines. Likewise, using proper psychological, individual, and social models immensely increase the adaptation and transformation of humans into stronger and more persistent organism. The chapter has greatly discussed and elaborated several theories of resilience and their adaptability to the daily lives of people. Likewise, the chapter has also covered various techniques that can be implemented by government and local bodies for the betterment of humans post COVID-19 pandemic.

Acknowledgements

No acknowledgment nor any funding sources are present.

Conflict of interest

The authors declare no conflict of interest.

Author details

Kanwar Hamza Shuja[1*], Arfa Mubeen[2], Sania Mazher[3] and Shazia Tariq[4]

1 Psychology Department, National University of Modern Languages (NUML), Islamabad, Pakistan

2 Capital University of Science and Technology (CUST), Islamabad, Pakistan

3 Quaid-I-Azam University (New Campus), Islamabad, Pakistan

4 National University of Modern Languages (NUML), Islamabad, Pakistan

*Address all correspondence to: kanwar.hamza@numl.edu.pk

References

[1] U.S. CDC. CDC COVID Data Tracker. US Centers Dis Control Prev [Internet]. 2022; Available from: https://covid.cdc.gov/covid-data-tracker/?CDC_AA_refVal=https%3A%2F%2Fwww.cdc.gov%2Fcoronavirus%2F2019-ncov%2Fcases-updates%2Fcases-in-us.html#cases_casesper100klast7days%0A https://covid.cdc.gov/covid-data-tracker/#vaccinations_vacc-total-admin-rate-total

[2] Qiu J, Shen B, Zhao M, Wang Z, Xie B, Xu Y. A nationwide survey of psychological distress among Chinese people in the COVID-19 epidemic: Implications and policy recommendations. Genetics Psychiatry. 2020;**33**:e100213

[3] Echegaray F. What POST-COVID-19 lifestyles may look like? Identifying scenarios and their implications for sustainability. Sustainable Production and Consumption. 2021;**27**:567-574

[4] Cohen MJ. Does the COVID-19 outbreak mark the onset of a sustainable consumption transition? Sustainability: Science, Practice and Policy. 2020; **16**(1):1-3

[5] Markard J, Rosenbloom D. A tale of two crises: COVID-19 and climate. Sustainability: Science, Practice and Policy. 2020;**16**(1):53-60

[6] Sikali K. The dangers of social distancing: How COVID-19 can reshape our social experience. Journal of Community Psychology. 2020;**48**(8): 2435-2438. DOI: 10.1002/jcop.22430

[7] Koide R, Lettenmeier M, Kojima S, Toivio V, Amellina A, Akenji L. Carbon footprints and consumer lifestyles: An analysis of lifestyle factors and gap analysis by consumer segment in Japan. Sustainability. 2019;**11**(21):5983

[8] The Economist. Covid-19 has led to a sharp increase in depression and anxiety [Internet]. 2021. Available from: https://www.economist.com/graphic-detail/2021/10/11/covid-19-has-led-to-a-sharp-increase-in-depression-and-anxiety. [Accessed: July 14, 2022]

[9] Gostin LO, Friedman EA, Wetter SA. Responding to Covid-19: How to navigate a public health emergency legally and ethically. The Hastings Center Report. 2020;**50**(2):8-12

[10] Martinelli L, Kopilaš V, Vidmar M, Heavin C, Machado H, Todorović Z, et al. Face masks during the COVID-19 pandemic: A simple protection tool with many meanings. Frontiers in Public Health. 2021;**947**(8):606635. DOI: 10.3389/fpubh.2020.606635

[11] Gostin LO. Life after the COVID-19 Pandemic. American Medical Association; 2022. p. e220323

[12] Leach M, MacGregor H, Scoones I, Wilkinson A. Post-pandemic transformations: How and why COVID-19 requires us to rethink development. World Development. 2021;**138**:105233

[13] Mathieu I. COVID-19 and the Crisis in Food Systems: Symptoms, Causes, and Potential Solutions. 2020. Retrieved from: https://policycommons.net/artifacts/2007245/covid-19-and-the-crisis-in-food-systems/2759688/

[14] Solnit R. A Paradise Built in Hell: The Extraordinary Communities That Arise in Disaster. Penguin; 2010

[15] Wiles JR. Overwhelming scientific confidence in evolution and its centrality

in science education—And the public disconnect. Science Education Review. 2010;**9**(1):18-27

[16] Stearns SC, Hoekstra RF. Evolution, an Introduction. Oxford University Press; 2000

[17] Charlesworth B, Charlesworth D, Barton NH. The effects of genetic and geographic structure on neutral variation. Annual Review of Ecology, Evolution, and Systematics. 2003;**34**(1):99-125

[18] Stearns SC. How the European Society for Evolutionary Biology and the Journal of Evolutionary Biology were Founded. Blackwell Publishing Ltd; 2008. pp. 1449-1451

[19] Greene RR, Galambos C, Lee Y. Resilience theory: Theoretical and professional conceptualizations. Journal of Human Behavior in the Social Environment. 2004;**8**(4):75-91

[20] Janas M. Build resiliency. Intervention in School and Clinic. 2002;**38**(2):117

[21] Luthans F, Vogelgesang GR, Lester PB. Developing the psychological capital of resiliency. Human Resource Development Review. 2006;**5**(1):25-44

[22] Bonanno GA. Loss, trauma, and human resilience: Have we underestimated the human capacity to thrive after extremely aversive events? The American Psychologist. 2004;**59**(1):20

[23] Southwick SM, Bonanno GA, Masten AS, Panter-Brick C, Yehuda R. Resilience definitions, theory, and challenges: Interdisciplinary perspectives. European Journal of Psychotraumatology. 2014;**5**(1):25338

[24] Rutter M. Psychosocial resilience and protective mechanisms. The American Journal of Orthopsychiatry. 1987;**57**(3):316-331

[25] Kim-Cohen J, Turkewitz R. Resilience and measured gene–environment interactions. Development and Psychopathology. 2012;**24**(4):1297-1306

[26] Panter-Brick C, Eggerman M. Understanding Culture, Resilience, and Mental Health: The Production of Hope. Springer; 2012. pp. 369-386

[27] Ungar M. Resilience across cultures. British Journal of Social Work. 2008;**38**(2):218-235

[28] Reed RV, Fazel M, Jones L, Panter-Brick C, Stein A. Mental health of displaced and refugee children resettled in low-income and middle-income countries: Risk and protective factors. Lancet. 2012;**379**(9812):250-265

[29] Ager A, Annan J, Panter-Brick C. Resilience: From conceptualization to effective intervention. In: Policy Brief for IRC Strategic Planning Meeting. May 6 2013;**2013**

[30] O'Leary A, Jemmott JB, Stevens R, Rutledge SE, Icard LD. Optimism and education buffer the effects of syndemic conditions on HIV status among African American men who have sex with men. AIDS and Behavior. 2014;**18**(11):2080-2088

[31] Garmezy N, Masten AS, Tellegen A. The study of stress and competence in children: A building block for developmental psychopathology. Child Development. 1984;**55**(1):97-111

[32] Andersson N, Ledogar RJ. The CIET Aboriginal youth resilience studies: 14 years of capacity building and methods development in Canada. Pimatisiwin. 2008;**6**(2):65

[33] Praputpittaya T, Yasri P. The COPE Model for Promoting Cooperative Learning in Classrooms. International Journal of Innovation Creativity. 2020;**12**(6):349-361

[34] Vogelgesang G, Clapp-Smith R, Osland J. The relationship between positive psychological capital and global mindset in the context of global leadership. Journal of Leadership and Organizational Studies. 2014;**21**(2): 165-178

[35] Masten AS. Ordinary magic: Resilience processes in development. The American Psychologist. 2001;**56**(3):227

[36] Coutu DL. How resilience works. Harvard Business Review. 2002;**80**(5):46-56

[37] Youssef CM, Luthans F. Positive organizational behavior in the workplace: The impact of hope, optimism, and resilience. Journal of Management. 2007;**33**(5):774-800

[38] Panzeri A, Bertamini M, Butter S, Levita L, Gibson-Miller J, Vidotto G, et al. Factors impacting resilience as a result of exposure to COVID-19: The ecological resilience model. PLoS One. 2021;**16**(8):e025

[39] Kolb DA. Management and the learning process. California Management Review. 1976;**18**(3):21-31

[40] Hunter JE. Cognitive ability, cognitive aptitudes, job knowledge, and job performance. Journal of Vocational Behavior. 1986;**29**(3):340-362

[41] Hunter JE, Schmidt FL. Intelligence and job performance: Economic and social implications. Psychology Public Policy Law. 1996;**2**(3):447

[42] Birdi K, Allan C, Warr P. Correlates and perceived outcomes of 4 types of employee development activity. The Journal of Applied Psychology. 1997;**82**(6):845

[43] Spreitzer GM, McCall MW, Mahoney JD. Early identification of international executive potential. The Journal of Applied Psychology. 1997;**82**(1):6

[44] Van Velsor E, Moxley RS, Bunker KA. The leader development process. Cent Creat Leadersh Handb Leadersh Dev. 2004;**2**:204-233

[45] Tugade MM, Fredrickson BL. Resilient individuals use positive emotions to bounce back from negative emotional experiences. Journal of Personality and Social Psychology. 2004;**86**(2):320

[46] Tugade MM, Fredrickson BL, Feldman BL. Psychological resilience and positive emotional granularity: Examining the benefits of positive emotions on coping and health. Journal of Personality. 2004;**72**(6):1161-1190

[47] DeRue DS, Ashford SJ, Myers CG. Learning agility: In search of conceptual clarity and theoretical grounding. Industrial and Organizational Psychology. 2012;**5**(3):258-279

[48] Eichinger RW, Lombardo MM. Learning agility as a prime indicator of potential. People and Strategy. 2004;**27**(4):12

[49] Neubert JC, Mainert J, Kretzschmar A, Greiff S. The assessment of 21st century skills in industrial and organizational psychology: Complex and collaborative problem solving. Industrial and Organizational Psychology. 2015;**8**(2):238-268

[50] Baran BE, Bible SC. Agility and Agile: An Introduction for People, Teams, and Organizations. SIOP White Pap Ser. 2019

[51] Gligor D, Gligor N, Holcomb M, Bozkurt S. Distinguishing between the concepts of supply chain agility and resilience: A multidisciplinary literature review. International Journal of Logistics Management. 2019;**30**(2):467-487

[52] Shuja KH, Aqeel M, Jaffar A, Ahmed A. Covid-19 pandemic and impending global mental health implications. Psychiatr Danubina. 2020;**32**(1):32-35

[53] European Centre for Disease Prevention and Control. Guidance on the provision of support for medically and socially vulnerable populations in EU/EEA countries and the United Kingdom during the COVID-19 pandemic Key messages [Internet]. 2020. Available from: https://www.ecdc.europa.eu/sites/default/files/documents/Medically-and-socially-vulnerable-populations-COVID-19.pdf

[54] Buheji M, Buheji A. Planning competency in the new Normal–employability competency in post-COVID-19 pandemic. International Journal of Human Resources Studies. 2020;**10**(2):237-251

[55] Ellwardt L, Präg P. Heterogeneous mental health development during the COVID-19 pandemic in the United Kingdom. Scientific Reports. 2021;**11**(1):15958

[56] Buheji M, Sisk FCW. You and the new normal: Jobs, pandemics, relationship, climate change, success, poverty, leadership and belief in the emerging new world. AuthorHouse; 2020

[57] Buheji M, Ahmed D. Foresight of Coronavirus (COVID-19) opportunities for a better world. American Journal of Economy. 2020;**10**(2):97-108

[58] Caza BB, Milton LP. Resilience at work: Building capacity in the face of adversity. Oxford Handbooks of Positive Organizational Scholarship. 2012:895-908

[59] Mishra P, McDonald K. Career resilience: An integrated review of the empirical literature. Human Resource Development Review. 2017;**16**(3):207-234

[60] Rochat S, Masdonati J, Dauwalder J-P. Determining career resilience. In: Psychology of Career Adaptability, Employability and Resilience. Springer; 2017. pp. 125-141

[61] Kossek EE, Perrigino MB. Resilience: A review using a grounded integrated occupational approach. The Academy of Management Annals. 2016;**10**(1)

[62] Lengelle R, Van der Heijden BIJM, Meijers F. The foundations of career resilience. In: Psychology of Career Adaptability, Employability and Resilience. Springer; 2017. pp. 29-47

[63] Adler A. The Practice And Theory Of Individual Psychology. Routledge; 2013

[64] Britt TW, Shen W, Sinclair RR, Grossman MR, Klieger DM. How much do we really know about employee resilience? Industrial and Organizational Psychology. 2016;**9**(2):378-404

[65] De Vos A, Van der Heijden BIJM. Current thinking on contemporary careers: The key roles of sustainable HRM and sustainability of careers. Current Opinion in Environment Sustainability. 2017;**28**:41-50

[66] Heslin PA, Keating LA, Ashford SJ. How being in learning mode may enable a sustainable career across the lifespan. Journal of Vocational Behavior. 2020;**117**:103324

[67] Lund EM, Forber-Pratt AJ, Wilson C, Mona LR. The COVID-19

pandemic, stress, and trauma in the disability community: A call to action. Rehabilitation Psychology. 2020;**65**(4):313

[68] Chudzikowski K, Gustafsson S, Tams S. Constructing alignment for sustainable careers: Insights from the career narratives of management consultants. Journal of Vocational Behavior. 2020;**117**:103312

[69] Akkermans J, Seibert SE, Mol ST. Tales of the unexpected: Integrating career shocks in the contemporary careers literature. SA Journal of Industrial Psychology. 2018;**44**(1):1-10

[70] Thompson MS, Cooper CL. A Rose by Any Other Name...: A Commentary on Hobfoll's Conservation of Resources Theory. Applied Psychology: An International Review. 2001;**50**(3):408-418

[71] Ferreira RJ. Predictors of social vulnerability: A multilevel analysis [Internet]. Vol. 75, Dissertation Abstracts International Section A: Humanities and Social Sciences. 2015. Available from: http://ovidsp.ovid.com/ovidweb.cgi?T=JS&PAGE=reference&D=psyc12&NEWS=N&AN=2015-99031-188NS-

[72] Hobfoll SE. Conservation of resources: A new attempt at conceptualizing stress. The American Psychologist. 1989;**44**(3):513

[73] Hobfoll SE. The influence of culture, community, and the nested-self in the stress process: Advancing conservation of resources theory. Applied Psychology. 2001;**50**(3):337-421

[74] Yi Y, Lagniton PNP, Ye S, Li E, Xu R-H. COVID-19: What has been learned and to be learned about the novel coronavirus disease. International Journal of Biological Science. 2020;**16**(10):1753-1766

Chapter 20

Self-Compassion and Personal Resources in Workers during the Pandemic: A Multidisciplinary View

Sara Palermo, Annalisa Grandi, Monica Martoni, Alessandro Giannandrea, Luisa Sist, Margherita Zito, Vincenzo Russo and Lara Colombo

Abstract

This chapter focuses on the importance of workers' personal resources during difficult times, such as the pandemic period. In particular, the role of self-compassion in the work context is examined as an important resource for maintaining psycho-physical well-being. Further attention will be given to the impact of self-compassion on neuroscience research and possible organizational interventions to develop and/or support self-compassion in workers.

Keywords: self-compassion, COVID-19, occupational health, interventions, neuroscience

1. Introduction

The recent pandemic has led to an unprecedented situation in terms of public health management, serious impact on the global economy, and also drastic changes in people's lifestyles. The effects on the psycho-physical health of the population have been widely documented internationally. The quality of the sleep-wake cycle has deteriorated [1], depression and anxiety have increased [2], as have symptoms of post-traumatic stress disorder (PTSD) [3]. As a result of the global pandemic, the world of work has changed and tried to adapt to the new scenario. Remote work became a useful tool to keep companies running, but also had an impact on workers' personal lives. The required constant availability, the difficult detachment from work and also the experience of social isolation [4, 5], indeed affected their mental health [6].

In a challenging context like that of the recent COVID-19 pandemic, it is essential to count on resources that can counterbalance negative consequences. These resources can be social, organizational, or—as we'll see in more detail in this chapter—of personal nature. First, we will deepen the theoretical frameworks that deal with personal resources and we'll show the evidence of the research with respect to the importance of maintaining and developing personal resources in workers. Second, we will look at a particular resource that has recently become the subject of occupational research, namely, self-compassion. Finally, we will address how self-compassion can be fostered in the work context and explore what types of interventions are most effective.

2. Personal resources in the work context

The reality of work has changed fundamentally in recent decades with new forms of contracts, demands for greater flexibility, and the introduction of information technology. Therefore, in order to understand these new work environments, it is essential to use lenses that allow an adequate reading of the relevant work-related factors. This is precisely the direction of the job demands-resources (JD-R) theory, proposed by Bakker and Demerouti [7] which has been widely validated by scientific evidence in the occupational field. This theoretical framework holds that each job has specific demands and resources that characterize it. Job demands deal with those aspects of work that require physical and/or psychological effort; whereas work resources are linked to those aspects of work that are functional for the achievement of professional goals, stimulate personal development and growth, and balance the negative effects of job demands [7]. Resources, in particular, can also be of a personal nature, other than work. The issue of resources and their importance in maintaining individual well-being is tackled by Hobfoll, who developed the conservation of resources (COR) theory [8, 9]. The COR theory states that individuals are inclined to protect their own resources (personal, social, and material) and acquire new ones [10]. According to the author, there are four basic principles that define this theory. The first principle holds that the loss of resources has a far greater and more rapid impact on the individual than their acquisition. This seems to have an evolutionary basis: even small losses can threaten survival from an evolutionary perspective. The second principle states that people must invest their resources to prevent the loss of resources, to recover from the loss of resources, and to increase resources. The third principle argues that in situations where the loss of resources is high, the gain of resources is more significant. The last principle states that when people consume their resources, they become defensive, aggressive, and irrational in order to preserve their self [11]. From this theoretical framework, it follows that people with more resources are less vulnerable to the loss of resources and are more able to obtain them in any case; since the loss of resources has a greater impact than the gain of resources and stress increases when resource loss occurs, individuals and organizations are in a loss spiral; finally, since the process of gaining resources has less impact and is slower, the spiral of gaining resources can develop slowly [11]. This framework states that resources can mitigate the relationship between demands (threats) and negative outcomes, which is consistent with the assumptions of the JD-R theory [12].

In accordance with the COR theory, personal resources are helpful because they can protect individuals from stressful events [9]. The role of personal resources in maintaining workers' well-being has been studied in various contexts, such as academia [13], education [14, 15], social work [16], health care [17–19], and mental health [20, 21]. Among the personal resources that have been most studied in the occupational context is optimism, i.e., a positive attitude toward life [22]. Optimists feel confident about meeting life's challenges and are more likely to maintain a balanced perspective during difficult times [23]. Research has shown that optimism is positively associated with work happiness [24], engagement [25], performance [26, 27], and job satisfaction [24, 28, 29], and negatively associated with occupational stress [30] and burnout [17, 18, 31]. The role of optimism in protecting against exhaustion has also been noted in recent studies related to work in the pandemic context [32, 33]. Another personal resource that has recently become of interest in the occupational context is humor, i.e., a lighthearted attitude toward ideas or life events [34]. Humor can be a useful coping strategy to relieve stress [35], and it can also facilitate communication when it would be too risky to be direct [36]. Relying on humor in situations of intense traumatic and emotional impact has been shown to be a functional coping strategy to maintain individuals' well-being among funeral professionals [37], emergency personnel [38], and body handlers [39]. In a meta-analysis on humor in the workplace, this personal resource was found to be positively associated with group cohesion, satisfaction, and job performance, while negatively associated with stress, burnout, and work withdrawal [40]. Humor was also found to be an important factor in balancing perceived stress and exhaustion during the COVID-19 pandemic [32, 41, 42].

There are many personal resources that are studied in the work context (e.g., social support, resilience, self-efficacy, and to name a few), but one particular resource has attracted research interest in recent years, namely, self-compassion, an attitude of kindness toward oneself when experiencing difficult moments.

3. Self-compassion: a recent interest for an ancient practice

The practice of self-compassion, which originated in Eastern culture, began to attract the interest of the West about twenty years ago. This practice is deeply rooted in the Buddhist tradition and has undergone some changes over the centuries. Originally—according to textual sources from the 5th to 3rd century BC—, this meditation process aimed at awakening compassion as a "radiation in all directions" [43]. The focus was thus on subjective experience, not toward a specific object. It was only in later times that the meditation practice became focused on individuals. In the *Sarvāstivāda* and *Theravāda* exegesis, as explained by Anālayo and Dhammadinnā [43], the suggested meditation pattern was to direct compassion first to a friend, then, progressively, to a neutral person, to a hostile or "difficult" person, and finally to all beings. In the *Theravāda* text, a reference to "oneself" also appears in the description of *mettā* [43], namely, a meditation aimed at cultivating loving-kindness [44]. The authors believe that the practice of *mettā* first directed toward oneself is due to a mistranslation of a Pāli word [43]: since meditation is considered a radiation, the practitioner should have achieved a certain level of self-acceptance to overcome aversion and ill will, therefore there is no need to direct *mettā* toward oneself. The distinction between compassion for oneself and for other people arises "accidentally," so to speak. Buddhist modernism, influenced by the *Theravāda* model, is much evident the importance to cultivate compassion toward oneself. Therefore, compassion to ourselves is considered the first step to a wider feeling of compassion to others [45, 46].

In Western society, compassion is often equated with the concept of empathy. When a person empathizes with another person, it means that he or she is experiencing the other person's emotional state, or in other words, that he or she is *feeling into* the other person's experience [47, 48]. Instead, an individual experiences the feeling of compassion when he or she sees the suffering of another person and desires to help in order to soothe that suffering [49]. In other words, there is a *feeling with* in the nature of compassion [48].

When we speak of self-compassion, as we have seen, we are referring to the practice of compassion directed toward ourselves. In recent years, Kristin Neff [50, 51] has begun to study self-compassion in order to explore what this concept entails and what kind of relationship exists between it and psychological functioning. According to the researcher, the construct of self-compassion is defined by three dimensions: self-kindness, common humanity, and mindfulness [50]. Self-kindness means showing gentleness and understanding toward ourselves instead of harshness and disapproval. Feeling connected to the world when we have experiences—especially unpleasant ones—is part of common humanity, namely, seeing our feelings as part of the human experience and not isolated. The third characteristic that qualifies self-compassion is being present to our feelings and thoughts—even the unwelcome ones—without identifying with them [50]. These three aspects, although different, can influence and reinforce each other. The detachment that mindfulness requires can promote self-kindness and reduce self-criticism in favor of self-understanding. In addition, because mindfulness leads to a more balanced perspective, it can help individuals feel more connected to the world rather than isolated from it. Self-kindness and common humanity can also promote mindfulness. When we are gentler with ourselves, we are more likely to accept ourselves and therefore less likely to be touched by negative emotions: these conditions can make it easier for us to consciously notice what we are experiencing without avoiding our feelings. Similarly, recognizing that pain and suffering are everyday human experiences helps to rebalance our perspective and to be mindful of our thoughts and feelings without identifying with them [50].

In defining the construct of self-compassion, it is also important to highlight from which concepts it differs. For example, research has shown a remarkable correlation between self-compassion and self-esteem [52, 53]. This correlation is likely due to the fact that both are positive self-attitudes [54]. The study by Leary et al. [52] showed that self-compassion—not self-esteem—was associated with a more positive evaluation of others and lower negative affect when receiving unpleasant feedback. Moreover, important differences emerged between the two constructs when compared to the attribution of negative events. People with high self-esteem tended to relate negative outcomes less to themselves, whereas people with high self-compassion tended to do the opposite. This result shows that people with high self-esteem may also have a selfish attitude to make themselves feel better, while people with high self-compassion are able to be gentle with themselves and also take personal responsibility [52].

Gilbert and Irons [55], instead, on the other hand, attribute the difference between self-compassion and self-esteem to the different physiological systems with which they are associated. According to the authors, self-compassion deactivates "the threat system,"—related to feeling insecure and defensive—and activates "the self-soothing system"—related to feeling safe. In brief, both self-compassion and self-esteem are associated with well-being, but while the first is useful to feel safe and secure, the latter makes individuals feel superior and self-confident. Thus, given the downsides of high of self-esteem, it would be useful to consider self-compassion as "a healthy attitude toward oneself," as Neff [50] suggests, in part because it is an easier resource to acquire.

Another concept from which self-compassion should be distinguished is self-pity. When people feel self-pity, they are absorbed in their troubles, feeling isolated from the rest of the world: they are the only ones who suffer. Self-pity is associated with egocentrism because people feel separate from others and overemphasize their painful feelings. Self-compassionate people, on the other hand, see their experiences in relation to others and do not over-identify with them, so they have the mental space to give kindness to themselves [50, 53].

Having defined what self-compassion is, we can address its relationship to the well-being of the individual. Indeed, several studies have shown the importance of this personal resource at different stages of the lifespan. Parents with self-compassion are better able to cope with shame and guilt, which are common in difficult parenting situations [56], and also with stress [57], improving their personal well-being. Adolescents who practice self-compassion show less perceived stress, fewer ruminative thoughts, and fewer depression symptoms, but higher positive affect and overall life satisfaction [58, 59]. In young adults—particularly students—self-compassion has been found to be associated with physical and psychological well-being [60, 61], psychological flexibility [62], and lower negative affect [63]. Research has also shown that self-compassion is associated with subjective well-being in older adults [64], even in elders with poor physical health [65].

As research widely demonstrates that self-compassion is a key concept in maintaining individual well-being [66], scientific interest has also increased in the occupational field to determine whether this personal resource can help workers cope with daily job demands. The role of self-compassion has been studied in various professions, such as health care [67, 68], education [69], social work [70, 71], mental health [72, 73], and construction [74]. In general, studies have shown that self-compassion is associated with lower levels of exhaustion—the core component of burnout—[68, 75–79] and higher job satisfaction [68, 78, 80]. Moreover, proactive coping is a promising research topic in the field of self-compassion. For example, it has been suggested that people with greater self-compassion approach life more proactively, which has implications for how people prepare for and cope with negative events [81].

Research on leadership has also found that self-compassionate leaders are perceived as more competent and politer [82].

The importance of self-compassion as a functional strategy has also been noted in challenging events, such as the recent COVID-19 pandemic. Cultivating self-compassion has been shown to be an important resource for protecting workers' mental health [32, 83, 84], mitigating feelings of loneliness in the workplace [85], and promoting occupational quality of life [86].

4. Neurobiological basis of self-compassion: preliminary findings

There is a lack of understanding of the structural and functional neural basis of self-compassion, despite its importance as a protective factor. Neural underpinnings of dispositional self-compassion have never been studied, but similar constructs have been studied in voxel-based morphometry studies [53]. Indeed, not only positive attitudes like self-compassion and self-esteem are highly correlated [50], but self-compassion is closely related to compassion as a more general concept [53].

This suggests that voxel-based morphometry studies of self-esteem and compassion could shed light on self-compassion's neural correlates. The anterior cingulate cortex (ACC), right dorsolateral prefrontal cortex (DLPFC), insula, and right temporo-parietal junction (TPJ) show greater gray matter volume when self-esteem and compassion are elevated [87–89]. Emotion regulation or empathic processes were thought to be associated with these regions [87, 88]. Moreover, according to Guan et al. [90], self-compassion is negatively correlated with gray matter volume in the left DLPFC, largely because self-judgment is reduced. The DLPFC has been previously associated with executive control [91, 92] and emotion regulation [93].

The identification of neural regions supporting dispositional self-compassion may also inform hypotheses about regions whose morphology can be associated with this trait via functional magnetic resonance imaging (fMRI). Several fMRI studies have found that dispositional self-compassion or self-kindness is associated with activation in the DLPFC, dorsal ACC, and posterior cingulate cortex (PCC)/precuneus, regions [94–96] believed to be involved in emotion regulation and self-referential processing [92, 97]. Studies suggest that self-compassion may depend on resources associated with the theory of mind and empathy (such as the insula and TPJ) as well as those responsible for emotion regulation and self-referential processing (such as the DLPFC, ACC, PCC, and Precuneus).

Researchers have therefore found dispositional self-compassion is associated with brain structure in areas that regulate emotion, process self-referential information, and process emotions, indicating possible cognitive and neural mechanisms that underlie self-compassion and shedding new light on how self-compassion works and how it contributes to health.

5. Interventions in the work context

Although research on self-compassion in the organizational field is quite recent, there are several studies in the literature that have allowed the construct to be outlined in this area as well.

According to a recent work by Dodson and Heng [98], the antecedents of self-compassion in the workplace are due to both individual and contextual characteristics. Regarding individual factors, some personality traits such as emotional intelligence [99] and attachment style [100] have been identified; some demographic characteristics also seem to be related to the level of self-compassion in workers, such as having more years of experience [101] and being men [102]. The work environment can also affect workers' self-compassion. For example, workload may be a barrier to the practice of self-compassion because it reduces the time available to engage in self-care strategies [103]. On the other hand, organizational support appears to be an element that facilitates the practice of self-compassion: working with supportive and compassionate colleagues helps workers engage more in self-compassion [103, 104].

The practice of self-compassion has been shown to have positive effects on the work environment. The greatest benefits are related to the psycho-physical workers' well-being: lower depression [74], lower exhaustion [68, 75–79], better self-reported physical health [105], and better sleep quality [106]. Among workers in close contact with suffering, self-compassion was also associated with lower compassion fatigue and greater compassion satisfaction [107].

Scientific evidence has amply demonstrated the importance of this personal resource for employee well-being. So how can self-compassion be developed and/or promoted in work environments? Although the use of interventions to enhance workers' personal resources is a relatively new trend [108], a number of training programs can already be identified that have produced effective results. Among the most widely tested interventions, even in work contexts, is Joh Kabat-Zinn's Mindfulness-Based Stress Reduction (MBSR) [109, 110]. The intervention was developed to reduce suffering in patients with chronic pain and consists of an 8-week program that includes both group work sessions and homework. The program consists of focusing attention on the here-and-now—that is, paying attention to the body's sensations, to emotions, thoughts, sounds, and breath—and taking distance from self-judgments and rumination. A recent systematic review considered more than 20 studies reporting the use of this methodology in work contexts [77]. Results show that this type of intervention benefits workers' well-being, particularly through lower levels of exhaustion, stress, depression, and anxiety, as well as increases in mindfulness, personal accomplishment, sleep quality, relaxation, and self-compassion [77].

Another widely used program, inspired by MBSR, is the Mindful Self-Compassion (MSC), developed by Neff and Germer [111]. It also consists of an 8-week commitment that includes learning both formal (sitting meditation) and informal (in daily life) practices of self-compassion. Compared to MBSR, this program is more focused on self-compassion and only secondarily on mindfulness [111]. While MBSR is systematic mindfulness training [112] and both MBSR and MSC programs focus on how to approach suffering with a mindful, non-overidentified attitude, MSC considers the experiencer rather than the experience. MSC emphasizes how to respond to personal suffering with kindness, acceptance, and caring during meditations but also in daily life by practicing "self-compassion in action" [113]. Results from samples of workers showed that after participating in the program, levels of self-compassion and mindfulness increased [107].

The approach proposed by Paul Gilbert should also be mentioned. The Compassionate Mind Training (CMT) was originally developed to help individuals with high levels of shame and self-criticism. The course lasts 8 weeks and is focused on developing compassion for oneself. The main practices and exercises for attaining mindfulness are focusing on the calming rhythm of breathing and the use of compassionate imagery. Six modules are provided, ranging from exploring the concept of compassion, to understanding how emotions work and how to manage them, to dealing with self-criticism through self-compassion [114]. Several studies have shown what benefits the adoption of this program can bring to the workers involved: less burnout, depression, anxiety, intrusion and avoidance symptoms, and self-criticism, higher professional life satisfaction, and self-compassion [78, 115–118].

Despite (i) the lack of comparability between studies due to differences in content, modes of implementation, and quality [98, 119–121], and (ii) fewer studies that explicitly focused on self-compassion as a primary outcome it has been recorded change in baseline self-compassion scores following compassion- or mindfulness-based interventions, raising the possibility that organizations can help employees improve their self-compassion skills.

6. Conclusions

Focusing on the role of personal resources is a very important issue for maintaining the well-being of workers, especially in a challenging period such as the COVID-19 pandemic. In order to support employees' psycho-physical health, improve their job performance and consequently increase productivity, employers can promote interventions aimed at developing and improving personal resources. Among these resources, self-compassion can be considered an adaptive strategy for well-being and positive psychological functioning, especially in stressful and demanding situations (i.e., assuming a role in the coping process) [81]. This type of improvement strategy/intervention aims to promote a culture of self-care in the work environment, i.e., a set of professional practices to promote personal well-being [122–124].

Conflict of interest

The authors declare no conflict of interest.

Author details

Sara Palermo[1,2*†], Annalisa Grandi[1†], Monica Martoni[3], Alessandro Giannandrea[4], Luisa Sist[5], Margherita Zito[6], Vincenzo Russo[6] and Lara Colombo[1]

1 Department of Psychology, University of Turin, Turin, Italy

2 Neuroradiology Unit, Diagnostic and Technology Department, Fondazione IRCCS Istituto Neurologico Carlo Besta, Milan, Italy

3 Department of Experimental, Diagnostic and Specialty Medicine, University of Bologna, Bologna, Italy

4 Department of Psychology, Sapienza University of Rome, Rome, Italy

5 Department of Biomedical and Neuromotor Sciences, University of Bologna, Bologna, Italy

6 Department of Business, Law, Economics and Consumer Behaviour "Carlo A. Ricciardi", Università IULM, Milan, Italy

*Address all correspondence to: sara.palermo@unito.it

† These authors contributed equally.

References

[1] Jahrami HA, Alhaj OA, Humood AM, Alenezi AF, Fekih-Romdhane F, AlRasheed MM, et al. Sleep disturbances during the COVID-19 pandemic: A systematic review, meta-analysis, and meta-regression. Sleep Medicine Reviews. 2022;**62**:101591

[2] Necho M, Tsehay M, Birkie M, Biset G, Tadesse E. Prevalence of anxiety, depression, and psychological distress among the general population during the COVID-19 pandemic: A systematic review and meta-analysis. International Journal of Social Psychiatry. 2021;**67**(7):892-906

[3] Zhang L, Pan R, Cai Y, Pan J. The prevalence of post-traumatic stress disorder in the general population during the COVID-19 pandemic: A systematic review and single-arm meta-analysis. Psychiatry Investigation. 2021;**18**(5):426-433

[4] Barone Gibbs B, Kline CE, Huber KA, Paley JL, Perera S. Covid-19 shelter-at-home and work, lifestyle and well-being in desk workers. Occupational Medicine. 2021;**71**(2):86-94

[5] Charalampous M, Grant CA, Tramontano C, Michailidis E. Systematically reviewing remote e-workers' well-being at work: A multidimensional approach. European Journal of Work and Organizational Psychology. 2019;**28**(1):51-73

[6] Grandi A, Guidetti G, Converso D, Bosco N, Colombo L. I nearly died laughing: Humor in funeral industry operators. Current Psychology. 2021;**40**(12):6098-6109

[7] Bakker AB, Demerouti E. Job demands-resources theory. In: Chen PY, Cooper CL, editors. Wellbeing: A Complete Reference Guide. New York: John Wiley & Sons, Ltd; 2014. pp. 37-64

[8] Hobfoll SE. Personal and social resources and the ecology of stress resistance. In: Shaver P, editor. Review of Personality and Social Psychology. Vol. 6. Beverly Hills, CA: Sage; 1985. pp. 265-290

[9] Hobfoll SE. Conservation of resources: A new attempt at conceptualizing stress. American Psychologist. 1989;**44**(3):513-524

[10] Halbesleben JRB, Neveu JP, Paustian-Underdahl SC, Westman M. Getting to the "COR": Understanding the role of resources in conservation of resources theory. Journal of Management. 2014;**40**(5):1334-1364

[11] Hobfoll SE, Halbesleben J, Neveu JP, Westman M. Conservation of resources in the organizational context: The reality of resources and their consequences. Annual Review of Organizational Psychology and Organizational Behavior. 2018;**5**:103-128

[12] Xanthopoulou D, Bakker AB, Demerouti E, Schaufeli WB. The role of personal resources in the job demands-resources model. International Journal of Stress Management. 2007;**14**(2):121-141

[13] Stelmokienė A, Genevičiūtė-Janonė G, Gustainienė L, Kovalčikienė K. Job demands-resources and personal resources as risk and safety factors for the professional burnout among university teachers. Pedagogika. 2019;**134**(2):25-44

[14] De Stasio S, Fiorilli C, Benevene P, Uusitalo-Malmivaara L, Chiacchio CD. Burnout in special needs teachers at kindergarten and primary school:

Investigating the role of personal resources and work wellbeing. Psychology in the Schools. 2017;**54**(5):472-486

[15] Lorente Prieto L, Salanove Soria M, Martinez Martinez I, Schaufeli W. Extension of the Job Demands-Resources model in the prediction of burnout and engagement among teachers over time. Psicothema. 2008;**20**(3):354-360

[16] Ben-Porat A, Itzhaky H. Burnout among trauma social workers: The contribution of personal and environmental resources. Journal of Social Work. 2015;**15**(6):606-620

[17] Contreras F, Espinosa JC, Esguerra GA. Could personal resources influence work engagement and burnout? A Study in a Group of Nursing Staff. SAGE Open. 2020;**10**(1). DOI: 10.1177/2158244019900563

[18] Garrosa E, Moreno-Jiménez B, Rodríguez-Muñoz A, Rodríguez-Carvajal R. Role stress and personal resources in nursing: A cross-sectional study of burnout and engagement. International Journal of Nursing Studies. 2011;**48**(4):479-489

[19] Lee H, Song R, Cho YS, Lee GZ, Daly B. A comprehensive model for predicting burnout in Korean nurses. Journal of Advanced Nursing. 2003;**44**(5):534-545

[20] Emery S, Wade TD, Mclean S. Association among therapist beliefs, personal resources and burnout in clinical psychologists. Behaviour Change. 2009;**26**(2):83-96

[21] Thompson I, Amatea E, Thompson E. Personal and contextual predictors of mental health counselors' compassion fatigue and burnout. Journal of Mental Health Counseling. 2014;**36**(1):58-77

[22] Carver CS, Scheier MF, Segerstrom SC. Optimism. Clinical Psychology Review. 2010;**30**(7):879-889

[23] Scheier MF, Carver CS, Bridges MW. Optimism, pessimism, and psychological well-being. In: Chang EC, editor. Optimism & Pessimism: Implications for Theory, Research, and P. Washington, DC, US: American Psychological Association; 2001. pp. 189-216

[24] Youssef CM, Luthans F. Positive organizational behavior in the workplace: The impact of hope, optimism, and resilience. Journal of Management. 2007;**33**(5):774-800

[25] Medlin B, Green KW. Enhancing performance through goal setting, engagement, and optimism. Industrial Management & Data Systems. 2009;**109**(7):943-956

[26] Luthans KW, Lebsack SA, Lebsack RR. Positivity in healthcare: Relation of optimism to performance. Journal of Health, Organisation and Management. 2008;**22**(2):178-188

[27] West BJ, Patera JL, Carsten MK. Team level positivity: Investigating positive psychological capacities and team level outcomes. Journal of Organizational Behavior. 2009;**30**(2):249-267

[28] Glass N. Investigating women nurse academics' experiences in universities: The importance of hope, optimism, and career resilience for workplace satisfaction. Annual Review of Nursing Education. 2007;**5**:111-136

[29] Kluemper DH, Little LM, DeGroot T. State or trait: Effects of state optimism on job-related outcomes. Journal of Organizational Behavior. 2009;**30**(2):209-231

[30] Avey JB, Luthans F, Jensen SM. Psychological capital: A positive resource

for combating employee stress and turnover. Human Resource Management. 2009;**48**(5):677-693

[31] Grau A, Suñer R, García MM. Burnout syndrome in health workers and relationship with personal and environmental factors. Gaceta Sanitaria. 2005;**19**(6):463

[32] Grandi A, Zito M, Sist L, Martoni M, Russo V, Colombo L. Wellbeing in Workers during COVID-19 Pandemic: The mediating role of self-compassion in the relationship between personal resources and exhaustion. International Journal of Environmental Research and Public Health. 2022;**19**(3):1714

[33] Özdemir Ş, Kerse G. The effects of COVID-19 process on health care workers: Analysing of the relationships between optimism, job stress and emotional exhaustion. International and Multidisciplinary Journal of Social Sciences. 2020;**9**(2):178-201

[34] Martin RA. The Psychology of Humor: An Integrative Approach. Amsterdam: Elsevier Academic Press; 2007

[35] Lefcourt HM, Martin RA. Humor and Life Stress: Antidote to Adversity. New York: Springer-Verlag; 1986

[36] Mulkay M. On Humor: Its Nature and Its Place in Modern Society. New York: Basil Blackwell; 1988

[37] Grandi A, Sist L, Martoni M, Colombo L. Mental Health Outcomes in Northern Italian Workers during the COVID-19 Outbreak: The role of demands and resources in predicting depression. Sustainability. 2021;**13**(20):11321

[38] Scott T. Expression of humour by emergency personnel involved in sudden deathwork. Mortality. 2007;**12**(4):350-364

[39] McCarroll JE, Ursano RJ, Wright KM, Fullerton CS. Handling bodies after violent death: Strategies for coping. American Journal of Orthopsychiatry. 1993;**63**(2):209-214

[40] Mesmer-Magnus J, Glew DJ, Viswesvaran C. A meta-analysis of positive humor in the workplace. Journal of Managerial Psychology. 2012;**27**(2):155-190

[41] Canestrari C, Bongelli R, Fermani A, Riccioni I, Bertolazzi A, Muzi M, et al. Coronavirus disease stress among Italian healthcare workers: The role of coping humor. Frontiers in Psychology. 2021;**11**:601574

[42] McFadden P, Ross J, Moriarty J, Mallett J, Schroder H, Ravalier J, et al. The role of coping in the wellbeing and work-related quality of life of UK health and social care workers during COVID-19. International Journal of Environmental Research and Public Health. 2021;**18**(2):815

[43] Anālayo B, Dhammadinnā B. From compassion to self-compassion: A text-historical perspective. Mindfulness. 2021;**12**(6):1350-1360

[44] Gethin R. The Foundations of Buddhism. Oxford: Oxford University Press; 1998

[45] Kornfield J. A Path with Heart: A Guide Through the Perils and Promises of Spiritual Life. New York: Bantam Book; 1993

[46] Wallace AB. Boundless Heart: The Cultivation of the Four Immeasurables. Ithaca, NY: Snow Lion Publications; 1999

[47] Stevens L, Benjamin J. The brain that longs to care for others: The

current neuroscience of compassion. In: Stevens L, Woodruff C, editors. The Neuroscience of Empathy, Compassion, and Self-Compassion. London: Elsevier Inc.; 2018. pp. 53-89

[48] Stevens L, Woodruff C. What is this feeling that i have for myself and for others? Contemporary perspectives on empathy, compassion, and self-compassion, and their absence. In: Stevens L, Woodruff C, editors. The Neuroscience of Empathy, Compassion, and Self-Compassion. London: Elsevier Inc.; 2018. pp. 1-21

[49] Goetz JL, Keltner D, Simon-Thomas E. Compassion: An evolutionary analysis and empirical review. Psychological Bulletin. 2010;**136**(3):351-374

[50] Neff K. Self-compassion: An alternative conceptualization of a healthy attitude toward oneself. Self and Identity. 2003a;**2**(2):85-101

[51] Neff K. Self-compassion and psychological well-being. Constructivism in Human Sciences. 2004;**9**(2):27-37

[52] Leary MR, Tate EB, Adams CE, Allen AB, Hancock J. Self-compassion and reactions to unpleasant self-relevant events: The implications of treating oneself kindly. Journal of Personality and Social Psychology. 2007;**92**(5):887-904

[53] Neff K. The development and validation of a scale to measure self-compassion. Self and Identity. 2003b;**2**(3):223-250

[54] Neff KD. Self-compassion, self-esteem, and well-being. Social and Personality Psychology Compass. 2011;**5**(1):1-12

[55] Gilbert P, Irons C. Focused therapies and compassionate mind training for shame and self-attacking. In: Gilbert P, editor. Compassion: Conceptualisations, Research and Use in Psychotherapy. London: Routledge; 2005. pp. 263-325

[56] Sirois FM, Bögels S, Emerson LM. Self-compassion improves parental well-being in response to challenging parenting events. Journal of Psychology: Interdisciplinary and Applied. 2019;**153**(3):327-341

[57] Neff KD, Faso DJ. Self-compassion and well-being in parents of children with autism. Mindfulness. 2015;**6**:938-947

[58] Bluth K, Blanton PW. The influence of self-compassion on emotional well-being among early and older adolescent males and females. The Journal of Positive Psychology. 2015;**10**(3): 219-230

[59] Galla BM. Within-person changes in mindfulness and self-compassion predict enhanced emotional well-being in healthy, but stressed adolescents. Journal of Adolescence. 2016;**49**:204-217

[60] Booker JA, Dunsmore JC. Testing direct and indirect ties of self-compassion with subjective well-being. Journal of Happiness Studies. 2019;**20**(5):1563-1585

[61] Hall CW, Row KA, Wuensch KL, Godley KR, Hall CW, Row KA, et al. The role of self-compassion in physical and psychological well-being: The role of self-compassion in physical and psychological well-being. The Journal of Psychology. 2013;**3980**(May):311-323

[62] Marshall E-J, Brockman RN. The relationships between psychological flexibility, self-compassion, and emotional well-being. Journal of Cognitive Psychotherapy. 2016;**30**(1):60-72

[63] Hope N, Koestner R, Milyavskaya M. The role of self-compassion in goal pursuit and well-being among university Freshmen. Self and Identity. 2014;**13**(5):579-593

[64] Homan KJ. Self-compassion and psychological well-being in older adults. Journal of Adult Development. 2016;**23**(2):111-119

[65] Allen AB, Goldwasser ER, Leary MR. Self-compassion and well-being among older adults. Self and Identity. 2012;**11**(4):428-453

[66] Zessin U, Dickhäuser O, Garbade S. The relationship between self-compassion and well-being: A meta-analysis. Applied Psychology Health and Well-Being. 2015;**7**(3):340-364

[67] Conversano C, Ciacchini Ŕ, Orrù G, Di Giuseppe M, Gemignani A, Poli A. Mindfulness, compassion, and self-compassion among health care professionals: What's new? a systematic review. Frontiers in Psychology. 2020;**11**:1683

[68] Raab K. Mindfulness, self-compassion, and empathy among health care professionals: A review of the literature. Journal of Health Care Chaplaincy. 2014;**20**(3):95-108

[69] Jennings PA. Early childhood teachers' well-being, mindfulness, and self-compassion in relation to classroom quality and attitudes towards challenging students. Mindfulness. 2015;**6**(2):732-743

[70] Miller JJ, Lee J, Niu C, Grise E, Molly O. Self-compassion as a predictor of self-care: A study of social work clinicians. Clinical Social Work Journal. 2019;**47**(4):321-331

[71] Miller JJ, Lee J, Shalash N, Poklembova Z. Self-compassion among social workers. Journal of Social Work. 2020;**20**(4):448-462

[72] Finlay-Jones AL, Rees CS, Kane RT. Self-Compassion, emotion regulation and stress among australian psychologists: Testing an emotion regulation model of self-compassion using structural equation modeling. PLoS One. 2015;**10**(7):1-19

[73] Kotera Y, Maxwell-jones R, Edwards A, Knutton N. Burnout in professional psychotherapists: Relationships with self-compassion, work – life balance, and telepressure. International Journal of Environmental Research and Public Health. 2021;**18**(10):5308

[74] Kotera Y, Green P, Sheffield D. Mental Health Shame of UK Construction Workers: Relationship with masculinity, work motivation, and self-compassion. Journal of Work and Organizational Psychology. 2019;**35**(2):135-143

[75] Barnard LK, Curry JF. The relationship of clergy burnout to self-compassion and other personality dimensions. Pastoral Psychology. 2012;**61**(2):149-163

[76] Hashem Z, Zeinoun P. Self-compassion explains less burnout among healthcare professionals. Mindfulness. 2020;**11**(11):2542-2551

[77] Janssen M, Heerkens Y, Kuijer W, Van Der Heijden B, Engels J. Effects of mindfulness-based stress reduction on employees' mental health: A systematic review. PLoS One. 2018;**13**(1):e0191332

[78] Matos M, Palmeira L, Albuquerque I, Cunha M, Pedroso Lima M, Galhardo A, et al. Building compassionate schools: Pilot study of a compassionate mind training intervention to promote teachers' well-being. Mindfulness. 2022;**13**(1):145-161

[79] Prudenzi A, Graham D, Flaxman PE, O'Connor DB. Wellbeing, burnout, and safe practice among healthcare professionals: Predictive influences of mindfulness, values, and self-compassion. Psychology, Health and Medicine. 2021

[80] Steinberg BA, Klatt M, Duchemin AM. Feasibility of a mindfulness-based intervention for surgical intensive care unit personnel. American Journal of Critical Care. 2017;**26**(1):10-18

[81] Allen A, Leary M. Self-compassion, stress, and coping. Social and Personality Psychology Compass. 2010;**4**(2):107-118

[82] Lanaj K, Jennings RE, Ashford SJ, Krishnan S. When leader self-care begets other care: Leader role self-compassion and helping at work. The Journal of Applied Psychology. 2022;**107**(9): 1543-1560

[83] Kotera Y, Mayer CH, Vanderheiden E. Cross-cultural comparison of mental health between German and South African employees: Shame, self-compassion, work engagement, and work motivation. Frontiers in Psychology. 2021;**12**:627851

[84] Lau BHP, Chan CLW, Ng SM. Self-compassion buffers the adverse mental health impacts of COVID-19-related threats: Results from a cross-sectional survey at the first peak of Hong Kong's outbreak. Frontiers in Psychiatry. 2020;**11**(November):1-8

[85] Andel SA, Shen W, Arvan ML. Depending on your own kindness: The moderating role of self-compassion on the within-person consequences of work loneliness during the COVID-19 pandemic. Journal of Occupational Health Psychology. 2021;**26**(4): 276-290

[86] Lluch-sanz C, Galiana L, Vidal-blanco G, Sansó N. Psychometric properties of the self-compassion scale — Short form: Study of its role as a protector of Spanish nurses professional quality of life and well-being during the COVID-19 pandemic. Nursing Reports. 2022;**12**(1):65-76

[87] Agroskin D, Klackl J, Jonas E. The self-liking brain: A VBM study on the structural substrate of self-esteem. PLoS One. 2014;**9**(1):e86430

[88] Hou X, Allen TA, Wei D, Huang H, Wang K, DeYoung CG, et al. Trait compassion is associated with the neural substrate of empathy. Cognitive, Affective, & Behavioral Neuroscience. 2017;**17**(5):1018-1027

[89] Leung MK, Chan CC, Yin J, Lee CF, So KF, Lee TM. Increased gray matter volume in the right angular and posterior parahippocampal gyri in loving-kindness meditators. Social Cognitive and Affective Neuroscience. 2013;**8**(1):34-39

[90] Guan F, Liu G, Pedersen WS, Chen O, Zhao S, Sui J, et al. Neurostructural correlates of dispositional self-compassion. Neuropsychologia. 2021;**160**:107978

[91] Diamond A. Executive functions. Annual Review of Psychology. 2013;**64**:135-168

[92] Sui J, Gu X. Self as object: Emerging trends in self research. Trends in Neurosciences. 2017;**40**(11):643-653

[93] Golkar A, Lonsdorf TB, Olsson A, Lindstrom KM, Berrebi J, Fransson P, et al. Distinct contributions of the dorsolateral prefrontal and orbitofrontal cortex during emotion regulation. PLoS One. 2012;**7**(11):e48107

[94] Berry MP, Lutz J, Schuman-Olivier Z, Germer C, Pollak S, Edwards RR, et al. Brief self-compassion training alters

neural responses to evoked pain for chronic low back pain: A Pilot Study. Pain Medicine (Malden, Mass.). 2020;**21**(10):2172-2185

[95] Liu G, Zhang N, Teoh JY, Egan C, Zeffiro TA, Davidson RJ, et al. Self-compassion and dorsolateral prefrontal cortex activity during sad self-face recognition in depressed adolescents. Psychological Medicine. 2022;**52**(5):864-873

[96] Williams K, Elliott R, McKie S, Zahn R, Barnhofer T, Anderson IM. Changes in the neural correlates of self-blame following mindfulness-based cognitive therapy in remitted depressed participants. Psychiatry Research: Neuroimaging. 2020;**304**:111152

[97] Yankouskaya A, Sui J. Self-positivity or self-negativity as a function of the medial prefrontal cortex. Brain Sciences. 2021;**11**(2):264

[98] Dodson SJ, Heng YT. Self-compassion in organizations: A review and future research agenda. Journal of Organizational Behavior. 2022;**43**(2):168-196

[99] Di Fabio A, Saklofske DH. The relationship of compassion and self-compassion with personality and emotional intelligence. Personality and Individual Differences. 2021;**169**(2020):110109

[100] Reizer A. Bringing self-kindness into the Bringing Self-Kindness Into the Workplace: Exploring the Mediating Role of Self-Compassion in the Associations Between Attachment and Organizational Outcomes. Frontiers in Psychology. 2019;**10**:1148

[101] Lianekhammy J, Miller JJ, Lee J, Pope N, Barnhart S, Grise-Owens E. Exploring the self-compassion of health-care social workers: How do they fare? Social Work in Health Care. 2018;**57**(7):563-580

[102] Yarnell LM, Stafford RE, Neff KD, Reilly ED, Knox MC, Mullarkey M. Meta-analysis of gender differences in self-compassion. Self and Identity. 2015;**14**(5):499-520

[103] Egan H, Keyte R, McGowan K, Peters L, Lemon N, Parsons S, et al. 'You Before Me': A Qualitative Study of Health Care Professionals' and Students' Understanding and Experiences of Compassion in the Workplace, Self-compassion, Self-care and Health Behaviours. Health Professions Education. 2019;**5**(3):225-236

[104] Killian KD. Helping till it hurts? A multimethod study of compassion fatigue, burnout, and self-care in clinicians working with trauma survivors. Traumatology. 2008;**14**(2):32-44

[105] Wayment HA, Huffman AH, Irving LH. Self-rated health among unemployed adults: The role of Quiet Ego, self-compassion, and post-traumatic growth. Occupational Health Science. 2018;**2**(3):247-267

[106] Kemper KJ, Mo X, Khayat R. Are mindfulness and self-compassion associated with sleep and resilience in health professionals? Journal of Alternative and Complementary Medicine. 2015;**21**(8):496-503

[107] Delaney MC. Caring for the caregivers: Evaluation of the effect of an eight-week pilot mindful self-compassion (MSC) training program on nurses' compassion fatigue and resilience. PLoS One. 2018;**13**(11):1-20

[108] Gilbert E, Foulk T, Bono J. Building personal resources through interventions: An integrative review. Journal of Organizational Behavior. 2018;**39**(2):214-228

[109] Kabat-Zinn J. An outpatient program in behavioral medicine for chronic pain patients based on the practice of mindfulness meditation: Theoretical considerations and preliminary results. General Hospital Psychiatry. 1982;**4**:33-42

[110] Kabat-Zinn J. Mindfulness-based interventions in context: Past, present, and future. Clinical Psychology: Science and Practice. 2003;**10**(2):144-156

[111] Neff KD, Germer CK. A pilot study and randomized controlled trial of the mindful self-compassion program. Journal of Clinical Psychology. 2013;**69**(1):28-44

[112] Crane RS, Brewer J, Feldman C, Kabat-Zinn J, Santorelli S, Williams JM, et al. What defines mindfulness-based programs? The warp and the weft. Psychological Medicine. 2017;**47**(6):990-999

[113] Germer C. The Mindful Path to Self-compassion: Freeing Yourself from Destructive Thoughts and Emotions. New York: Guilford Press; 2009

[114] Gilbert P, Procter S. Compassionate mind training for people with high shame and self-criticism: Overview and pilot study of a group therapy approach. Clinical Psychology & Psychotherapy. 2006;**13**(6):353-379

[115] Beaumont E, Durkin M, McAndrew S, Martin CR. Using compassion focused therapy as an adjunct to Trauma-Focused CBT for Fire Service personnel suffering with trauma-related symptoms. Cognitive Behaviour Therapist. 2016;**9**:e34

[116] Hollins Martin CJ, Beaumont E, Norris G, Cullen G. Teaching compassionate mind training to help midwives cope with traumatic clinical incidents. British Journal of Midwifery. 2021;**29**(1):26-35

[117] Maratos FA, Montague J, Ashra H, Welford M, Wood W, Barnes C, et al. Evaluation of a compassionate mind training intervention with school teachers and support staff. Mindfulness. 2019;**10**(11):2245-2258

[118] Matos M, Albuquerque I, Galhardo A, Cunha M, Lima MP, Palmeira L, et al. Nurturing compassion in schools: A randomized controlled trial of the effectiveness of a Compassionate Mind Training program for teachers. PLoS ONE. 2022;**17**(3):1-36

[119] Kotera Y, Van Gordon W. Effects of self-compassion training on work-related well-being: A systematic review. Frontiers in Psychology. 2021;**12**:630798

[120] Rudaz M, Twohig M, Ong C, Levin M. Mindfulness and acceptance-based trainings for fostering self-care and reducing stress in mental health professionals: A systematic review. Journal of Contextual Behavioral Science. 2017;**6**(4):380-390

[121] Wasson R, Barratt C, O'Brien W. Effects of mindfulness-based interventions on self-compassion in health care professionals: A meta-analysis. Mindfulness. 2020;**11**(8):1914-1934

[122] Barnett JE, Cooper N. Creating a culture of self-care. Clinical Psychology: Science and Practice. 2009;**16**(1):16-20

[123] Bressi SK, Vaden ER. Reconsidering Self care. Clinical Social Work Journal. 2017;**45**(1):33-38

[124] Maltzman S. An organizational self-care model: Practical suggestions for development and implementation. The Counseling Psychologist. 2011;**39**(2): 303-319

Chapter 21

Perspective Chapter: Cultural Competence and the Education of CSD Professionals in Times of COVID-19

Fernanda Dreux M. Fernandes, Maria Vitoria do Amaral and Cibelle La Higuera Amato

Abstract

This manuscript aims to discuss the experiences and expectations regarding the cultural competence of Brazilian CSD students and the challenges brought by the COVID-19 pandemic. Cultural awareness has been one of the competencies focused on by CSD programs in Brazil. However, travel and face-to-face contact with persons from different cultures and environments is just one of the possible ways of experiencing cultural awareness. The interruption of these opportunities due to the COVID-19 pandemic did not reduce the interest in learning and improving cultural abilities. It is possible to think about alternatives for embedding discussions and experiences regarding cultural sensitivity in students' routine studies and practice.

Keywords: COVID-19 PANDEMIC, cultural competence, communication sciences and disorders, Brazil

1. Introduction

This chapter aims to bring information and consideration regarding cultural competence as part of the education of the professionals that work with Communication Sciences and Disorders in Brazil. The first important information is that this professional is called Phonoaudiologist and has habilitation both in Speech and Language and in Audiology.

> Phonoaudiologist is the professional with higher education that works in the area of Communication Sciences and Disorders. In all Latin America the areas of Audiology (assessment and rehabilitation of hearing and hearing disorders) and Speech-Language Therapy (assessment and intervention with communication, voice and swallowing disorders) are the professional field of Phonoaudiology.

Another major aspect that must be brought to attention is the complexity of the country. The authors will present some information about Brazil as a country and the current issues that are most relevant to the discussion of how cultural competence is considered in the education of Phonoaudiologists and the impact of COVID-19 in this regard.

It is easy to understand that the overview about Brazil will be superficial and incomplete, as would happen with any other attempt to synthesize important aspects such as the history, geography, and economy of a country in just a few paragraphs.

2. Brazil: some information about the country

What is nowadays the country of Brazil was a Portuguese colony from the sixteenth century until the nineteenth century. The formation of its people and society was the result of the genocide of the original population, the enslavement, and forced immigration through the kidnapping of African individuals aiming to boost the colony's economic workforce based on the extractivist agriculture [1]. During the three centuries of slavery, almost 4 million persons were forcibly brought from Africa to Brazil [2]. These groups, added by the European colonizers, brought different cultural elements that are now an intrinsic part of Brazilian culture in areas such as food, religion, music, and language [3].

When slavery came to an end there was no official segregation, but structural racism still can be observed. It is clear in the small numbers of African descendants in universities, or higher positions in the workforce or political posts—when the topic is black women, the lack of possibilities is even bigger. Albeit several debates have been dedicated to the racial question in Brazil, including the famous idea of a racial democracy [4], this is still a sensitive issue generating social gaps in different and complex levels of the Brazilian society in major cities as well as in small and distant towns.

> Structural racism is defined as a social, economic and politic system where institutional and public policies reinforce and maintain the segregation and inequities of social groups based on ethnicity, race or "color."

The "whitening" process that the Brazilian population went through during the nineteenth and twentieth centuries, with the arrival of different groups of immigrants, mainly from Europe, the Middle East, and Japan, was a National State Policy and helped in the deepening of racial and social inequalities. Its reflexes are seen until the present day. **Figure 1** shows the origins of the 4.3 million immigrants that arrived in Brazil during the nineteenth century.

Brazil is the 5th largest country in the world and there are also enormous geographic contrasts. The largest cities are located in the southeast, a very industrialized region that concentrates almost 55% of the country's entire gross product and 42% of the population. For example, São Paulo is the largest city, with over 12.3 million inhabitants; Rio de Janeiro has a demographic density of over 5.6 thousand inhabitants per square kilometer. The north and central regions are the most rural and preserved areas, despite the recent reduction of environmental preservation policies. In the Amazon region, the state of Roraima has the lowest demographic density in the country, with 2.33 inhabitants per square kilometer.

Immigration and migration processes are also different in different regions and at various moments, with different cultural impacts. During the last decade, the number of

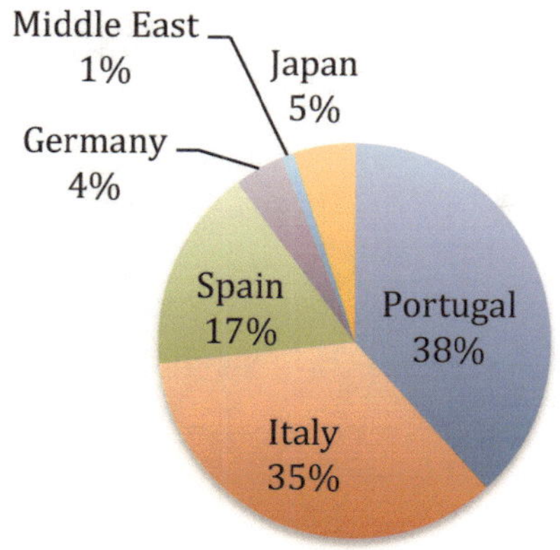

Figure 1.
Imigrants during the nineteenth century.

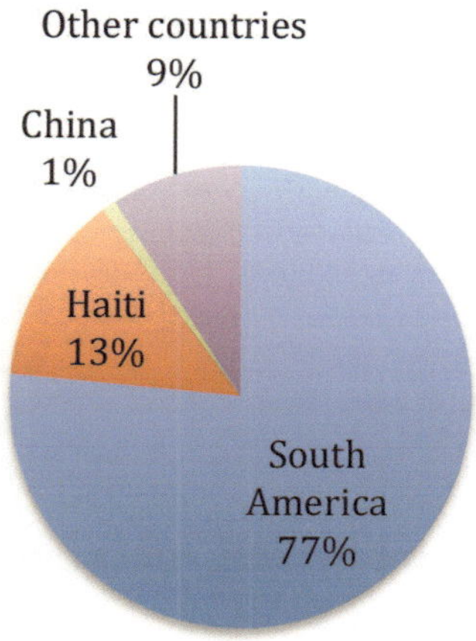

Figure 2.
Immigrants in the last decade.

immigrants arriving in Brazil has increased from 17,188 in 2010 to 117,037 in 2020 [2]. **Figure 2** shows the origins of the largest groups of immigrants to Brazil in the last decade.

Their distribution in the different regions of the country is shown in **Figure 3**.

Brazil has many and large cultural, social, environmental, economic, and educational differences. Portuguese is the official language, spoken by the whole population (over 213 million), but there are large differences associated with specific regions of the country, traditions, age groups, and other aspects.

The original populations are still another aspect of Brazilian diversity. Of the almost 1 million persons of indigenous origin, 60% live in protected areas designated by the federal government. The North region has the largest indigenous population and there are 305 different ethnic groups that speak 274 different languages [5].

It becomes clear that cultural differences are, historically, a relevant part of Brazilian society. Therefore, all the major universities have "Culture and Extension" offices that encourage and support initiatives directed toward the integration between the universities and the specific society where they are located. This way, different actions are carried out in different universities aiming to better reach the different groups. This includes the programs in the areas of communication sciences and disorders.

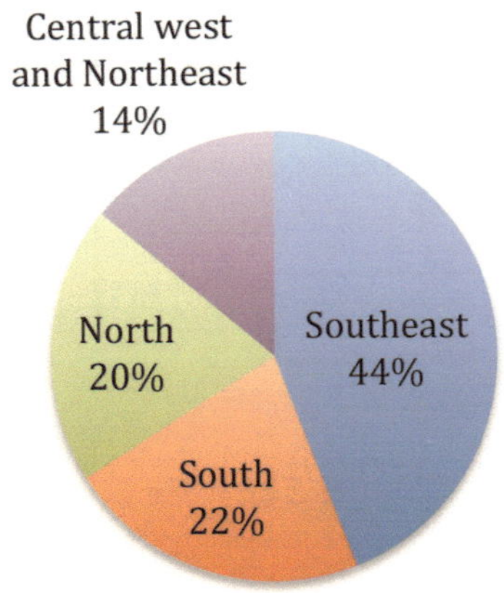

Figure 3.
Distribution in the different regions.

Culture and Extension offices in the universities usually have a mission statement of bringing together the university and the environment and community where it is located. The activities are usually as diverse as developing educational experiences to children of different groups to expand sports technology, or from providing health assistance to facilitating cultural shows of developing environmental systems for pollution control.

3. Phonoaudiology—CSD professional education in Brazil

Out of approximately 48,000 *phonoaudiologists* in Brazil, 16.5% are specialists, 7.3% have a Master's degree, and 3% have Ph.D. degrees. The phonoaudiologist has habilitation in both Speech-Language Pathology and Audiology, after completing a bachelor's program with an average workload of 4000 h, including supervised practice. Presently there are 81 bachelor's programs in Phonoaudiology, with a total of approximately 8000 students.

The Ministry of Education determines education guidelines for phonoaudiologists that guarantee basic standards for the whole country. The guidelines allow different programs address specific needs and characteristics associated with different regions, cultures, and institutions. The number of programs in the different regions of Brazil is roughly associated with the size of the population therein, as can be observed in **Figure 4**. Programs include a minimum of 800 h of supervised practice in clinical schools and school hospitals, with supervision by professors [6]. These services are offered free of charge. They include populations that are usually underserved in all the regions of the country.

The first programs were developed in Brazil in the 1950s decade. One of them was part of the education department of a catholic university and the other was part of the otorhinolaryngology department of a school of Medicine. As expected, there are clear differences regarding how each program approaches cultural competence in professional education. In both programs, as is the case in all Phonoaudiology education, the opportunities for supervised practice involve contact with a very diverse population.

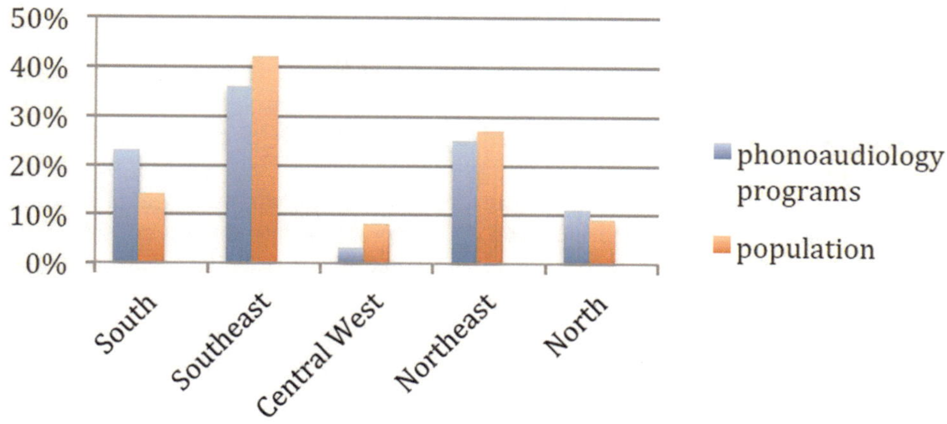

Figure 4.
Distribution of Phonoaudiology bachelor programs and of the population in the different regions of Brazil.

> Cultural Competence refers to a continuously evolving process that involves self-awareness regarding our actions with individuals from cultures that are different from our own. It includes considering the culture, beliefs and values of students, clients and patients in any decision-making and intervention processes.

Therefore, fostering competencies of cultural awareness, respect and empathy is part of the supervisors' routine work. However, there is not a uniform approach to this content by the different programs; there is a constant search for improvement, based on specific institutional aims and policies.

For example, in one of the oldest programs mentioned above, 5 years ago, after ample discussions by the faculty, a new educational project was approved. According to the project, students started observing supervised practice during the first semester of the program. This activity enabled the early start of discussions about cultural diversity and exercises of cultural competence. These experiences continue to develop, involving different activities and experiences in all the 10 semesters of the program, with effective practice in various scenarios in the last four semesters.

Regarding reach-out projects, depending on the specific pedagogical plan of each program, before the COVID-19 pandemic, actions from various programs focused on cultural diversity in different contexts. They involved, for example, screening for hearing and communication disorders in regular visits to riverside communities in the Amazon region by students from the state of Sao Paulo. Other groups could be involved in programs developed in small towns in the Southeast region, or reaching refugees that arrived from countries such as Venezuela, Haiti, or Colombia.

Cultural competence has been part of the different programs, with different intensities and approaches, for several years. There is not a specific policy about it, determining how or at which moment of the program the issue should be addressed. Therefore, each program can place the focus on cultural competence according to the specific academic context.

The process of getting access to academic education in Brazil is a process mostly based on the results of specific academic exams. Therefore, usually, the groups of students are also comprised of individuals from different social, economic, and cultural backgrounds. Dealing with these differences is an important issue in academic programs, and most important in areas that deal with human communication and interaction, such as Phonoaudiology.

4. Changes and challenges presented by the COVID-19 pandemic

Brazil has public systems that guarantee integral health care and 9 years of fundamental education to the whole population. However, these systems do not eliminate the severe inequities that can be observed everywhere. The COVID-19 pandemic had a major impact in several areas of health care delivery. Despite a vaccination system that otherwise works very efficiently and a population that was willing to be vaccinated, the distribution of vaccines was delayed and the process was very slow. The health system collapsed in all regions of the country, with overloaded ICUs and even a shortage of oxygen at some moments.

As occurred in several countries, the Brazilian central government was slow to respond to those challenges, failing to provide leadership aimed toward unified and collaborative actions. All decisions were transferred to state and city authorities, resulting in disjointed efforts and few positive results.

More than 650,000 persons perished, millions were infected, and continue to struggle with the consequences. Economic impacts continue to be observed in unemployment, increasing numbers of bankruptcies, hunger, and homelessness. These consequences are evident in all regions and affect either rural or urban populations.

Now, more than 1 year after the start of the vaccination in Brazil, a significant proportion of the population is vaccinated and the number of infections and deaths are decreasing. Several restrictions are being suspended, face-to-face activities are starting, and schools are re-opening. However, the consequences of the COVID19 pandemic will probably continue to affect the educational, health, and economic systems for a long time. It is not possible to think that things will be "back to normal" within a short period. It is important to think, for example, not just about children that were sick with COVID-19 and the long-term consequences of long hospitalization periods with, eventually, reduced oxygen amounts provided to the brain. Health, educational, and social security systems will have to deal with a great number of children that were orphaned and how to guarantee equal chances and compensating intervention. There are several challenges that will have to be met in the near and farther future.

4.1 Phonoaudiology education and the pandemic

Since the onset of the pandemic, in the first semester of 2020, it became clear that social distancing was one of the most effective ways of avoiding the spread of the COVID-19 pandemic. Authorities and stakeholders proposed several strategies to reduce human physical contact while trying to maintain most of the activities we used to consider "normal." Most of the universities either enhanced or implemented online classes, study groups, and supervisions. However, it was believed that this situation would last for a few weeks or a few months at the most. During those first weeks, there was a somewhat relaxed approach to the new challenges with expectations such as "*we will do what we can*"; "*when we go back to normal we will solve it*" or even "*we should stop everything and wait it out and then see what needs to be done.*"

As a result, different groups proposed and organized different responses. Some universities interrupted completely their activities, while others continued with online theoretical courses but interrupted all practice. Still, others built on previous experience and expertise in telehealth in order to continue to offer services. This also facilitated the establishment of clinical competence for future practice.

> Telehealth or telepractice is the use of digital information and communication technologies, such as computers and mobile devices, to access and provide/receive health care services remotely.

Access to the Internet and digital equipment varies widely among students. In some cases the public university provided equipment and Internet packages to students, aiming to improve equity of access to tele-practice, tele-supervision, and distance education among students. The same was not true for many patients. It was not as easy to reduce the differences between patients from different social and cultural backgrounds, who did not have access to such technologies. Barriers to providing services through remote technologies also included the parent's education level, their proficiency in the use of digital technology, and involvement with the intervention process.

> Remote technologies can include, personal computers, notebooks, tablets and mobile phones.

As weeks, months and a year went by it became clear that those who started adapting their practices earlier had more effective results and better outcomes. This applied to teaching activities involved in theoretical courses as well as interventions associated with supervised practice.

The COVID 19 pandemic made even more evident another unwanted kind of social distancing. Differences in access to basic health resources highlighted social differences. As a result, discussions with students about alternatives to address the various and specific difficulties became frequent topics of classes and supervision meetings. Through such discussions, access to technology emerged as another challenge to be addressed in the process of increasing the equality of chances and opportunities for all.

Even considering that there are an increasing number of Internet users, there is still a large proportion of the population without any access to the web. Concerns about the use of digital technology in school environments, which have yielded poor results despite some public policies supporting accessibility to persons with special needs, are reported [7].

Research conducted before the pandemic revealed that, with 71% of the Brazilian population responding, 28% of the households did not have access to the Internet; 25% of the population did not use the Web and only one-third of the participants did any kind of work through the Internet. People living in the rural area (79%) or with lower income (85%) reported using the Internet exclusively on their cell phones [8].

A study focused on children and adolescents before the pandemic informed that there were 3 million children and adolescents that did not have access to the Internet in Brazil; of which 1.4 million never had access to the Web either in school, at work, or at home. Besides that, 4.8 million children and adolescents between 9 and 17 years (18% of the population) did not have access to the Internet at home [9]. Considering the use of digital technology in the schools, the study reports that 58% of the students from urban schools used cell phones to perform school activities and only 33% of the teachers had some kind of instruction about the use of the Internet. In rural environments, only 40% of the schools had at least one computer with access to the Internet and 9% could access the Web via other devices [10].

Telehealth resources have great potential to address barriers such as the lack of professional experts in a specific area, and physical distance, besides saving transportation time and costs. However, not all families have access to the best technology devices to allow for the best services of online therapy. Professional education programs should include competencies regarding the resources available in different contexts.

It seems that the alternative strategies that had to be used in the implementation of tele-practice represent an important experience to be considered in offering SLP services to underserved or unserved populations and to in-training professionals that will be able to use them [11]. A study [12] conducted in 2020 assessed the reactions of final-period undergraduate students after 10 weeks of supervised telepractice with children with ASD in Sao Paulo, Brazil. Results indicate that 70% of them reported being self-confident and encouraged and that it was possible to continue the learning process. They considered that the improved contact with the families was the most positive aspect of telepractice, while the negative aspects were the lack of personal contact and the dependency on technology. This same publication [12] reports on 552 sessions of online language therapy with 83 children with ASD. These data highlight the importance of flexibility in the use of the available technology. More than 50% of the contacts occurred through WhatsApp. This surely is not the best way to provide a speech-language therapy session, but the alternative was no therapy. Overall, in 76.3% of the sessions, the therapists (supervised students) reported that the specific goals were met. These preliminary results seem to indicate that even in a situation where the resources are not the best ones, telehealth seems to be a viable alternative to the delivery of SLP services to children with ASD and their families.

5. Cultural awareness and cultural competence

Cultural differences and characteristics are not just observed in the minorities represented by migrants, refugees, and persons that frequently lack adequate access to basic housing, health, and education services [11]. They can also be observed in everyday life in small attitudes, and in regional popular sayings and customs that involve social, cultural, and economic aspects. Critical thinking is necessary to understand cultural differences that may reflect power differences associated with cultural identity. The notion of cultural humility [13] involves a better understanding of health issues regarding the context in which they occur.

Cultural awareness is essential to all SLPs in everyday situations [14], but more so when the service is provided through technological resources that "put the therapist inside the client's home."

This is the situation either when the therapist proposes to work with the client with the assistance of an adult at home or if "guiding" activities that are to be conducted at home by a familiar adult. Anyway, we are "invading" the client's home (and probably the whole family), by being part of the routine of other family members, sharing routines and habits. Regardless of how productive it can be for the work itself, allowing the inclusion of tasks and abilities in the child's routine and environment, we are entering their homes and it is easy to consider that this "participation" maybe a little (or too much) more than the families anticipated. The same may be true about online teaching. The study setting for the student may not be appropriate; or the student may feel uncomfortable and exposed, sharing their home environment or a disrupted routine during a class or supervision. It can happen anywhere, with anyone. Building the notion that improving cultural competence will be a never-ending task for any professional that deals with people, education, or communication should be part of the aims of education regarding remote access in education and intervention for the future.

The pandemic interrupted projects of modernity previously proposed and the need for changes has emerged. The ruptures created by the pandemic may represent an important opportunity for society to overcome barriers imposed by prejudices, lack of coherent information, and other elements that can harm the action of the speech therapist within the clinical practice. The notion of telepractice as the only mode of access between the phonoaudiologist and the client/patient during a long period and the cultural aspects involved has never been discussed like this before. Cultural competence in remote practice is now an essential part of the equation.

The concept of cultural competence has already been studied by several specialties within the area of health, addressing how it can benefit both the professional and the patient. One of the studies highlights that culture is not only something that people have but also something present in every human being, in its roots, which influences all their actions. In the literature, cultural aspects have already been defined as a set of values, beliefs, and norms that guide the thinking and decision-making processes of a certain population group about the actions it takes [15, 16]. Then, if the culture in which individuals are born can determine the thought and actions of each individual and the group, the expansion of this culture and the encounter, clash, and confluence with other cultures, can modify complete mental processes as well as personal, professional, and group decision-making mechanisms [17].

The phonoaudiologist is the professional trained to assist the language and communication skills of individuals of all ages. The assistance, however, should consider all complex issues regarding cultural sensitivity in all aspects involved in the integration of knowledge, competencies, and attitudes that influence therapeutic practice. Betancourt et al. [18] pointed out that the health professionals' awareness of these complex dimensions that relate to cultural competence incorporates the understanding of the influence of social and cultural issues on beliefs and behaviors, taking into account their interaction with health providers. For these reasons, the COVID-19 pandemic and the need to transform all intervention, supervision, and education activities to remote access, made it clear that cultural competence must include these resources as part of the discussions during the speech-language pathologist's training.

The understanding of the multicultural aspects of clients with speech, language, and hearing problems is essential to the professional's ability to perform their best practices, providing a high-quality service for the population.

A small study conducted online interviews with 54 undergraduate and graduate students of Phonoaudiology and questioned their positions on the relevance of cultural competence in their professional training and their ability to work with individuals from different cultures. The results indicate that only 20% of the participants considered they had good knowledge about different cultures and 70% would be interested in different cultural experiences. This is important feedback regarding teaching strategies. Faculty needs to address how to bring cultural awareness as one of the competencies that are focused in several academic activities so students would be able to recognize and value the experiences they are already having with persons from different cultures. Different strategies may be used to achieve this goal, such as lectures, online discussions, or classroom activities [19]. The challenges imposed by the pandemic, restricting personal contact, will demand the continuity of the search for the best strategies.

6. Considerations

The small study reported above confirms the expectations of Brazilian students in the area of communication sciences and disorders regarding the impact of experiences with different cultural groups on the development of cultural competence. The limitations imposed by the COVID-19 pandemic delayed all planning about face-to-face contact in the short term. However, there are many alternatives for distance meetings and communication. Developing communication partnerships among students and universities from different regions, environments, and even countries can foster interaction between students and improve general cultural sensitivity. Hopefully, the return to more mobile possibilities will allow the continuity and improvement of previous experiences.

Even different languages should not be barriers if communication is the true aim. Learning how to understand each other and reducing differences and distances may be the kind of soft skill that contributes to the development of empathy. It can surely be interesting for a CSD student to experience the role of not being able to communicate efficiently and needing to overcome linguistic and cultural barriers and becoming more flexible in different settings. It may be said that empathy is not enough, but it can be an important intrinsic motivator to the development of cultural competence.

Author details

Fernanda Dreux M. Fernandes[1]*, Maria Vitoria do Amaral[1]
and Cibelle La Higuera Amato[2]

1 Department of PT and OT, School of Medicine CSD, Universidade de Sao Paulo, São Paulo, Brazil

2 Developmental Disorders Graduate Program, Mackenzie Presbiterian University, São Paulo, Brazil

*Address all correspondence to: fernandadreux@usp.br

References

[1] Holanda SB. Roots of Brazil. Notre Dame, Indiana, United States: University of Notre Dame Press; 2012. (First published in 1936)

[2] Portal da Imigração. 2021. Available from: https://portaldeimigracao.mj.gov.br/images/dados/relatorio-anual/2020/Resumo%20Executivo%20_Relat%C3%B3rio%20Anual.pdf

[3] Ribeiro D, Ribeiro GL. The Brazilian People: The Formation and Meaning of Brazil. Florida: University Press of Florida; 2000

[4] Freyre G. The Masters and the Slaves—A Study in the Development of Brazilian Civilization. California: University of California Press; 1986

[5] Survival Brasil. 2021. Available from: https://www.survivalbrasil.org/povos/indios-brasileiros

[6] Fernandes FDM, Wertzner HF. Competence-based curricula for the education of speech-language pathologists and audiologists in Brazil. Folia Phoniatrica et Logopaedica. 2014; **66**(4–5):176-182. DOI: 10.1159/000366129

[7] United Nations Education, Science and Culture Organization. Assessing Internet Development in Brazil: Using UNESCO's Internet Universality ROAM-X Indicators NIC.BR/CETIC.BR. 2019. Available from: https://cetic.br/publicacao/assessing-internet-development-in-brazil-usingunesco-s-internet-universality-roam-x-indicators/

[8] Centro Regional de Estudos para o Desenvolvimento da Sociedade da Informação. Survey on the Use of Information and Communication Technologies in Brazilian Households: ICT Households. 2018. Available from: https://www.cetic.br/publicacao/pesquisa-sobre-o-uso-das-tecnologias-de-informacao-e-comunicacao-nos-domicilios-brasileiros-tic-domicilios-2018/

[9] Centro Regional de Estudos para o Desenvolvimento da Sociedade da Informação. Survey on Internet Use by Children in Brazil: ICT Kids Online Brazil São Paulo. 2017. Available from: https://cetic.br/publicacao/pesquisa-sobre-o-uso-da-internet-por-criancas-e-adolescentesno-brasil-tic-kids-online-brasil-2017/

[10] Centro Regional de Estudos para o Desenvolvimento da Sociedade da Informação. Survey on the Use of Information and Communication Technologies in Brazilian Schools: ICT in Education. 2017. Available from: https://cetic.br/publicacao/pesquisa-sobre-o-uso-das-tecnologias-de-nformacao-e-comunicacao-nas-escolas-brasileiras-tic-educacao-2017/

[11] Levey S, Moonsamy S. Unserved and Underserved Populations: New Approaches to Inclusivity. New York: Peter Lang Publisher; 2021

[12] Fernandes FDM, Sun IYI, Rodrigues BF, Cabral CP, Tosetto C, Segeren L. Speech language therapy for children with ASD and their families during the Covid-19 pandemic: Considerations about professional training and service delivery on a majority country. Highlights on Medicine and Medical Research. 2021;**4**:32-38. DOI: 10.9734/bpi/hmmr/v4/7594D

[13] Greene-Moton E, Minkler M. Cultural competence or cultural humility? Moving beyond the debate. Health Promotion Practice. 2020;**21**(1):142-145. DOI: 10.1177/1524839919884912

[14] Hyter YD, Salas-Provance MB. Culturally Responsive Practices in Speech, Language, and Hearing Sciences. San Diego, California: Plural Publishing; 2018

[15] Leininger MM, McFarland MR. Culture Care Diversity and Universality: A Worldwide Nursing Theory. Burlington, Massachusetts, United States: Jones & Bartlett Learning; 2006

[16] Luquis RR, Pérez MA. Cultural Competence in Health Education and Health Promotion. Hoboken, New Jersey, United States: John Wiley & Sons; 2021

[17] Clauss-Ehlers CS, Sood AB, Weist MD. Introduction: An urgent call to understand the status of children and young people within a social justice paradigm. In: Clauss-Ehlers CS, Sood AB, Weist MD, editors. Social Justice for Children and Young People: International Perspectives. UK: Cambridge University Press; 2020. pp. 3-19

[18] Betancourt JR, Green AR, Carrillo JE, Ananeh-Firempong O. Defining cultural competence: A practical framework for addressing racial/ethnic disparities in health and health care. Public Health Reports. 2003;**118**(4):293-302. DOI: 10.1093/phr/118.4.293

[19] Chae D, Kim J, Kim S, Lee J, Park S. Effectiveness of cultural competence educational interventions on health professionals and patient outcomes: A systematic review. Japan Journal of Nursing Science. 2020;**17**(3):e12326. DOI: 10.1111/jjns.12326